*B*REASTFEEDING MATTERS

What we need to know about infant feeding

MAUREEN MINCHIN

Alma Publications 1998

Alma Publications aims to make well-researched materials about maternal and child health and nutrition available to parents and professionals. The realities of publishing and bookselling are such that our recommended retail prices must allow everyone concerned to make a living. However, we make books available on favourable terms to parent self-help groups; we provide special discounts for disadvantaged persons and groups; we give away many books to key individuals and groups around the world. Alma Publications profits are used in the cause of the protection, promotion and support of breastfeeding. Our main objective is not to make money but to inform the community and so help make needed changes. If this retail price is beyond your means, please write directly to us.

Recommended retail price: $25. Prices direct from Alma Publications: 2-5 copies: $20 plus postage; 6-10 copies, $17.50 plus postage. Bulk orders please write for rates. Trade discounts available to booksellers and parent self-help groups.
Alma Publications, 14 Acland St., St. Kilda Vic 3182. Tel/fax: (03) 9537 2640; and 6 Thear St., East Geelong Vic. 3215 Australia.

Printing history: First published January 1985 by Alma Publications, second edition Alma Publications and George Allen & Unwin Australia Pty. Ltd 1986; third, revised edition published November 1989; fourth revised edition June 1998.

Minchin, Maureen K. (Maureen Kathryn)
Breastfeeding Matters: what we need to know about infant feeding.

4th rev. ed.
Bibliography.
Includes index.
ISBN   0 9593183 3 X   (Pbk.)

1 Breastfeeding. 2. Breastfeeding –social aspects. 3. Infants –nutrition. I. Title.

649.3

Edited and typeset by Philip Minchin
Cover design John Van Loon; photo James Maher Photography.
Printed by McPherson's Printing Group
An All Australian Book.

C ONTENTS

*L*IST OF ILLUSTRATIONS

ACKNOWLEDGMENTS

A special acknowledgment is due to my son Philip, without whom this book would never have been written, and now, without whom this edition would never have been published. One of the joys of working in this field is watching our breastfed babies grow up into responsible, loving, caring and highly intelligent adults, also passionate about the harms being done to the world's children. Philip's skills have made my life a great deal easier in the last decade! And he has edited this revised version through many changes and done so cheerfully and well. Of all the editors I have dealt with, he is the best.

Authors always rely upon the input and assistance of others, many of whom cannot be named publicly. Space would not permit me to list all those to whom I am indebted: the parents, NMAA counsellors, midwives, doctors, scientists, and others from many disciplines with whom I have discussed ideas and who have freely shared information. Special thanks must go to the staff of the NMAA Lactation Resource Centre, as well as the librarians at Deakin University, Geelong Hospital, and the Center for Food Safety and Nutrition, Washington, who have helped in ways that go beyond the strict call of duty, together with the ever-obliging Keith Smith of Corporate Printers, and Luke Matthews who proof-read diligently and provided much constructive criticism, improving the readability of the text. It's great to work with those who share one's concerns about the issues. Thanks too, to those who have supplied illustrations, acknowledged elsewhere, particularly John van Loon, Prue Carr, Chele Marmet, James Maher, and the staff of the Deakin Media Unit and Sovereign Hill Historical Park. As always, thanks to my whole family, who have all had to make many accommodations to the fact that working in this field takes huge inputs of time and money and provides few monetary rewards. And thanks to my now adult daughters, Catherine and Lizzie, for indexing and filling in where work needed to be done, and in Catie's case, together with James, providing a refresher course in babies and young mothers via young Brigit, who adorns the cover in a typical playful pose! Particular thanks must go to my dear friend Professor Mary Renfrew, whose contributions have been woven into its fabric, and to many other lactation consultants and friends and students who have all helped to keep me learning over the past two decades.

I do really want to thank all my friends, colleagues and correspondents over that time. It has not been an easy run for many of us, but we have come through with principles and honour intact, still (relatively!) sane and still determined to work for justice and dignity for women and children in a world that frequently denies it. In our different ways and spheres, we are all feminists: we want women to take responsibility for their lives, and not be defined or trapped by other people's expectations; we rejoice in the power of women to be creative forces in our society; and we believe that this reproductive sphere is one of the crucial areas where women must take control of their lives. We want to provide women with the information needed to make the best possible choice, and the support to carry through that choice.

Many women – far too many – have suffered greatly because of difficulties with infant feeding. Many have shared their private agonies in the hope that others could benefit. As they struggle to repair the damage done to their identity, their lives, and their children, they deserve our support and respect. This book is thus dedicated to such mothers, and to the hope we share that in future there will be far fewer casualties of mismanaged infant feeding. And it is dedicated with great affection to Dr. Mavis Gunther. Her contribution to maternal and child health has been immense. Without her I should never have begun to look critically at the "slovenly terms used by those who have not troubled to see what the injury is". She changed my life and that of my children, and so of all those whom I have reached via teaching and writing.

Permission to reproduce copyright material was kindly granted by the following: Toni Adams; Margaret Bell; Enid Beck; Prue Carr; Sarah Danner; Chloe Fisher; Helen Grigg; INFACT Minneapolis; the Lactation Institute, Encino; Helen Lawrenson; Mapa GmbH, manufacturers of NUK teats; James Maher; Neil Matterson; Methuen Books Pty. Ltd.; Viv Greasley and Mike Woolridge then of the Oxford Lactation Research Group; the trustees of the Sovereign Hill Historical Park, Ballarat; Rhonda Styles. Other material quoted and attributed seems to fall within the limits of copyright laws; however should anyone feel that more formal permission is required I apologise for any oversight.

And a final thank you and dedication...

In loving memory of Dave Wells,
an honest lawyer,
a good friend,
a great character,
the man who quietly funded the very first Minchin publication in 1982,
an inveterate sparring partner,
a true believer in justice and law,
a brave man.

"Law is not about making money, but about justice and the proper order of things."

"The first duty of the lawyer is to the court."
(JDB Wells, 1941-1996)

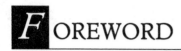OREWORD

There is a proverb - "learning is not so much the filling of a pail as the lighting of a flame." Maureen Minchin's book *Breastfeeding Matters* is testament to this adage.

Global research is daily confirming what far-sighted writers such as Maureen have been saying for decades - that human breastmilk is an essential and perfect food for human babies, not only in the first few weeks, but over many months, even years.

As an experienced midwife (who secretly thought she possessed a reasonable understanding of breastfeeding) I was aghast at my lack of knowledge when I first read Maureen's work. The words tumbled from the pages - each chapter bringing further revelations. As I read on I could not help thinking "Why did I not know this? Where was a book such as this when I first studied midwifery?" Maureen's book demonstrates to those involved in infant feeding how crucial it is to have current research-based practice when dealing with such a vital aspect of early life. It is a clarion call to excellence in practice and a fervent defence of the birthright of all humans to be fed species-specific milk. She speaks to us with a passionate intelligence, while at the same time presenting her compelling evidence in a clear reasoned prose. Her scholarly attention to detail and skilful use of language makes this book an absorbing read. Maureen is not afraid to challenge ritualistic and out-moded approaches to infant feeding management. Moreover, she backed each assertion with a thorough reference source at the end of each chapter - an essential embarkation point for those of us interested in pursuing the subject further.

It should not be too much to expect that a well-thumbed copy of this work will be on the desk of all health care professionals who are daily dealing with the complexities of breastfeeding management in our community. This marvellous book should become an essential text for every midwife, nutritionist, pharmacy and medical student. It is commended to all those interested in promoting human rights, improving community health and pursuing "best practice" in health care.

Heather Harris, B. Ng., M. Mid. Studies, IBCLC.
Clinical Nurse Consultant - Lactation
Royal Women's Hospital Melbourne, Australia.
June 1998

*I*NTRODUCTIONS

Author introduction 1998

Revising *Breastfeeding Matters* has been a convoluted process. I will address the practical issues in the afterword (see p. 376) Here I wish to be brief and state the most important take-home message, the conviction that has crystallised after more than twenty years of working for better infant health.

There are many small things we can all do to protect promote and support breastfeeding, which will make small differences to breastfeeding rates and to the health of women, children, and society. We need to do these as best we can. But there are two large things we need to do, to make a huge difference to breastfeeding rates.

These are quite simple. First we need to inform everyone of the inherent risks of the "qualitative dysnutrition" that is artificial feeding, which remains, as I said in 1984, the largest uncontrolled in vivo experiment in human history. We also need to count and publicise the cost to mothers and fathers in particular, and society in general, of that strangest of anti-social practices, artificial feeding.

Secondly, we need to convince policy-makers that these inescapable risks justify social support that enables women genuinely to choose whether to return to the paid workforce while their child is under three. If the financial imperative to take paid work were removed, I believe most women would choose to be with their young children, and could organise to create social networks supportive of both mothers and children, such as I enjoyed only twenty years ago in rural Australia. Naturally, any such support should not jeopardise the right of women to continue in the paid workforce, and such women should be be guaranteed the whole range of workplace conditions that allow breastfeeding to continue. Both groups of women –working at home or in a paid job - need to be advocates for the needs of all women, not merely their preferred group.

I believe now that if we cannot achieve these two goals in so-called developed nations, other than in Scandinavia, we will watch breastfeeding duration, and then initiation, decline under the economic pressures of modern society.

I know that only those concerned for infant and maternal health are likely to be reading this. I take this opportunity to thank you, and urge you to continue working to end the unconscionable death toll of millions of infant lives lost to improper feeding and its consequences. To paraphrase one rabbi's response after presentation at the 1993 World Conference on Religion and Peace joint meeting with UNICEF, 'It is sad that a world which has condemned the Holocaust can tolerate such a holocaust every year of infant lives.' That comparison does not belittle either human tragedy.

Maureen Minchin, January 1998

Breastfeeding Matters is a classic which altered perceptions of breastfeeding management, so that much which seemed controversial in 1984 is now common -place. Completed in 1983 and published in January 1985, it was the first affordable book to create awareness of the risks artificial feeding poses, not just to poor people somewhere else, but to people living in every society. It has helped make its readers aware of the need not to demonise industry as the sole cause of all our infant feeding woes, but to see that there have been other factors, including the ignorance of health professionals. They were trained in a bottle-feeding culture where they had little exposure to breastfeeding, and as a result did not know how to support women who were learning o breastfeed, and often gave advice that resulted in women wean-ing. This book clearly described the basis for supportive breastfeeding practices, and made accessible material by earlier writes that had been overlooked or forgotten. Other factors conspiring against breastfeeding have been the pressures from an increasingly consumerist middle class, combined with a hostile social environment – long working hours, expensive childcare of variable quality – in which women with babies and paid jobs find themselves. And women have been slow to support each other in this. It is only in recent years that feminism has come to realise that women who have babies, and who breastfeed, need support, not blame from their sisters.

This book has sparked many research studies, inspired other writers, and brought about fundamental change in advice to breastfeeding women, in areas ranging from infant suckling to mastitis. It has stood the test of time remarkably well. In many ways it deserves to remain as it is, a piece of early 1980s writing.

But there was a need to update it. In the last 15 years, breastfeeding rates have not improved as we then thought they might. In the UK there has been no improvement in either initiation or discontinuation rates. In many countries, the women who still breastfeed least are those who because of their adverse social circumstances, have most need to do so. There remains a fiercely ambivalent attitude to breastfeeding across the lay and professional communities – "breast is best but bottle-feeding is just (well, almost) as good, and breastfeeding is really rather embarrassing, especially in public." Little has changed in those years in many countries.

When I came to re-read the chapter I wrote in 1983, I was surprised by how little it needed to be changed. Many of the problems and challenges remain. Given the extent to which other health and social issues have developed in this time – communication (faxes, e-mail, the internet, mobile phones), technology (computing, 'smart' cards), health care (informed choice, evidence-based care, diagnostic techniques), the status of women (paid maternity leave, more women in senior roles), education (university-based midwifery education, equal sex ratios of medical students), we might well have expected breastfeeding problems to be behind us. But we would be wrong.

So this book includes, with only minor adjustments, the chapter I wrote in 1983. I hope that in another 15 years time, I will be able to say that most of these problems were left behind us in the old millennium.

Professor Mary J. Renfrew (formerly Houston)
Director, Mother and Infant Research Unit,
University of Leeds, UK

Author introduction 1984: Why this book?

O n my shelves are dozens of books about breastfeeding – books for doctors, lay counsellors, nurses, health-care administrators and, above all, for parents. Most are in total agreement with one another, recycling the accepted wisdom. Can another book on such an overworked topic be justified?

I believe so. This book represents a departure from the usual breastfeeding publication, because it has as many questions as answers, and many of its answers differ from accepted wisdom, or seek to provide some rational basis for current practice. It raises neglected issues and examines many of the (mostly avoidable) problems of breastfeeding. A lot of women find breastfeeding difficult, unpleasant and a thankless task, so if we are to advocate universal and exclusive breastfeeding for a baby's first half-year – and I believe the scientific evidence demands this – we need better management of problems and greater support from social structures before exhortations to breastfeed cease being merely another stick to beat women with.

To succeed at breastfeeding, women need two things: adequate motivation and management. In Australia at this time, a woman's motivation is undermined by the widespread fallacy that "while breast is best, the bottle nowadays is nearly as good" (discussed in Chapter 1). And the management of breastfeeding and its difficulties ranges from reasonable to abysmal – why bother when substitutes are available? No one seems interested in explaining the logic of a particular practice, so that women must make blind stabs at getting it right – whether the 'it' be what creams to use on nipples or how to hold your first-born. Women have been forced to rely on word of mouth between friends and on the suggestions of lay organisations. These have many virtues and have done a great job overall, but the ability to scientifically evaluate the rationale of recommended practices has so far been beyond their resources of personnel and income. Of course this sort of evaluation should be the task of scientifically trained professionals, hence my promotion of Breastfeeding Clinics.

The art of breastfeeding is a specialised aspect of the science of lactation. Too often those concerned with the science know little of the art – and vice versa. This results in a failure of nerve for both. The professional, aware of the importance of breastfeeding, may be hesitant to speak out about its importance when she knows that she cannot help mothers succeed, and to emphasise its importance may make 'failed' breastfeeders feel anxious, or guilty, or worse. The amateur, who may be better at the art, is under-confident about the science and hesitates to speak out strongly for fear of looking foolish, or causing controversy which might reflect adversely on any group with which she is associated. Both are aware that standard advice about breastfeeding problems does not help a minority of women. This is usually (and unscientifically) ascribed to some defect in the mother, rather than in the advice. Take the mother who has tried through weeks of constant suckling, to increase her milk supply to meet her baby's needs. I see red when someone says "If that hasn't worked, then she really doesn't want to feed and we'll help her wean"; or "Well, you must be one of the 5% who can't breastfeed adequately". As will be made clear in Chapter 5, there are dozens of other avenues to explore before making those unprovable spot diagnoses.

In travelling and talking with experienced midwives and lay counsellors, I have come to see that breastfeeding knowledge is very patchy. At present what is known in the United Kingdom is unheard of in the United States, and vice versa. So if you wonder why I bother emphasising the non-infective nature of most mastitis, for example – when you have accepted that for years – it is because other people still equate infection and mastitis.

I see the need for a two-pronged attack on the problems of breastfeeding. First, we need professional and community education as to the incredible complexity of human milk and an outspoken acknowledgment of the hazards – yes, hazards – of any alternative. Concomitantly, because we believe all that, we need to take breastfeeding problems seriously, and provide rational detailed diagnosis and treatment. I hope this book helps in both areas. It will be seen by some as radical, because when dealing with sensitive topics, it's traditional to try to keep everyone happy. (One author of a book on infant care, when asked why he had compromised so heavily on the formula-feeding issue, while in private he thought formula extremely hazardous, replied simply: "The book would have no market if I said that in print.") Radical I hope this book is, in the sense of getting down to the roots of the issues – and I suppose, in my willingness to break with that tradition of soothing everyone, despite my dread of the likely reaction of those who consider that I have no business raising these questions. But it must be stated that my position is the only sane conservative one. I am simply arguing that until we can prove that artificial formulae are safe, in both the short and long term, only human milk is good enough for babies.

The onus of proof must always be upon those who want to promote or legitimise artificial substitutes for a natural product or process. So far very little scientific proof has been offered. In condemning the use of dairy whiteners for infant feeding, the American Academy of Pediatrics asserted, quite rightly, that "popularity, extravagant claims, and special marketing practices cannot make white liquids nutritionally equivalent to infant formula". I would submit that our acceptance of infant formula as satisfactory substitutes for human milk is based far more upon "popularity, extravagant claims, and special marketing practices" than it is upon rigorous testing. Just as dairy whiteners are inferior to formula, so is formula inferior to human milk. But the confusion of all three as white liquids, therefore suitable for infant feeding, is hardly surprising when a century ago some then leading babyfood companies were selling virtually pure starch and water by means of extravagant claims and special marketing practices!

The latest batch of artificial substitutes may well prove adequate to sustain growth within normal bounds for very many children, though the phenomenal growth in sales of specialised and hypo-allergenic formulae during the 1970s should make it clear that regular formula will not suit at least a significant minority, and attempts to improve the 'normal' infant formula should continue. But no one could maintain that the 1970s formulas now used as normal feeding are not an enormous improvement over the first "perfect infant foods". No one could maintain that such formulas and their precursors have not proved useful to women in this century: formulas would never have been so widely used had they not met with eager acceptance from women seeking to escape the confines of tradition. No one could maintain that present manufacturers are not sincere in their efforts to make a quality product, and in their belief in the necessity for, and the benefits of, their product. Administrators and salesmen are not scientists, and may be genuinely unaware of the problems I have outlined in this book. They may genuinely believe that industry did not lead, but merely followed cultural changes; they may see the need for their product as a necessary part of a modern lifestyle, rather than as an artefact created by nineteenth-century advertising and reinforced by cultural and social practices and organisation – all of which can be changed.

I do not see all past manufacturers as unscrupulous villains, who must bear all the blame for the movement away from maternal breastfeeding. While it was naïve 19th Century businessmen who, by creating and widely advertising their products, brought about a situation in which the idea of infant feeding choice seemed reasonable, that choice was taken up by middle-class women for reasons beyond the manufacturers' control. Professionals and writers too, were heavily implicated in this process. The little knowledge they had – so much more than in past times – was a dangerous thing, in that it gave a semblance of scientific certainty to experiments in infant feeding that today could not be countenanced. It is not at all unusual for scientific progress to have such unfortunate side-effects, and twentieth-century science is not immune. As Valman stated so clearly, "A major advance in the care of the newborn has often followed the observation that an accepted method of treatment has killed or maimed babies."

I do not see all present manufacturers as ruthless businessmen, willing to sacrifice any number of babies to shareholders' profits. But neither do I see them as philanthropists, willing to go bankrupt in the cause of child health. Their own colossal commercial interests will make them interpret reality in ways favourable to their own cause. They will be the last to accept that there are any substantial health risks inherent in a product they have been selling – they, and the researchers they have been employing. They cannot be relied upon to provide truly objective data, and the money they provide for advertising and cocktail parties and other professional 'perks' must be seen as contributing to infant malnutrition by increasing the price of their expensive product. No one should pretend that this desire to serve the medical profession and all others dealing with childbearing women is pure altruism. The basic concept underlying help to professions is that "if we do this job well, the health professional will choose Ross brand", as the Vice-President of Ross Laboratories said in 1981. Professionals need to be more aware that they are the target of an immensely expensive, sophisticated marketing strategy. If they believe that this cannot influence their attitudes, beliefs and behaviour, they are simply naïve. Many concepts in professional literature come straight from the pen of an advertising copy-writer or company employee. (The strenuous nature of breastfeeding, or the insufficient milk syndrome, or the value of nipple shields...) There is, and must be, an inherent tension and at times conflict of interest between professionals and commercial salesmen, when a better product is available free.

I do not expect industry to like this book, raising as it does for popular attention the question of the potential and actual risks of their products. Industry's greatest success has been to create a climate of opinion in which breast milk and formulae are thought to be much the same, and true conservatives like me are deemed to be radical extremists. If manufacturers feel that I have been unfair in my treatment, I should be delighted to hear from them. Their response will help to determine their credibility as people whose 'goal, as it always has been, is to find ways to improve the nutritional status of the young child', as one very senior executive stated. Since this book is likely to result both in more women breastfeeding and a more careful use of infant formula, I believe I can expect from them enthusiastic support. I shall report any interesting responses.

There are those who will find this book disturbing; others will find it infuriating. Some people feel comfortable only with the apparent objectivity and neutrality of scientific language; stating absolutely no more than can be incontrovertibly demonstrated, having 'six bob each way' in any area of controversy; refusing to expose themselves to the possibility of being proved wrong. Personally, I too would feel more comfortable if this were such a book. As I prepare it for publication, the tensions between academic and activist sometimes reach intolerable levels. The academic me urges caution, to wait until I can document every single point beyond the possibility of argument. The activist me considers that such a delay is morally unacceptable; that 'objectivity' is as much a value judgement and a political choice as is commitment; and that common sense is on my side. Many women and not a few men are irritated by 'objectivity' and identify strongly with books that combine information with commitment, even passion. This is such a book. I'm aware that I may be proved wrong on specifics, but absolutely positive that I'll be proved right on essentials – so the risks are worth taking when balanced against the risks of doing nothing.

I believe that most people working with breastfeeding mothers will find that this book, unlike many others, does more than reiterate standard advice; that there is much that is 'new' in these pages. But if anyone reads it and finds that there is nothing new to her or him, please write to me instantly. I've been looking for people like you all over the world!

Maureen Minchin, June 1984
Geelong, Australia

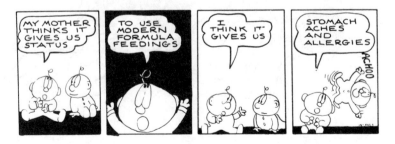

Status or stomach ache? (cartoon by Brunner, courtesy UNICEF)

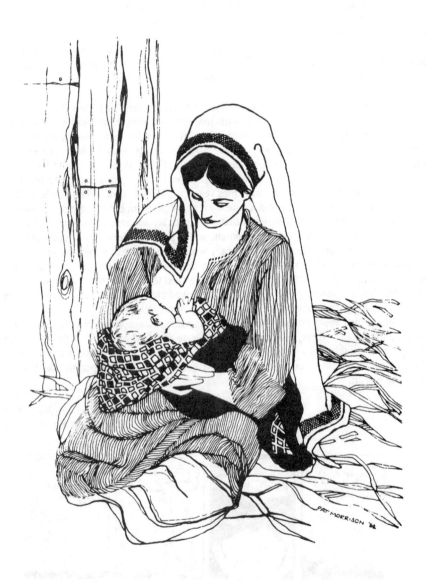

1. WHY BREASTFEEDING MATTERS

I am eager that the medical profession broaden its approach to infant feeding in relation to a broad spectrum of diseases. Among epidemiological factors the method and type of feeding should be included... in trying to activate interest in breastfeeding among those who are reluctant to change or even to consider change, it may be necessary to point out dangers to Western technological society, which has come to accept bottlefeeding as a completely adequate substitute for breastfeeding. Even if we have no answers at present, simply to ask questions that provoke unease might spark the action which will lead to systematic enquiry into these problems.

R. G. Hendrickse, in *Breastfeeding and the Mother*
(Ciba Foundation Symposium, 1976) p. 247.

It is not possible to manufacture this volume of [infant formula] without some mistakes occurring during their manufacture. It is not possible to legislate perfection in production or anything else.

Proceedings of AOAC conference
on infant formula production, 1985, p. 6.

"It's hard to come out and say, 'Your baby is going to be stupider or sicker if you don't breastfeed'," says Dr. Lawrence Gartner, chair of the American Academy of Pediatrics' working group on breastfeeding. "But that's what the literature says."

Your Child from Birth to Three
Newsweek special edition, April 1997, USA, p. 32.

Mother's milk is always best. Artificial substitutes are always risky. And infant feeding affects every child for life, in a multiplicity of ways known and as yet unknown.

Though all parents want their special child to get the best start in life, not all babies do. There will always be some situations in which the optimal is not practical, and people must settle for the inferior. But that is no excuse for allowing the distinctions between best and second best to become so blurred that parents actively 'choose' the inferior, believing the differences to be trivial. That is where we still are today in relation to the so-called choice of infant feeding method. Despite all that has been learned, even in 1998 the average doctor, midwife, nurse and parent truly believe that among the blessings of modern science is a recipe for infant formula so close to mothers' milk as to be virtually indistinguishable. While this belief persists, the

9

concept of informed choice in infant feeding is a nonsense. Informed choice involves knowing and evaluating risks and benefits, and the myth persists that there are no real risks to artificial feeding.

The truth about infant feeding is very different. What follows is a little of what could be said as long ago as 1984 about the hazards of artificial feeding. It was by no means the end of the story, and at the end of the references I will indicate later compilations which took this chapter as their starting point and updated it.

Yet gradually things are changing. Some doctors who once thought extreme my passionate concern about infant formula are saying things as plainly and as strongly as Larry Gartner, in the opening quotation to this chapter. What is more, *Newsweek* would never have published such plain speaking in 1984. We are not yet at the stage where all healthworkers will say bluntly that all babies need to be fed women's milk for optimal development physically and mentally, although scientific research makes it plain that if babies were not reliant on their parents to 'choose' for them, breastmilk would be their undisputed choice. But that day is coming: unless, yet again, politics and economics wins out over science and health. This book is an attempt to ensure that parents do not allow the almighty dollar and social convenience to deprive their children of optimal health for life.

What I wrote in this chapter in 1984 disturbed and angered some healthworkers and some women who bottlefed their children. Yet the anger women felt was not directed at me for telling the truth, but at healthworkers who had failed to do so when women indicated that they didn't want to breastfeed. As one woman said, "Did the doctor think I was such a selfish person and rotten mother that such information wouldn't have made a difference, or was he just ignorant?" The element of free and informed choice has been largely lacking in decisions about infant feeding, due to inadequate knowledge and poor management and support of the pregnant and post-partum woman. It stands to reason that guilt is therefore quite inappropriate: we deserve to feel guilty only when we make poor decisions knowingly, ignoring our informed conscience. The guilt issue is discussed further elsewhere in this book.

What follows should not be taken as a complete account of significant differences between human milk and substitutes, nor a complete record of problems that have occurred with artificial substitutes, even up until 1984. It is intended rather to illustrate the kinds of problems that we know or can reasonably expect to occur when we interfere with extraordinarily complex physiological systems. In 1998 we know even more about the consequences, and I have added at the end of this chapter a few resources summarising some of what we now know about this area, including some of my own later writing.

Nutritional differences between human milk and substitutes

Breastmilk is an incredibly complex collection of all the nutrients necessary for optimal infant development: metabolically, immunologically, and neurologically. It is also a great deal more than that, as will be discussed later. Not even the most optimistic or foolhardy infant formula salesperson claims that formula can compete in these regards. But in the area of *nutritional adequacy* substitutes for breastmilk (hereafter formula) are widely believed to be "very close" to women's milk – so let's assess that claim.

How do we measure the nutritional adequacy of any diet? By seeing whether it provides enough nutrients for apparently normal health and growth in the individual. How do we measure that? First, by analysing the composition of the diet and checking it against what is currently known/believed about human needs; next, by monitoring the growth and health of the individual and measuring the individual's progress against what is known about growth and health in this particular society at this particular time in history. So we rely heavily on established standards. But how can we be sure that our reference standards are indeed valid?

Some artificial formulae sold in some nations are made to meet various national and international standards of composition, hygiene, and so on. These standards are originally derived from an analysis of human milk. Many people think this a simple matter of measuring what's in breast milk, then seeing that the same amounts go into a can; much advertising encourages this simplistic belief. Problems begin with measuring breast milk. Researchers have only recently begun to develop techniques and equipment sensitive enough to begin the task of analysing breast milk. Whole meetings have been devoted to the question, "what constitutes a representative sample of breast milk?"[1] After researchers decide when and how to take the sample, it must still be accurately analysed and decisions made about how to average out the sometimes wide discrepancies observed between the milk of mothers with equally thriving babies. Since the 1960s many new discoveries have been made. Many changes to formula have been necessary, and have been instituted at varying rates by different companies. Some of these changes, though well intentioned, have proved disastrous, just as some of the earlier omissions and inclusions were later realised to be. We can never have a guarantee that this process of new discoveries is ended: the role of micro-nutrients such as trace elements, for instance, is largely unknown, yet these are increasingly processed out of formula; almost certainly the total protein content of formula will be lowered[2] in the not-too-distant future.

Before considering specific problems, let it be remembered that we are not dealing with Infant Formula, a standardised and totally consistent product. Formulae vary widely in their composition. They almost all claim (in violation of the World Health Organisation's Code of Marketing) to be closest to mothers' milk in some respect. All these claims can be 'true': one formula may be closest to human milk protein levels, another closest to the levels of particular minerals, a third closest to the types of essential fatty acids in human milk. All may be equally distant in other respects, and those other differences may invalidate the earlier claim: it is little use to have the right amounts of linolenic acid in formula if the baby cannot absorb it. In the last decades, authorities in a few countries have begun to specify what the ingredients of formula should be. However, standards are most often written by committees dominated, numerically or technically, by formula industry expertise. Further, most standards specify ranges: 'not more than this, not less than that' for most ingredients. Consider the mathematical possibilities for differences between formulae with 20 or 30 variables. Both the standards and the formulae are of very recent origin, so the significance of these differences is quite unknown. Only long-term clinical experience could indicate which formulae are the most suitable (or least unsuitable, perhaps). Yet how many doctors, as a routine part of all paediatric consultation, record in detail the formula and other infant diet? Who knows when a particular brand of formula is reconstituted slightly differently? Why is the long-overdue comparative research between brands rarely done?

Why can't requirements and standards (where they exist) be more precise?

The answer is that we don't know enough about human milk (the basis of the standard) and about bioavailability of nutrients in different combinations. Many people do not realise that human milk can be very variable: within a feed, over a day, from one breast to another, one woman to another, and over time.[3] There are excellent reasons for this flexibility, and the baby's characteristics help to determine it. If the baby is born prematurely, for example, the milk the mother makes will be higher in many of the growth factors and other nutrients[4] the baby needs for adequate growth. If living in a cold climate, there will be more fat for energy;[5] in a hot climate, more water to prevent dehydration.[6] If the baby suckles strongly, as big babies tend to, the infant may obtain more fat to meet growth needs.[7] If the mother is slightly malnourished, the total volume of her milk may drop slightly, but the amount of protein and fat will not,[8] and her baby will grow beautifully. Of course there can be less positive reasons for human milk variability, such as derangement of the maternal-infant interaction by arbitrary rules about feeding; extreme over- and under-nutrition in the mother; drugs given to mother or baby, and so on. But in the usual course of things, milk composition continues to change to keep pace with the infant's needs: so much so that the milk of the mother of a three-month-old is not ideal for a newborn baby, any more than the premature infant can thrive solely on the milk of a mother who gave birth to a full-term baby.[9] So what milk do we measure in trying to get an average; what age of baby do we set standards for? Formulae for premature infants are different from those for premature babies. Should formula for the first week be identical in composition with formula for the third month? Imagine the costs involved in variable formulae. Yet human milk adjusts constantly throughout the whole lactation period.

Standards for formulae are based on data about pooled human milk, which is potentially very different from what any individual baby would thrive on. To the average figure obtained by analysis, a certain percentage is added for safety – better too much than too little being a general assumption. For some ingredients this extra is indeed necessary, because so much of the nutrient content of the formula is not able to be digested by the baby (see p. 15). But how much extra; how much is too much; how can one anticipate a baby's response to the extra? Does one aim at putting in enough to achieve the levels of absorption achieved from breast milk?

To give an example, this has meant putting into formulae more than ten times the amount of iron in breast milk.[10] Breast milk contains very little iron, which is well-utilised thanks to a transfer factor which makes iron unavailable to gut bacteria.[11]

Bacteria in the bottlefed infant's gut use much of the iron in formula; this encourages the growth of particular bacteria which can cause gut damage and disease.[12] Large amounts of iron act as an irritant, and may cause blood loss from obvious or hidden bleeding in the baby's gut. For some babies, the result of added iron was thus iron deficiency anaemia, and secondary infection due to low antibody production.[13] Babies on soy formulae may have additional problems absorbing iron.[14]

According to eminent paediatrician Frank Oski,[15] there has never been much logic about the amounts of iron in formulae. One company had been marketing a formula with 6mg. per 100kcal: the same amount of iron is absorbed from this as from 12mg. per 100kcal. The company was aware of this, but made available a formula with 12mg. in order not to suffer losses in the marketplace due to its competitor being seen as providing more of a good thing. It would seem that manufacturers have come to agree with Professor Oski: by mid-1984 they were suggesting an iron level of 3mg. per 100kcal, or a quarter of the amount many babies currently receive. Evidence about the role of iron in gastrointestinal bleeding has steadily mounted.

Iron status of bottlefed infants remains a matter of professional concern. Too little will cause anaemia (more common in the bottlefed). Too much will also cause anaemia, and much more. Zinc deficiency can be caused by too much iron; widely divergent zinc/iron; zinc/copper; iron/manganese ratios in infant formulae have unknown consequences.[16] (But 2000 times the amount of manganese as in breast milk does not seem a good idea!) Nutritional authorities are now setting maximum levels for nutrients in formula, as they begin to worry about such things. Industry usually resists the introduction of maxima.

Ironically, mistaken concern about the small quantities of iron in breast milk led some doctors to advocate the early introduction of iron-containing solids to the breastfed baby's diet. By interfering with the iron transfer factor, or reacting to produce insoluble iron compounds,[17] these foods brought about the anaemia they were given to prevent, thus confirming the doctors in their view of breast milk as inadequate nutrition. It now seems clear that exclusive breastfeeding is adequate to maintain excellent iron status for at least 6-9 months,[18] if not longer, provided that the baby is not premature and does not bleed heavily from any cause, and the mother is not severely malnourished.

Human milk is also very low in protein compared with formulae, but it contains other readily-absorbed nitrogenous compounds for nutrition and for protection against infection. The forms of protein in alien milks are not so well-utilised, therefore more protein must be put into the formula. The body must break down all this extra protein and then excrete the wastes: an additional stress for the immature liver and kidneys. The breakdown products accumulate in the blood when the baby cannot dispose of them fast enough. We understand why babies must be tested for phenylketonuria (PKU): a specific enzyme defect means that the child cannot break down and excrete phenylalanine, one amino acid. But tyrosine and other amino acids, the break down products of protein, can also reach toxic levels if babies receive more than they can manage. One researcher states that perhaps 80 per cent of bottlefed neonates have blood levels of tyrosine "high enough to cause concern about brain damage, impairment of intelligence, and later learning disabilities."[19] Some babies will manage perfectly well. (But how can parents ever know whether a child might have been brighter, or better able to concentrate and learn?) Other babies, maybe with lower enzyme levels, with inbuilt defects, or stressed by other factors, may be affected. No one does tests to monitor blood levels of amino acids in normal babies on normal formulae: the assumption is that all average babies should be able to cope. But tyrosine, interestingly, is the precursor of dopamine, a neurotransmitter found in abnormal amounts in the brain of babies dying of SIDS, or 'cot death'.[20]

The change to whey-based formula was designed to more closely approximate the whey-casein ratio of human milk, with its pattern of amino acids. This is much featured in advertising material, and the problems of whole cows' milk accentuated. (Protein structure and blood levels, as well as mineral load.) Yet what is better in theory may not always be better in practice. Perhaps because of differences in bioavailability, whey predominant formula actually result in higher plasma amino acid and serum urea nitrogen levels than do the older whole milk formulas. Researchers who discovered this concluded that present infant formulas are providing excessive quantities of protein, and that "feeding bovine whey to the full-term infant is not more desirable than feeding bovine casein."[21] This is not what advertising says!

The problem of limited knowledge

What goes into formula is what is believed to be essential at the time of creating the standard.[22] Researchers are increasingly questioning the standards. For example, until quite recently, the recommendations for amounts of calcium, phosphorus and magnesium were based on data published in 1953. A study of 102 women showed that their thriving infants' intake was considerably less, and so in April 1984 the minimum allowable levels were revised.[23] Prior to this some doctors regarded human milk as inadequate to meet the recommended daily allowance of these elements. It is something of a joke for human milk (the basis of the RDAs) to be judged deficient because it contained less than necessarily-inflated standards derived from inadequate data. At the same time, maximum levels for iron and iodine were set: both are now recognised as harmful in excess, and iodine is a common (though illegal above certain limits) contaminant of cows' milk due to the use of iodophor disinfectants. Some years ago zinc was not thought to be essential for babies: we learned that it is because zinc-deficient infant formula caused retardation, sub-optimal growth, and skin lesions in babies.[24] But when hypo-allergenic formulae were first marketed, we had to learn the importance of zinc all over again as babies suffered from zinc deficiency.

Nor are those the only examples that come to mind. A few years ago, biotin was not in some infant formulae: it now is because researchers uncovered the fact that animals dying of a SIDS-like syndrome were biotin-deficient.[25] Were some contemporary cot-death babies biotin-deficient? Cysteine, another amino acid, was until recently not regarded as essential for term babies because it was assumed that, like adults, they could synthesize it from other dietary components. Their capacity to do so proved to be limited; cysteine is now on the essential list.[26] Were there specific derangements of infant metabolism as a result of its absence? Similarly, taurine, essential for the myelination of the central nervous system and brain after birth, was almost totally absent from many formulae until late 1984. Studies have shown significant differences in brain size of rats fed taurine-deficient formula, with corresponding intelligence deficits. Other studies show damage to the retina of the eyes of cats and monkeys and retinal changes in children with low plasma taurine levels.[27] One wonders too about how multiple sclerosis victims and others suffering from demyelinating diseases were fed as infants. Did inadequate nutrition result in an abnormal myelin layer, more susceptible to insults such as viral attacks? There is now research to show higher rates of infant bottle-feeding in MS sufferers.

To cysteine and taurine one could add carnitine,[28] another amino acid now suspected of being essential for the newborn. Concern has also been expressed about the bottlefed baby's selenium intake, which is much less than the breastfed baby's;[29] or the much higher intake of fluoride (see p. 206). There are controversies about virtually every nutrient presently known. But researchers have learnt to be cautious about simply adding another ingredient. As the base product to which they are added is extensively processed, unexpected interactions can occur, resulting in further problems: for example, adding vitamin D to prevent rickets (partly due to the poor absorption of calcium from earlier formulae) resulted in hypercalcaemia. It will be decades before nutritional scientists can reliably predict the outcome of manipulations of formula.

I should illustrate this by describing the worst known example to date of this sort of mishap. The first infant formulae contained far too much salt, which was responsible for virtual epidemics of hypernatraemia[30] – babies convulsed and sometimes suffered kidney and brain damage. Scientists had expressed concern about these high salt levels since the 1960s;[31] the impetus to change to lower levels was not overly urgent in the United Kingdom until Dr. Mavis Gunther's intention to publish comparative figures in a book for mothers became known. The manufacturers rapidly made the change,[32] and so-called 'low-solute' formulae became standard before the book was finally published. The 1970s were the time when the apparent link between salt intake and hypertension (high blood pressure) became widely accepted. US manufacturers lowered or eliminated salt from infant foods. (Though in 1985 the FDA was still engaged in debate with one major babyfood manufacturer over this very issue.) Over 1978-9, one US formula company, Syntex, therefore eliminated chloride from some of their products. Infants being fed Neo-Mull-Soy and Cho-free developed metabolic alkalosis – failure to thrive, constipation/diarrhoea, vomiting, dehydration, kidney problems, developmental delays. Years later, the children still suffer from "consistently delayed speech, slow gross motor development, increased convulsion rates, rotting teeth, kidney defects, mild retardation and cerebral palsy."[32] Those few children who were identified as victims had often been wrongly diagnosed. What consumer protection agency brought this to light? Only the persistence of parents, and the curiosity of a doctor who saw six cases of a supposedly rare kidney disorder in a short time, and who did not dismiss as neurotic the grandmother who suspected the formula. By March 1980, 120 children had been identified as suffering from this problem. What proportion this is of those actually affected is anybody's guess. Between 20,000 and 50,000 children were fed these formulae in any one week; any child whose parents used this (as recommended) as the child's only source of nutrition would have been damaged. Indeed among the 120 there are some whose condition is less severe because they were not solely reliant on the formula, but got other foods as well. Many of the children were identified as the result of publicity given to two mothers who have trenchantly criticised the political manoeuvring that has prevented the Center for Disease Control in Atlanta from carrying out studies that might have located other victims and other problems; prevented anyone from ascertaining whether and to whom the defective formulae were exported; and prevented prosecution of the company despite a recommendation from the FDA for prosecution. It is certain that Cho-free was in use in some Melbourne hospitals in 1980 because I received a phone call asking if I could help a baffled supply officer locate further supplies for premature babies: all he had discovered was that the firm no longer existed. I later received assurances (but no proof) that this was not from the defective batches, but as Syntex formulae were defective for so long a period, if they were not defective they may have been very old stock. Without an agency such as the FDA used to be pre-Reaganisation, it is difficult to follow through such incidents. Syntex was no backyard operation: its chief scientist was actually on the AAP committee on nutrition. That such a stupid mistake could occur says much about infant formula manufacturing.

This incident illustrates vividly how good intentions may lead to great harm when tinkering with infant formula. No one stopped to consider what those electrolyte changes might mean to babies with cystic fibrosis,[33] either. But not all changes are deliberate; some are accidental. A new type of processing led to the destruction of B vitamins in one formula in the 1950s.[34] Result? Brain damage. For years no one was concerned about the lead in soldered cans, although lead is a cumulative poison that damages the brain. When researchers asked questions, they found frightening answers.[35] One Washington study showed lead levels of 5-50mcg. per 100ml. of formula; 29-36 mcg. per 100ml. of evaporated milk. Assuming a daily formula intake of 550 ml. (and assuming, often erroneously, that water used in making up the formula was lead-free), babies would receive a staggering 28-275mcg. per day from formula alone. Breastfed babies were receiving 0-25 mcg. per day, which is below the 30mcg. then arbitrarily set as the threshold of risk from lead intake, but which could still be improved. Discussions between manufacturers and the FDA were spine-chilling: manufacturers seemed to see this (and other issues such as nitrosamines) as being of no great urgency.[36] They got their way: in the US they were given until 1985 to fully convert to welded cans. Other countries have had stricter regulations about fruit juice! The world's first published list of further accidents – a very incomplete one – can be found towards the end of this chapter.

Commercial considerations

The choice of food sources from which to compose a formula is as wide as the world itself. Decisions about which to use will be based on both nutritional and commercial facts. When corn oil became expensive, soy oil was added to corn and coconut oil; when arrowroot became difficult to obtain tapioca starch and corn syrup replaced a mixture of maltose/sucrose, dextrins and arrowroot starch.[37] Perhaps these changes were a nutritional improvement or made no difference, but the logic behind them was commercial. If sunflower seed oil is too expensive this year, and coconut oil much cheaper on the world market, the cheaper product may be chosen and blended with other ingredients to replace the expensive one. In fact, coconut oil is widely used in infant formulae because it is a saturated fat that is readily absorbed, so that babies gain weight well on it, according to two US paediatricians. They went on to state that "coconut oil is actually toxic and has been demonstrated to cause serious problems in laboratory animals and normal human adults", and expressed concern about "the possibly dangerous inclusion of oxidised fatty acid molecules, a component never tested, yet commonly found in commercially prepared formulas."[38] Similar queries have been raised about the safety of carrageenan.[39] When the safety of trans fatty acids made from soybeans was elsewhere questioned, the reply was that to restrict their use would be "to destroy the biggest cash crop in the US."[40] How reassuring.

The infant formula industry is very big business. In 1981 world sales were estimated at $2 billion[41] (by 1997, the US market alone was reportedly worth this much). More than half of this 1981 market was in developing countries, where sales growth often averaged 15-20% annually, compared with 5% or less in developed nations. This industry exists primarily to make money for its investors. Its products are as subject to human error, chance, and technological failure as are those of any other industry. We would be naive to expect anything different, simply because the product is for babies. If a mistake looks like being too costly to rectify, any manufacturer must be tempted to take short cuts in an attempt to limit losses. Drug companies are certainly alleged to do so,[42] and their products are at least as sensitive as formula. On the whole, formula products are probably safe enough, and probably nutritionally adequate for most babies – i.e., children can usually survive and grow on these mixtures, just as many did on the past mixtures now condemned as totally unsuitable but then accepted. However, an element of risk must remain in the use of substitutes. Where this differs from the risks we daily accept in living is in the fact that it is too often an unnecessary risk which *we* choose, *not for ourselves, but for our children.*

My instinctive reaction on learning such things was 'Surely government checks exist?' We have come to expect regulation of sensitive areas such as this. The plain fact is that there are no special regulatory agencies, no systems of inspection or random analysis, outside the US, and even the FDA is beleaguered. Britain and Australia operate gentlemens' agreements with industry, which is believed to be responsible and trustworthy. Within the medical community the specialisation of research ensures that there are few people to call upon with detailed expertise about both infant formulae and human milk; very often industry representatives know far more about formula than anyone else, and are deferred to for want of information with which to challenge their perspective. Industry representatives would like more independent expertise to consult themselves! While they naturally make public claims of absolute rectitude and fail-safe testing, privately they can afford to be more honest about their product. Do they always produce that perfect product every mother trusts so blindly? Consider this excerpt from 1982 a book by a notable formula apologist: "A recent survey indicated some rather wide variations in the level of certain mineral and trace mineral components of infant formula. Both excessively high and excessively low concentrations of given mineral elements were reported for some products. A number of factors could be responsible. In general, consistent standardisation would have to take into account variations in initial concentration in formula ingredients and the influence in dairy-based products of feed, medications, and udder health. In addition, technologies of protein separation and refinement may add to or deplete from these components more or less of a variety of minerals and trace minerals. Quality control would require a rather exact accounting prior to fortification, if indeed fortification is needed."[43] That 'rather exact accounting' was not happening in the US in 1981: is it happening in Britain and Australia, not to mention less affluent societies? Note too, that while the influence of the human mother's feed, medication and health is constantly in the news, one hears little about just such variables in cows whose milk is used for human babies.

I exaggerate, you say. Surely in matters so important to Australian babies we have consumer protection. Let me tell you a 1990s story from a large maternity hospital with a special care nursery. A midwife rang me in distress to say that all the babies in special care had been sick, and the problem had been traced to the formula used for all of them, even the breastfed ones. (Why?) She told me that the hospital had rung the manufacturers and they intended to take away all the remaining formula and replace it with a better batch; and that the hospital was not going to report the matter to the Health Department: could I do so? I asked why she did not, and was told the staff had been warned to keep the matter quiet for fear of legal action by parents of the damaged babies. She was certain she would lose her job if she were identified as the source of the information. So I rang the Health Department and spoke to the senior doctor in charge of this area of public health. Very serious, he agreed: tell the midwife to report it, or get the hospital to, and a recall of the whole batch from every hospital could be arranged. I explained again why I was ringing rather than the midwife. No, it must be reported by the hospital: the Health Department could not go into a public hospital asking questions on the basis of an outside report. I asked what protection there would be of the informant if I were able to persuade the midwife to contact him. None, her name would go on the files and be accessible under Freedom of Information legislation. I rang the midwife: she could not afford to lose her job. I had promised her I would do nothing without her agreement. So babies were injured, some developed necrotising enterocolitis, and perhaps some died in hospitals that were slower to recognise the formula as the source, which would be very likely in small units. Parents never knew, and the Health Department did not want to. There is no protection for whistle blowers in the state of Victoria, perhaps because the Health Department responsible for the hospitals does not want parents to know: like the hospitals the Health Department too could be at risk of a lawsuit. Check the procedures in your state or nation: are they any better?

Problems of use, water and containers

With any manufactured product there is always the possibility not only of company error, but of user error. This has ranged from over-concentration (leading to hypernatraemia and brain damage, even in a hospital nursery)[44] to over-dilution (leading to failure to thrive, even starvation); bacterial overgrowth due to inadequate hygiene and storage; accidental salt poisoning when salt was mistaken for sugar. By now the world appreciates that where mothers are poor, uneducated about formula use, lacking abundant fuel for sterilising, clean water, and refrigeration, the results of using artificial formulae are disastrous. Over a million infants die for want of breastmilk annually. On a smaller scale such tragedies continue in every country, including Britain, Australia and the US, particularly among native peoples and the poor, but the rich are not protected completely.

Further problems arise from the fact that many formulae must be reconstituted with water, when variations in the mineral and trace elements in water can be considerable. A formula with added fluorine, mixed with fluoridated water, may contain toxic amounts of an element known to interfere with enzyme activity. But no warnings are put on the label because the dental benefits are thought too important, and parents thought so stupid that they could not understand that what is true for the infant whose sole diet is formula is not true for an older, bigger child drinking less water. Who monitors the water used at home? Prolonged boiling will further concentrate the mineral load. Are there parents relying on bore waters, very hard water, or on mineral water for infant feeding? In the UK and elsewhere mineral waters have been advertised as safe for babies;[45] some may be (the very low-solute ones) but mineral waters generally are not, and in 1996 Israeli babies were dying of hypernatraemia because of the use of high-solute mineral water. Conversely, are parents using distilled water, or processing water through a water softener?[46] Neither can be recommended. Companies too, must monitor their water supplies, particularly if they market liquid formulae. In 1983 one formula manufacturer found that two of its four wells were contaminated with dangerous chemicals.[47] These were then tested for, and found, in the formula, but at levels thought insufficient to justify any recall, although there was considerable debate about this by consumer groups. The company installed better filtration systems, and removed those wells from use. However, this vigilance was a little late. The discovery was a purely inadvertent one, the result of the local county's program to determine the extent of groundwater contamination. If no one thinks to check for such problems, should we assume that none exist? The American Academy of Pediatrics would prefer to know a little more: in June 1985 they wrote to the FDA requesting "comprehensive screening" of groundwater and other foodstocks used in formula, as well as a survey of the "extent of industrial compound contamination of other infant foods currently available".[48] Current EPA regulations require sampling only once every 3 years, and then not for the most common contaminants. As AAP President Dr. Frank Young stated, "It is evident that greater vigilance over the purity of infant formula ingredients, both water and food materials, must be instituted." Sampling of water *near known toxic disposal sites* has begun, and some analysis of infant formula was promised although no results have been published. But readers of the expensive trade journal, *Food Chemical News*, which is the main source for such interesting information, would know that such increased vigilance flies in the face of all that the Reagan and Bush Administrations did in the area of food regulation. There is profound anxiety among members of Congress over the extent of the politicisation of the FDA, and its willingness to protect industry rather than consumers; even long-established progressive measures such as full label disclosure are threatened.[49]

Between the manufacturer and the user there is the problem of distribution and storage. It is clear that formula sealed in air-tight cans does deteriorate; the FDA has spelled out some of the problems. Still one sees cans of formula exposed to direct sunlight for weeks or months. What effect might this have on nutrient availability? What monitoring exists to expose the effects of careless handling and storage on the best of formulae?

As well, there are real problems associated with the use of cans, feeding bottles and teats, rather than breasts. Conscientious manufacturers will talk candidly off the record about the rough interiors (perfect for trapping stale milk and breeding bacteria) of some very expensive, much advertised models. Only certain plastics are suitable for use in contact with food: are all the cheaper models, imported from countries without comprehensive food regulations, made from safe plastics? What checks have been made on migration of chemicals into milk, or fruit juices? There has been a great deal of concern about the levels of nitrosamines (chemicals known to cause cancer) in bottle teats. West Germany set a standard of no more than 3 parts per billion (ppb); the US, under heavy pressure from the Rubber Manufacturers Association, initially allowed 100ppb for domestic use and 150ppb for hospital use teats (subjected to greater stress).[50] Then in March 1984 parents were urged by the FDA to boil bottle teats several times before use, discarding the water each time, to lower nitrosamine levels.[51] The irony of this advice is that nitrosamines and other stabilisers are added to prolong the life of the rubber; boiling rapidly shortens that life. A US standard of 10ppb was to be phased in by 1985; this has been changed to 10ppb of any individual nitrosamine, rather than the total. It is said that smaller amounts are impossible to monitor accurately. Yet some teats are now being marketed as totally free of nitrosamines. If they are using the same raw materials, one wonders why all manufacturers cannot produce nitrosamine-free teats. If they are using different materials, one wonders whether all potential problems from those new materials have been thoroughly investigated.

Clearly some manufacturers are more conscientious about these issues than others. The migration of hazardous compounds from bottle or teat into infant food is a trivial risk compared with some aspects of formula feeding. But have those investigating stomach cancers asked about this aspect of very early exposure to the carcinogens known to produce stomach cancer?

It may seem extreme to question the harmlessness of bottles and teats. But in chapter 5 you can see examples of technology once advertised as positively beneficial, but now obviously harmful. Researchers in the 21st century may be equally critical of our safe products. The leaching of lead into formulae was discussed earlier. Other problems are on record. Tin-alloy cans 'can impart variable but often substantial amounts of tin into food. In Ghana, a progressive leaching of tin into locally produced evaporated milk resulted in a tin content of over 100mg. per litre... after storage.' This can cause zinc deficiency.[52] Excessive quantities of the plasticiser used to line some formula cans were found in the product after a conveyor belt malfunctioned. What level of testicle-shrinking phthalates[53] can be found in formula and what are the consequences? Why has the concern about this focused only on soy formulae when cow's milk formulae also contain significant levels of such compounds?

No matter what type of container is used to store infant formulae, there will be some interaction between container and contents. This is why some materials are known to be unsuitable for certain purposes, and some are forbidden altogether. But regulatory bodies are realists. What they permit or proscribe is what is technically feasible and politically acceptable at that moment in history. If manufacturers argue that crippling expense would be involved in meeting certain standards, the standards are very likely to be re-drafted in collaboration with them. This is inevitable; it is not unique to manufacturers concerned with baby goods. Indeed, I expect that they are more careful than many others, because babies more readily get sick, and when consuming only one product, more easily expose the problem. This is simply the way of things when goods must be processed. My point is that the best infant feeding product is not stored in cans, but processed on demand by mothers.

Similarly, the mechanics of feeding from a bottle may have deleterious effects. The increased interest in hypoxaemia (oxygen lack) during bottlefeeding[54] is disturbing; and the oral mechanics of feeding may affect some children's facial structures. (See chapter 9.)

To summarise this section on the nutrient content of artificial formulae:

- we don't know what ought to be in them;
- we can't guarantee that what we intend to put in will be what we do put in;
- we don't know how to put it there in such a way that it will still be there when prepared for the child;
- nor can we guarantee that it will be made up by the user as it should be; and
- we don't have any real idea of the consequences of using these very variable mixtures exclusively for months, as we are now urged to do.

It seems to me fairly obvious that had all mothers breastfed until 1980, and scientists then began to formulate a substitute, any product they suggested would have been subjected to rigorous double-blind controlled prolonged testing before being allowed on the market. The pity is that this is all too late. Yet the business of deciding on the 'right' ingredients is in many ways the simplest bit of an impossible task.

Bioavailability of nutrients

It used to be assumed that to be well-fed one simply had to ingest nutrients. "Because there's plenty of calcium and iron in our formula baby won't be deficient in either." As we've seen for iron, things are much more complicated. Small quantities, well-absorbed because of transfer factors, are preferable to large quantities. Human milk is known to contain transfer factors for iron, zinc, folic acid, and vitamin B_{12}.[17] The fats in human milk come partly pre-digested by some of the 60-70 enzymes recently discovered; this provides the baby with an instant energy source at little metabolic cost.[17] By contrast, the formula-fed baby must metabolize a variety of sometimes quite foreign fats.[55] Protein digestion is assisted by some of the thirteen nucleotides found in human milk;[56] just a few nucleotides added to formula may not work in the same way and may even be harmful. Iron absorption is dependent upon the presence of adequate amounts of vitamin C; some soy formulae are thought to be deficient in both.[14] The particular ratios between nutrients are also important to proper utilisation: as we have seen earlier, these ratios in formula have been obviously wrong. And so on: it would require a proper academic course to cover all these interactions adequately – and by the time the course was finished it would need revision.

Lactose is a good example of a simple nutrient with complex effects on many areas of the body. The high lactose content of human milk enhances the absorption or retention of several minerals,[57] and is vital in maintaining an acid pH in the gut favourable to helpful bacteria that manufacture vitamins. Lactose is also a crucial nutrient in brain growth.[58] Yet corn syrup solids, sucrose, and other carbohydrates replace lactose in some formulae. These other sugars can be fermented by common yeasts to produce alcohol, which in some people results in the 'Auto-Brewery Syndrome': the person can be intoxicated without drinking alcohol. Louisiana researchers have stated that further studies are needed "to determine if there is a relationship between ethanol production in the gastrointestinal system and the Sudden Infant Death Syndrome."[59] Needless to say, human milk has anti-fungal activity, so that yeast overgrowth and fermentation is unlikely. No studies have been published.

As a result of these and other nutritional differences, the breastfed baby's endocrine responses differ from those of the formula-fed child.[60] The long-term significance of those differences has not been uncovered, although it is interesting to see some researchers stating that breastfeeding protects against the development of childhood diabetes.[61] Researchers studying adult endocrine disorders rarely consider childhood diet as a variable; because of the specialised nature of Western medicine, they may even be unaware of the profound differences between human milk and substitutes.

Other factors in human milk make its nutritional impact even greater. Researchers have discovered that human milk contains high concentrations of identified and unidentified growth factors, which "may be important in the differentiation and proliferation of infant tissues";[62] these are particularly high in the milk of mothers who give birth prematurely.[63]

So women's milk can nourish babies where a formula made to exactly the same specifications would be deficient. We know in fact that healthy breastfed babies have an energy intake much less than previously suspected. Even when additional solids are given, at four months of age, average intake remains at 70-80kcal per kg. and babies thrive.[64] (Contrast this with the 120kcal per kg. which has been accepted as necessary for so long.) According to the tables by which breastmilk has in the past been deemed inadequate, babies on such low intakes would have no energy for any activity.

Obviously the tables were wrong for breastfed babies.

Thus our second criterion for judging nutritional adequacy is exposed as shaky. Growth tables derived from mixed populations of artificially fed and breastfed babies are simply inappropriate for judging the health and growth of the fully breastfed infant, although standards based on the growth of the fully breastfed infant could be used to judge the adequacy of formula-fed babies' growth in a very crude fashion. (Weight and length tells one little about body composition: it is known that the type and distribution of body fat of artificially fed infants is different from that of breastfed infants, for example: findings that suggest distortion of normal development) The patterns of growth emerging from studies of breastfed children are different from the older tables.[65] As Garza said at the US Surgeon General's Workshop on Breastfeeding and Human Lactation, "Human milk is a highly complex mixture with a nutrient balance that may promote a level of metabolic efficiency unattainable by the formula-fed infant... If the energy consumed by bottlefed infants represents a true excess, are there any positive or negative long- or short-term consequences?"[66] Over-nutrition is usually associated with negative consequences, of course.

Bioavailability does not depend on merely the interaction between ingredients. The baby's body is also involved. There are considerable differences in the amount of energy digested and absorbed by individual babies on an identical diet. The reported energy content of formulae is not their actual caloric content, but rather what is believed to be their 'metabolisable' energy: what baby can use. As one researcher has pointed out, these estimates are based upon studies in young adults[67] fed mixed diets, and therefore may not be generally applicable to all neonates. Here again, the inflexible nature of formula is a disadvantage. Using the same formula, one baby may be overfed because of his high metabolic efficiency, while another may be underfed because of his relatively low metabolic efficiency (which had the baby been breastfed, could have been assisted by the other properties of human milk, and by the baby's ability to regulate his intake.) The consequences for either baby would not be immediately obvious, because we can never be sure whether children should be growing differently, unless they are grossly over- or under-weight.

All these differences in nutrient composition and bioavailability do add appreciably to the stress and waste products the infant must cope with. Thus many experts insist that any already-stressed neonate ought to be fed human milk alone.[68] Ironically, it is these babies – those born prematurely, twins, multiple, caesarian births, difficult births – who have been most at risk of being given artificial formula. This can sometimes be necessary at present. But what proportion of the later disturbances common in these children might be the result of such a curious use of formula? We should explore better options, such as human milk formulae, when mother's milk is unavailable or inappropriate. As an interim measure, we could at least insist on the use of less highly allergenic formulae for stressed neonates,[69] while being aware that by the next generation allergic reactions even to these will have sky-rocketed.

Other deficiencies of artificial substitutes

The differences outlined in the above section should make it clear that those who are concerned about the widespread use of infant formula have good reasons for their concerns. Unfortunately, this is only the beginning; there are many more differences between breastmilk and formula which have negative implications for babies fed artificially. It needs to be said that the breastfed baby is the biological norm: insofar as any baby is different from what he/she would have been if breastfed, that baby is abnormal. And insofar as any substitute fails to provide what women's milk provides, it is deficient. Infant formula has many inescapable deficiencies.

Immunological differences

Human milk is not simply food. It is a living tissue, including many substances that affect not only the body's use of nutrients but also its immune capacity. Nutrition and immunity are inextricably interwoven in either a healthy or vicious cycle.[70] Good nutrition means plenty of components for the immune system; high immunity means good ability to absorb and utilise nutrients. Poor nutrition leads to immune deficiency, which allows infection, which robs the body of nutrients. Even a lack of one specific nutrient can cause immune deficiency: we have mentioned the role of lactose, iron and zinc in this regard, but many other milk components are actively involved in the immune response – vitamins, minerals, essential fatty acids, and so on. Enzymes are not only active as aids to digestion: they are also extremely active against bacteria. Human milk contains over 3000 times the lysozyme (one such enzyme) found in cows' milk.[71] Of course live cows' milk is itself a very different substance from processed dehydrated formula. Although it cannot be recommended for infant feeding for many good reasons, there have been, and probably always will be, a few children who can cope with one particular cow's fresh milk and not the pooled pasteurised mixtures; probably because of factors such as enzymes. By 1984 scientists had isolated and identified 60-70 enzymes in human milk. The function of some is still unknown; hence it is impossible to guess what their absence from formula might mean, and to test that possibility. A similar paragraph might be written about the many hormones in human milk, which has become another area of exciting research.

Transfer factors mentioned earlier also serve an immunological purpose. Lacto-ferrin, the iron transfer protein, inhibits staphylococci, E. coli and thrush, unless the baby is overloaded with iron. Similarly the B_{12} transfer factor starves harmful bacteria of nutrients essential for growth. By contrast, cows' milk is designed to encourage the bacterial growth a ruminant animal needs for digestion. Formula derived from it thus provides the ideal culture medium for the growth of bacteria harmful to humans. Breastmilk does not.

Human milk also contains almost as many live cells – macrophages, lymphocytes, neutrophils, and epithelial cells – as blood itself.[72] It has been called 'white blood' in one culture. These cells can actively destroy bacteria, fungi, and intestinal parasites and help to regulate the immune response to other excitants such as foods and inhalants. Not until the late 1970s was it realised that if the mother was exposed to some antigen, specially primed cells would migrate to the breast and excrete antibodies in her milk. This means that if mother and baby are exposed to some infection, the baby's under-developed immune system does not have to fight infection unaided. The mother's milk will soon provide a dose of the specific antibody needed, as well as all the usual non-specific antibiotic factors. More recent research indicated that as well as this enteromammary axis,[73] there is a bronchomammary[74] one as well – that is, if the mother is exposed to infection via her respiratory tract, cells will migrate to the breast, and antibody be fed to the baby. Mother's milk is good medicine, as well as good food.

Not surprisingly, every study of the relative health of breast and formula-fed babies comes out with fewer infections among the breastfed ones,[75] even if in some cases these can be later explained away by statistical analysis. The differences were much more dramatic earlier in this century, which is usually taken as proving that formula is now safe. There are numerous other possibilities to explain that observation, not least of them the appalling methodology of many studies. Until recently almost none controlled for the impact of foods[76] other than breast milk given to the breastfed baby: before babies in hospital were given the free complementary feeds so obligingly provided by manufacturers, they may well have been healthier.[77]

These live cells, among them antibodies, are widely recognised as existing in colostrum. Hence one still hears, 'yes, it's important for babies to get the colostrum, but after that the milk gets watery and it doesn't matter so much.' It's certainly true that colostrum contains high levels of antibodies, among them secretory IgA, which is thought to act as a local 'paint' for the intestines, preventing the entry of foreign molecules that might set up allergic reactions. (It has since been shown that some antibody is absorbed to provide systemic protection as well.[78]) But newborns cannot handle large volumes of fluid very well; their kidneys must adjust to this task. Colostrum is concentrated milk of a kind best designed to getting all systems working well: its laxative properties have been known for decades. Later milk is just as well suited to the child's needs at that time, and contains just as many antibodies overall,[76] although they are less concentrated in the larger volumes the older baby receives. In fact, during gradual weaning (safest for both mother and child) as the volume of milk decreases once again, the level of antibody rises,[79] helping to protect both the breast and the weanling from infection. If the child becomes ill during weaning, as many do in conditions of poor hygiene, or in food intolerant families, he or she usually reverts to the breast alone, and benefits from this once-again-concentrated milk. (Additional water is sometimes needed by the baby as the mother's supply builds up.)

The formula industry has become very aware of the importance of this immunological argument in persuading mothers to breastfeed. They are now actively seeking ways to add immune factors to formula. In the 1990s the addition of a few nucleotides is being misleadingly advertised as follows:

- Immunity is naturally conferred by breastmilk. [True.]
- Nucleotides occur naturally in breastmilk. [True.]
- Nucleotides help maintain a baby's immune system. [True.]
- Our brands are now fortified with nucleotides.

QED what? That 'our brands' confer the immunity that breastmilk does, because we've added a few of the 13 nucleotides which are only one of the dozens of breastmilk factors affecting infant immunity? It is equally possible that adding a few immune factors will cause an imbalance in the immune system that leads to greater reactivity and hypersensitivity, without having positive effects at all. Where are the studies showing clinical benefits from these formulas?[80]

Some researchers, working with children admitted to hospital with gastroenteritis, have dosed cows with human infectious agents, then collected the cows' colostrum and fed that to children.[81] This worked quite well, and could prove to be useful: but no one mentioned the possibility of breastfeeding, let alone vaccinating the mothers. Had those children been breastfed, many would not have been in hospital. In one Australian hospital between June and December of 1979, 168 children were admitted with gastroenteritis.[82] Not one was fully breastfed at the time of admission, 15 were partially breastfed: none of these 15 was severely ill, despite the fact that these were younger babies and the more severe disease with dehydration occurred with greater frequency in infants less than 6 months of age. In a similar study in England,[83] only 2 of 608 children admitted with gastroenteritis were receiving any breast milk. The community's breastfeeding rate was 14 per cent, which should have meant another 80 or more sick children had breastfeeding not been protective. In a study in the US,[84] only one of 107 infants was being breastfed. As the author of that paper said, "The data in this study strongly indicates that breastfeeding plays a major role in the protection against intestinal infections. *The effect is almost as dramatic in a modern, middle-class US community as in a developing country.*" [My emphasis.] Israeli experience is similar.[85] Indeed, human milk is being used as therapy in cases of chronic intractable diarrhoeal disease in older children,[86] and is protective even against cholera,[87] that most dreaded intestinal infection.

If drug companies were able to do what we lactating women do automatically – rapidly produce significant quantities of specific antibodies to whatever threatens our children – hospital wards would empty. They have in Baguio, in the Philippines, where 100 per cent of babies are now fed human milk. (The number of abandoned children has also decreased dramatically.) There are no effective, specific anti-viral drugs on the market. Interferon was unrealistically hailed as a possible cure-all – the interferon family is only one of many anti-viral factors in human milk, which is known to be active against many different viruses[88] as well as other pathogens, including giardia lamblia[89] and other intestinal parasites.[90] For this reason, weaning during maternal illness is not sensible: the baby has already been exposed to the pathogen, and maternal antibodies are providing some protection. Every summer hospitals fill with cases of gastroenteritis, and every winter with bronchiolitis, and no one points out that few of these babies are fully breastfed. Being artificially fed increases a baby's chances of hospitalisation, or of sickness in day care, quite significantly.

Allergy and intolerance

No discussion of the immunological benefits of breastfeeding would be complete without considering this question. It has been conclusively demonstrated that prolonged exclusive breastfeeding will significantly reduce the incidence of food allergy and intolerance, even among families with a strong tendency to allergy.[91] It has also been shown that the time of exposure[92] to cows' milk correlates well with subsequent problems: the younger the child, the greater the risk. (This would be true of any food – it just happens that cows' milk is the food most commonly given.) Premature babies given any pre-term formula showed significant differences in their serum response to cows' milk challenge, when compared with breastfed infants.[93] But not all formula-fed children are allergic, and not all breastfed children free of allergy, although a very interesting study showed that no breastfed child without a family history of allergy became allergic, whereas many formula-fed infants without a family history did develop allergy *de novo*.[94] In some cases breast milk merely delays the onset and/or mitigates the severity of the allergic response; in other cases it may even be the proximate cause of symptoms in the child. I have written at length about this elsewhere,[95] and the issue is no longer really controversial for those who read the literature which I have reviewed, so here I shall confine myself to general comments.

Clearly, the incidence of food intolerance has increased in Western societies during this century, and it increases in less-affluent societies along with urbanisation and formula-feeding. It seems reasonable to suppose that in disrupting complex physiological systems[75] never designed to be exposed to foreign foods, difficulties in handling those foods might follow. Like Glaser, I too believe that 'the apparent rapid increase in the development of allergic diseases can be attributed largely to the abandonment of breastfeeding when safe pasteurised milk became available fifty years ago.'[96] But I would not expect exclusive breastfeeding in one generation to undo the harm that has been caused. It was very evident from the parents I have dealt with that food intolerance problems in breastfeeding babies were related to maternal childhood sensitivities and/or to pregnancy diet. Each generation must be born out of the bodies of the last. It has become clear that intra-uterine sensitisation is possible,[97] and that antigen transmitted via breast milk[98] can cause symptoms ranging from colic to hyperactivity, eczema, and problems with virtually every part of the body. Modifying the diet of a food-sensitive mother can bring instant relief, but does not undo the sensitisation that has occurred; her child may have to take care with food throughout life, particularly when subjected to stress of any kind, including pregnancy. The return to breastfeeding has been led by the social classes most commonly exposed to earlier, grossly inadequate formulae, and possibly damaged by that exposure: how much improvement can we realistically expect? Finnish studies suggest a strong protective effect:[88] perhaps formula did not become so pervasive over so many generations in Finland? And how can we quantify the role of early exposure when there are other variables to consider, such as the increased survival and therefore procreation of immune-deficient or highly allergic people, the extraordinary proliferation of chemicals affecting the immune system, changes in drug habits (nicotine, alcohol, caffeine, prescription drugs), increased stress loads, and changes in formula and processing techniques? The bottom line, however, remains this – in a family with a history of allergy, artificial feeding dramatically increases the risk of severe life-long disease, and exclusive breastfeeding for 6 months by a mother who has avoided her individual allergens during pregnancy, and who avoids them in lactation, will result in a much healthier child, perhaps even an allergy-free child.

Problems of human milk and formula

But can maternal milk be shown to be harmful, and less suitable than a formula, in particular cases? Yes, but rarely. The medical literature is dotted with case reports such as that of the Californian vegetarian mother whose baby was B_{12} deficient. From this case formula advocates may leap to concern about the B_{12} status of milk of mothers in developing countries,[99] despite the many possible health, medical, dietary and environmental differences between the Californian and other mothers. (Factors such as oral contraceptive, antibiotic and other drug use, smoking, alcohol intake: all would be relevant.)

Similarly, the discovery that many women excrete viral particles (as well as anti-viral factors and specific antibodies) in their milk has led to exaggerated fears as to the risks of using any but the individual mother's milk for her own baby. This may be due to ignorance of the probable immunising effects of such transmission, as well as ignorance of the flourishing milk banks that have existed in many countries for decades, with a far better record for protection against infection than any other altern-ative food source. (It is in Scandinavian countries, where infant mortality is lowest,[100] that human milk has been most widely used.) In some hospitals, nurses clearly believe that it is highly unsafe to use donor breast milk, even when the mother requests it. Certainly there are hazards,[101] all manageable. What amazes me is the fact that these risks are not balanced against the intrinsically greater hazards of using the physiol-ogically inappropriate, often contaminated, industrially manipulated, milk of an alien species. Babies die as a result of this ignorance and naivete.

Similar one-sidedness is a hallmark of any discussion of chemical contamination of human milk. Nowhere was this more evident than in the Report of the Task Force assessing the scientific evidence relating to infant feeding and infant health.[102] While the hazards of chemicals in breast milk were clearly delineated, there was no mention at all of chemical pollution of formula. Yet we know that the pasture,[103] the feed,[104] the milk,[105] the tanker that transports it,[106] the water used in manufacture and preparation, the cans that store it,[107] not only are at risk but actually have been seriously contaminated in the past. My basic conclusions are these:

1. Mothers have more control over their own pesticide and drug intake than they have over that of dairy animals, and they are deluded if they believe Australian regulatory agencies exercise such strict controls as to provide any assurance of safety. It is possible for milk to be produced and sold without ever being checked in any of the infrequent "market basket surveys" that the government conducts.

2. Simple control measures can reduce a mother's chemical exposure. These include obtaining food from relatively unpolluted sources; careful washing and peeling; reducing animal fat and organ meat intake; reducing overall meat intake, especially from battery-produced animals, fish at the top of the food chain (shark, for example);

and shellfish or fish from contaminated waters such as bays with heavy industry effluent discharges; eliminating household pesticides (particularly slow-release fat-soluble chemical compounds such as are found in pest strips, and long-lived toxins such as dieldrin, aldrin, and related substances); avoiding cigarette smoke.

3. A baby's exposure to toxins may be increased if his mother diets sufficiently to break down body fat during lactation, as fat-soluble chemicals may be excreted in milk. Hence mothers should not aim at rapid weight loss during lactation. (The only way some compounds can ever leave the body is through breast milk. Perhaps mothers with known high residues in body fat should be assisted to exercise sufficiently to lose weight and lactate *after weaning*. This might significantly lower body stores before the next pregnancy).

4. Even in extreme cases of chemical pollution, the scientific consensus is that it remains safer to breastfeed than not to do so. The Firemaster Incident in Michigan[101] (when PCB-contaminated stock-feed poisoned milk and meat, and thus people) was one such disaster, but mothers were not advised to use formula. Long-term follow-up of breastfed infants showed no effect on cognitive development.

5. Farmers producing milk as their livelihood are under pressure to sell their milk, even when they suspect it to be dubious. Dyes have been added to penicillin to reduce the loss to cheesemakers that occurs when farmers do not withhold penicillin-contaminated milk: this would not be necessary if all farmers could be trusted to be scrupulous in observing rules about chemical use. That farmers are unaware of the hazards of many chemicals they use is a fact causing increasing concern around Australia, but one which is hardly surprising to anyone who has seen TV commercials for pesticides on country channels. Some farmers scoff at the idea that residues *could* cause problems, and see their task as being to outwit the bureaucrats who make petty rules. When DDT-contaminated meat from a river area in New South Wales was quarantined, there was an outcry from farmers, directed not at the sources of contamination (apparently rice-growers in the area) but against high-handed destruction of good beef. Reading the reports in *Food Chemical News* of a major US meat packer slaughtering diseased and dying cattle for use in school lunch programmes reminds us that the world is full of people wanting to make money at other people's expense, and none too scrupulous about the means.

6. Formula too can be contaminated, as this chapter makes obvious. *The Age* newspaper has uncovered the fact that 'filthy' milk tankers were used to carry milk after transporting (in breach of regulations) chemicals and tallow;[103] and the further fact that the matter was hastily covered up rather than fully investigated by the appropriate authorities. In theory this could not happen. But what formula company would test for every possible contaminant? Why should they suspect the existence of "widespread malpractice in the trucking industry"? Or by any of their suppliers of pre-mixes? No doubt they have quality control systems that reduce the risk somewhat. But confidence in infant formula rests upon the presumed adherence of *everyone* involved in a complex production and manufacturing process to the highest possible standards of practice. Yet there is little evidence of such impeccable behaviour in other areas of society.

Psychologically it would be incredibly difficult for mothers concerned about potential toxins in their milk to succeed at breastfeeding, despite the accumulating evidence that compounds which are harmful to a foetus during gestation have few effects when exposure is solely via breastmilk. Women who have reason to be concerned about toxins – those known to have been heavily exposed, in industry or agriculture – should be able to have tests done so that their fear can take definite shape, and reasonable decisions made. Such a decision will almost always be to breastfeed, but occasionally levels may warrant the use of donated breastmilk while the mother lactates and loses weight to reduce her body stores, perhaps breastfeeding after a couple of months expressing and discarding milk. The rest of us should do the sensible things that reduce our exposure, then forget all about the problem, confident that breastfeeding is less risky than formula feeding in almost every conceivable case.

To bolster that confidence, here is some unequivocally good news. All babies begin to accumulate radioactive strontium in their bones before birth. "In the baby who is being breastfed, the body content of strontium diminishes [the baby excretes more than he or she takes in] but the bottlefed infant has increased strontium in his bones, as cows' milk may contain six times as much strontium as breastmilk" and the mineral balance of cows' milk ensures that it is deposited in baby's bones.[108] The dangers of strontium have decreased in the UK as atmospheric pollution with strontium is less in the northern hemisphere. But the conclusion that that "the consumption of human milk should reduce radioactive exposure" must be a comfort for those of us who live with the aftermath of British tests in Australia, or French tests in the Pacific.

Infant feeding matters more than most people realize. Ebrahim, a senior lecturer at London's famous Institute of Child Health, summarises some areas of concern: "Artificial feeding carries risks. Infants who are fed artificially are biologically different from those who are breastfed. Their blood carries a different pattern of amino acids, some of which may be at levels high enough to cause anxiety. The composition of their body fat is different. They are fed a variety of carbohydrates to which no other mammalian species is exposed in neonatal life. They have higher plasma osmolality, urea and electrolyte levels. Their guts are colonised by a potentially invasive type of micro-flora, at the same time as they are exposed to large amounts of foreign protein resulting in an immunologic response. In addition they are deprived of the various immune factors present in human milk. All these factors need to be taken into account every time a decision is made not to breastfeed an infant, for inherent in that decision are known and unknown risks to the infant."[109]

We have touched upon some of the known risks: greater risk of anemia, infection, gastroenteritis, selective malnutrition and its consequences, allergy in all its forms: these may be more common in socially deprived groups, but affect even the children of the affluent. (Indeed, allergy is more likely to be diagnosed in affluent families because such parents do not tolerate the patronising dismissal of their concerns about colic and other 'minor' symptoms.) It is also highly likely that certain types of heart disease are related to infant feeding.[110] (This may prove to be a form of immune-mediated disease, or food intolerance, or both.) Links between artificial feeding and serious disorders include childhood diabetes,[111] childhood coeliac disease,[112] ulcerative colitis,[113] and Crohn's disease.[114] Worst of all, evidence exists for the involvement of artificial feeding in some cases of SIDS, or cot death. As two eminent UK paediatricians stated, "SIDS is too common; it is much rarer in breastfed infants; and the best prophylactic action a mother could take for this major cause of death in infancy is to breastfeed her baby."[105]

As well, interesting new benefits of having been breastfed continue to be reported. In 1984, researchers reported that this 'dramatically' improved the success rate of kidney transplants from donors related to the mother of the recipient.[115] Despite Australia's high incidence of kidney disease, this was not newsworthy. Yet it clearly indicated that there are long-term immunological consequences of being breastfed, and is important to anyone involved in transplantation as a researcher or patient.

It should be clear by now that breastfeeding offers significant protection against disease of all kinds to children everywhere. My overview is incomplete, partly because there is no room to cover controversial topics such as intellectual development, SIDS, and AIDS. More importantly, it is incomplete because only now are scientists asking those questions that Hendrickse outlined (see p.1). The results are sometimes confused by methodological mistakes, and by the now-epidemiologically-biased populations studied. But I am confident that the more we ask such questions, and the higher our index of suspicion of anything that disturbs normal functioning, the more likely it is that in time everyone will agree that *the risks of formula are unacceptable except where truly unavoidable.*

This broad picture of the advantages of breastfeeding must be qualified in two ways. Firstly, it is theoretically not beyond human ingenuity to eventually devise the perfect infant formula. It is theoretically even possible that this could be better than human milk in some ways. Possible, but not likely. It is doubtful whether parents would accept the idea of anyone's babies being used as guinea pigs for experimental formulae, once the news about breast milk is circulated. It is certain that the costs involved in creating this perfect formula will make it prohibitively expensive, another piece of technology for the rich while poor families either buy and dilute it or use less satisfactory products. This should be morally repugnant to any caring person. It is also certain that there will be major technical problems in developing such a formula. As Gaull said, "It is conceivable that a departure from it [human milk] may represent nutritional improvement, but how to establish that this is a real improvement, without a later price to pay, is a major scientific problem."[116] So this theoretical possibility beloved by Dugdale[117] is of no social significance, and is morally abhorrent.

Secondly, while I am adamant that women's milk is the best possible choice at present, enthusiasm for the product in general should not lead to uncritical advocacy in every individual case. Because of variations in nutrition, health, exposure to toxins and so on, it is possible that a particular mother's milk may be less than ideal for her baby's health and growth. In such cases, weaning (even on to formula, although other human milk is preferable) may be necessary; in others, supplementation of breast milk will be the best choice. Such cases will be rare when mothers are adequately helped with breastfeeding. The first line of investigation ought to be improvement of maternal health status and a careful investigation of the techniques of breastfeeding. If these prove fruitless (very rare), the baby may be better off bottlefed. As Gunther said, 'Breastfeeding is for the baby, not the baby for breastfeeding.' But too often babies are arbitrarily weaned, and are not better off. The widespread assumption that giving formula solves breastfeeding problems is utterly infuriating. The breastfeeding problem may worsen, and so may the mother and infant's physical and psychological health.

Sometimes not, of course. Many babies develop normally (as this culture defines normal, which of course has been affected by the consequences of widespread bottle-feeding) when formula-fed, just as many did on those earlier mixtures now considered so dreadful by the very groups that once promoted them. To my mind, this is a tribute to the marvellous adaptability of the human body, rather than to the formulae. Yes, those we now have sustain adequate growth; they probably are an improvement on earlier ones; but they are still very crude approximations of what women's bodies produce. As Hambraeus wrote, "It is of course a truism to state that proprietary milks should be made to resemble human milk to the greatest possible extent. However, as long as it is based on milk obtained from other species it can only be humanised to a degree. It is obvious that it is impossible to compose a formula with optimal nutritive value for the human infant as long as the composition of breast milk and its physiological variations are still incompletely known. Another basis for the composition of an optimal formula might be a thorough knowledge of the nutrient requirements of infants. Here also our knowledge is limited, partly due to large individual variations between healthy infants. Most data on nutrient requirements are based on indirect evidence obtained from observations of the intake of the known essential nutrients in infants totally breastfed with normal growth".[118] But remember that we are not yet certain what is normal growth for breastfed infants in every culture, and that nutrients in human milk behave differently!

Formula advocates sometimes challenge all this science as having no clinical significance, and all the epidemiological associations as being statistically invalid, or contradicted by other studies. (The flaws in which may be glaringly obvious on close scrutiny, but which serve to reassure some professionals that the topic is still debatable, so change is not needed.) Says Professor Dobbing, "From the purely nutritional, or compositional viewpoint, [why?] there is no evidence whatsoever that in real life (as opposed to the laboratory) modern formulas are nutritionally inadequate or dangerous." Strong words. He goes on to say that "they are likely to get closer to the human product as time goes on. Indeed further expensive modification is likely to result in rather more profit for the manufacturer than for the baby."[119] Other researchers are less confident of the nutritional adequacy of infant formula, and the safety of tinkering with it: "Manufacturers of cows' milk formulas have been mainly concerned with attempting to market a product resembling as closely as possible, the proximate principles of breast milk. Not unexpectedly, manifestations of disease have occurred among infants fed formulas deficient in certain nutrients... Other deficiency syndromes may appear in the future as the process of further 'humanizing' milk will promote manipulation of certain nutrients at the probable expense of micro-nutrients, the presence and importance of which may not as yet be fully appreciated. As research into the composition of breast milk continues, new nutrients are constantly being discovered."[120] A paediatric gastroenterologist stated that "There is little doubt that with our increased technological sophistication the further refinement of nutritional products will exceed our knowledge of the intricacies of nutritional metabolism. The sickest of infants are of course at greatest risk. We should be careful, however, not to unknowingly place our well infants at risk also. With our limited knowledge, we must be careful to adhere to the maxim, 'First do no harm.'"[121]

Settlements of millions to damaged children tend to suggest that harm has been done. Perhaps Dobbing was genuinely unaware of the many problems on record: the information is mainly American, and mostly not from medical sources. (This is not to suggest that such problems were or are more common in America: merely that it is easier to find out about them in a country where citizens are litigious, whistle blowers are protected, and consumer organisations have been active for longer.)

It will be regarded as alarmist of me to list these incidents; breastfeeding advocates are supposed to concentrate on the good things about breast milk, and not the nasty things that formula has done to babies. But I think that is rather like trying to stop people smoking by emphasizing all the positive pleasures of not smoking while never mentioning the harm that smoking has done. Both smoking and artificial feeding profoundly derange body systems *in everyone*, although *not all* those who smoke or who are bottlefed will have serious illness as a result. Both are obnoxious because decisions made by one person are likely to do harm *to others who have no choice in the matter*. The analogy cannot be pushed too far, because smoking is always and only harmful, while artificial formula has allowed many children to survive in the absence of breastmilk, even if it may also have damaged them. Even so, I think it's time for healthworkers to take off the kid gloves and state plainly to parents *that they cannot make an informed decision about feeding choice until they have discovered to what risks other people inadvertently subjected their babies.*

Formula mishaps: a preliminary list (as at 1984)

Before the 1960s babies were fed on varieties of dried, evaporated, condensed, and whole milk modified according to various methods; with cod liver oil, juices, and other supplements given to make up for the obvious deficiencies of cows' milk. Brand name products such as SMA, Similac, Lactogen, and others existed but were nothing like the complicated mixtures they now are; nor were they used by any but a minority of families. The results of these inadequate feedings included high morbidity and mortality from infection, malnutrition and brain damage, anaemia, and much else. Some of this was less obvious than it now would be because the death rate declined over this period due to improved living standards, sanitation, antibiotics, and so on. Specific problems included:

- Low levels of folic acid and lack of vitamin C caused megaloblastic anaemia;[122]
- pyridoxine deficiency caused fits, cerebral palsy and retardation;[123]
- Excessive protein loads caused dehydration, uremia and brain damage;[124]

- protein imbalance in some formulae caused brain damage;[125]
- Vitamin E deficiency caused haemolytic anaemia;[126]
- Insufficient iron caused anaemia and increased infections;
- Excessive iron caused gut bleeding, anaemia and immunological disorder;[10]
- Excessive vitamin D caused convulsions and kidney damage due to hypercalcaemia;[127]
- Excessive phosphorus caused convulsions due to hypocalcaemia;[128]
- Vitamin C deficiency caused scurvy;[129]
- Zinc deficiency caused retardation, failure to thrive, and distressing skin disorders (acrodermatitis enteropathica);[130]
- Essential fatty acid deficiency caused skin, gut, and eye disorders, and failure to thrive;[131]
- Vitamin A deficiency[132] caused diarrhoea, facial palsy, and symptoms in liver, spleen, breast and elsewhere.

These were obvious problems, clearly physiological in origin, and were thus recognised more quickly than subtle problems will be. Companies modified their products at different rates; some of these problems continued into the next decade. No regulations existed to monitor what happened to defective formulae: there were no legal impediments to continued sale on domestic or foreign markets.

Problems recognised in the next decades included:

- Lactobezoars (tough indigestible curds) caused bowel obstruction requiring surgery to relieve it; most commonly this occurred in premature infants on the early high calorie prem formulae;[133]
- Neonatal hypocalcaemic fits occurred "at the end of the first week in about one per cent of bottlefed babies, but are not seen in breastfed babies".[134] Late hypocalcaemia also developed in some;
- Hypomagnesaemic fits were found to occur "only in bottlefed infants";[131]
- Lead and other heavy metal contamination (which is cumulative and can result in brain damage) was realised to be a matter for concern;
- Neonatal metabolic alkalosis with failure to thrive in the second and third weeks of life occurred in infants fed the early 1970s formulation of Nutramigen, despite the fact that this formula met 1974 guidelines for composition;[135]
- Goitre occurred because of improperly heated soy formulae and/or lack of iodine;[136]
- Prolonged prothrombin time due to vitamin K deficiency led to acute epidermal and retinal bleeding in some infants;[132]
- Bacterial contamination of some American and Australian formulae caused salmonellosis, vomiting and diarrhoea;
- Necrotising enterocolitis was reported in infants fed formula with very high osmolarity.[137] The mortality rate is high, and artificial feeding increases the risk *1000%*, although it can happen rarely in breastfed infants;

- High solute loads in formulae led to hypernatraemic dehydration; consequences included 'permanent brain damage, gangrene and disseminated intravascular coagulation.'[19]

Particular formulae involved 1978-1985 include:

1978 Enfamil with iron was contaminated with bacteria (E. coli)

1979 SMA was recalled because improper homogenisation had led to gastrointestinal upsets;

- Neo-Mull-Soy and Cho-free were deficient in chloride, causing metabolic alkalosis. Other formulae were checked and some were too low in (but not totally lacking) chloride;

1980 Soy-a-lac and I-Soy-a-lac contained excess vitamin D;

- Enfamil with iron was recalled because some had curdled and was green, sour, and contaminated;

1981 Enfamil with iron (ready to use) was recalled because some was contaminated with solvents from excessive can-lining material;

1982 SMA and Nursoy were recalled (more than 2.3 million cans) because they lacked vitamin B_6;

- SMA Concentrate (Maine) contained black foreign matter;

- SMA Concentrate (Maine) had a bad odour, and the fat had separated. After three days of vomiting, one child stopped immediately the formula was changed;

1983 Soy-a-lac recalled because of problem with vitamin A stabilisation;

- Naturlac recalled because lacking in thiamine, copper, and B_6;

- Similac and Isomil were found to contain carcinogens due to contaminated well water; levels were not high enough for recall;

1984 Holes were found in formula cans stored in one New York warehouse. Sabotage was suspected.

- Neo-Ag-U, a Taiwanese formula, was deficient in calcium, causing tetany.

- De-Lact Infant contained calcium caseinate, an ingredient which could have been fatal to infants. It proved difficult to trace all cans.

- New York hospital nursery staff noticed that a sealed bottle of Enfamil looked coagulated; culture revealed Enterobacter cloacae. The staff who reported this in a medical journal suggested that prepared formula should be carefully inspected and heat-treated before re-use. This, however, would damage some nutrients.

- In 1984 the FDA discovered a loophole in the Act in relation to the microbiological safety of formula powders. It was reported that the "manufacturer can (and routinely does) refuse to allow FDA access to records not directly related to nutritional quality."[138] This was to be rectified in 1985; but to read that manufacturers refused access until forced to provide it does not increase one's confidence that they have nothing to hide.

1985 Ross Laboratories were ordered to cease distribution of formula manufactured on a new production line which was wrongly supposed to be identical to an existing line, until elaborate testing had been carried out. FDA argued that by law such a change should have been reported to the FDA as it constituted a 'major' change in processing which "experience alone would indicate [could have] a possible significant adverse impact on levels of nutrients"[139] Inspection subsequently revealed some major differences between the processing lines.

- Recall of Kama-Mil Powder, and Nutra-Milk Infant Formula, deficient in folacin, zinc, and Vitamin D, and defective in several other ways. The FDA had great difficulty locating the manufacturers, ascertaining how much and where the products were sold.
- Gerber Meat Base Formula recalled because of excess vitamin A
- Pamphlets suggesting Edensoy drink was suitable for infant consumption were recalled after reports of rickets, vision problems, and malnutrition in a baby fed the product as its sole source of nutrition
- Carnation Evaporated Milk (Australia) was mislabelled as Prosobee (a soy brand), a potentially fatal mistake for severely milk-intolerant babies.

Talking to senior FDA officials about the effectiveness of the 1980 Act makes it clear that many more defective batches of formula are being stopped from reaching the market because of better quality control in the face of so much consumer anxiety, and some very expensive legal settlements. The official concerned agreed that prior to 1980 there must have been innumerable batches of defective formula that slipped through to the market and whose effects were never traced. Where there are no stringent controls, this probably still occurs.

These problems are not confined to capitalist or affluent countries. Russia has continuing problems with formula quality; high copper levels in Indian formula are causing childhood liver disease: these and other problems cannot all be dismissed as not really intrinsic problems of artificial feeding. As Lynn Pilot and Carol Laskin wrote, "Blind trust and confidence in infant formula is a thing of the past. From our experience we know that the simplistic responses that 'this was an isolated incident and we have an excellent record' are not acceptable."[140] There never has been, and never will be, a formula that is free of the risk of nutritional imbalance, accidental contamination, or other deficiencies. This is true of all processed foods, and it is the reason we adults are urged to reduce our risk by varying our diet. What makes formula different (and in my view, an unacceptable risk whenever breastmilk can be used) is firstly, that it is recommended as an infant's sole diet for months; and secondly, that a better product, with fewer risks, is available more cheaply.

Naturally formula advocates reply that human milk is also risky. *There are two crucial differences rarely mentioned in discussions of comparative risks.* A woman can have a great deal of control over potential problems with her milk. But even if she cannot, or chooses to ignore obvious precautions, and the quality of her milk is poor (unlikely, as breastmilk quality is remarkably stable), *only her baby is affected.* She is not producing millions of cans for thousands of babies. Secondly, in almost all cases where breast milk is deficient, *there will be some clue in the mother's health to that possibility*, and a careful doctor will have some leads to follow up. Looking at a can of formula rarely suggests what problems may occur! *Problems of infant formula are thus of a different order and scale than those of human milk, despite politically and commercially motivated attempts to reassure the public that they are really equivalent.*

When I had my children, I believed, as most mothers do, that modern formulae were almost as good as breastfeeding, and that only poverty, ignorance, or carelessness made artificial feeding hazardous. I religiously used formula as a weaning supplement, rather than crude cows' milk; for my third, I even used soy formulae despite the expense. (Nothing but the best for my children! I might add that the third is the only soy-intolerant child in the family.) What I believe now is very different. As I searched for information about breastfeeding problems, I came across so many pieces of information about bottlefeeding and illness that I began to look at how formulae had been created. Instead of seeing these problems as unrelated incidents, I came to realise that *infant formula had never been proven safe before it was marketed*; rather, it had grown by a process of trial and error involving other people's babies. The terms in which the American Academy of Pediatrics condemned the use of dairy whiteners as infant food seem to summarise it well: "Popularity, extravagant claims, and special marketing practices cannot make white liquids nutritionally equivalent to infant formula."[141] *Nor can they make infant formula equivalent to human milk.* Do parents know this when they 'choose' to artificially-feed?

I agree with Vahlquist, another eminent nutritionist, who wrote in 1976: "Obviously the new discoveries have widened the gap between human milk and even the most ambitious and sophisticated of formulae. No doubt the formula industry will make every effort to produce new formulae which come closer, at least superficially, to human milk. But attempts to bridge the gap will remain futile since we are dealing here with such complex systems and such species-specific substances that even very costly models cannot be foreseen to reach the ideal model. Thus the new discoveries in the field of the species-specificity of human milk will serve to underline very strongly the uniqueness and biological superiority of this produce of Nature, and will provide new arguments for ardent action to retain the age-old breastfeeding tradition. We can be sure, too, that the discoveries of the last decade will not be the last in this context."[142] How right he was.

Notice two things here. The prediction of new discoveries has been validated endlessly since 1976. A brief review of some of the latest developments would include further lists of defects and recalls, further proof of poorer health and cognitive development in artificially-fed children, and further concern about negative effects on women's health. These are summarised by some of the references at the end of this chapter. But remember, we could have known this when Vahlquist did, and millions of babies have been needlessly bottle-fed since then. When will we see artificial feeding as a health hazard as serious as tobacco smoking? When will we stop talking about breastfeeding's "benefits", and start talking about artificial feeding **RISKS**?

Notice too that Vahlquist said *ardent* action. So what action is needed? This book will next examine in-hospital management of the breastfeeding mother and child.

NOTES
CHAPTER 1: WHY BREASTFEEDING MATTERS
[1] Report on a workshop, "Methodologies in Human Lactation", chaired by Dr M. Neville, *J. Pediatr. Gastroent. Nutr.*, 1984, 3, 268-99.
[2] L. Hambraeus, "Proprietary milk versus human milk for infant feeding", *Ped. Clin. N. Am.*, 1977, 24, 17. See also *Lancet*, 1984, ii, 167-8, where Hambraeus and others question the whole approach to protein and its utilisation, and the validity of recommendations for formula feeding.
[3] M.C. Neville et al, "The mechanisms of milk secretion", in M.C. Neville and M.R. Neifert, *Lactation: Physiology, Nutrition and Breastfeeding.* (Plenum Press, 1983); G.A. Harzer Changing patterns of breast milk lipids in the course of lactation and during the day. *Am. J. Clin. Nutr.* 1983, 37, 612-21.
[4] J.A. Lemons et al, "Differences in the composition of pre-term and term milk during early lactation", *Pediatr. Res.* 1982, 16, 113-7; J.Bitman et al, "Comparison of the lipid composition of breast milk from mothers of term and pre-term infants", *Am. J. Clin. Nutr.* 1983, 38, 300-2.
[5] This occurs in all mammals, the extremes being those living in polar regions. The differences are less marked in humans who build shelter and wear clothes.
[6] N. Goldberg; E. Adams, "Supplementary water for breastfed babies in a hot and dry climate: not really a necessity", *Arch. Dis. Child.* 1983, 58, 73-4.
[7] Some breast pumps are known to create such pressure that "excessive mammary tissue lipids may be removed that would not be available to the infant under normal nursing conditions." A.M. Ferris; R.G. Jensen, "Sampling and determination of lipids in human milk", *J. Pediatr. Gastroent. Nutr. 1984*, 3, 111-3. 'Barracuda' babies seem to have the same effect.
[8] R.A. Lawrence, *Breastfeeding: a Guide for the Medical Profession.* (C.V. Mosby, St. Louis, 1980) p. 135.
[9] C.E. Casey; M.K. Hambidge, "Nutritional aspects of human lactation", in Neville and Neifert, reference 3, p. 236-8.
[10] N. Campbell, "Nutritional and immunological aspects of breastfeeding", *Austr. Nurses' J.* 1981, 10, 11, 40-7.
[11] J.J. Bullen, "Bacteriostatic systems in human milk", in A.W.Wilkinson (ed.) *Immunology of Infant Feeding.* (Plenum Press, 1981)
[12] C.L. Bullen, "Infant feeding and the faecal flora", ibid.
[13] B. Kochanowski; A.R. Sherman, "Decreased antibody formation in iron-deficient rat pups – effect of iron repletion", *Am. J. Clin. Nutr.* 1985, 41, 278-84.
[14] M. Gilloolly et al, "The relative effect of ascorbic acid on iron absorption from soy-based and milk-based formulas", *Am. J. Clin. Nutr.* 1984, 40, 522-7.
[15] F.A. Oski, "Nutritional anemias of infancy", in F. Lifschitz,(ed.) *Pediatric Nutrition* (Marcel Dekker, 1982); Sadowitz and Oski, "Iron status and infant feeding practices in an urban ambulatory center", *Pediatrics* 1983, 72, 1, 33-5.
[16] Lonnerdal, B et al, "Iron, Zinc, Copper and Manganese in infant formulas", *Am. J. Dis. Child.* (1983) 137: 433-7.
[17] G.E. Gaull et al, "Human milk as food", in A. Milunsky et al (ed.) *Advances in Perinatal Medicine* vol.2. (Plenum Press, 1982) p. 59; F.A. Oski, S.A. Landow, "Inhibition of iron absorption from human milk by baby food", *Am. J. Dis. Child.* 1980, 134, 459-60.
[18] McMillan, J.A. et al, "Iron sufficiency in breastfed infants and availability from human milk", *Pediatrics* 1976, 58, 686.
[19] C.G. Neumann; E.F.P.Jelliffe, "Effects of infant feeding", in D.B. Jelliffe and E.F.P. Jelliffe (eds.) *Adverse Effects Of Foods.* (Plenum Press, 1982) p.544.
[20] D.G. Perrin et al, "Sudden infant death syndrome: increased carotid body dopamine and

noradrenaline content", *Lancet* 1984, ii, 535-7.

[21] L.M. Janas et al, "Indices of protein metabolism in term infants fed human milk, whey-predominant formula, or cows' milk formula", *Pediatrics* (1985) 75, 4, 775-84.

[22] The US Food and Drug Administration has failed to affirm the safety of particular ingredients permitted by the 1976 Codex Alimentarius, for example.

[23] Feeley et al, "Calcium, phosphorus and magnesium contents of human milk during early lactation", *J. Pedatr. Gastroent. Nutr.* 1983, 2, 262-7; FDA Consumer, July/August, 1984, p.5.

[24] E.M. Moynahan, "Acrodermatitis enteropathica: a lethal inherited zinc deficiency", *Lancet* 1974, ii, 399-400.

[25] R.L. Hood; A.R. Johnson, "Supplementation of infant formulations with biotin", *Nutr. Rep. Int.* 198021, 727-31.

[26] R.A. Lawrence, (reference 8) 1985 edition, p.316-7.

[27] G.E. Gaull et al, "Taurine and cholesterol supplementation of formulas in preterm infants", *Pediatr. Res.* 1980, 14, 499.

[28] H.L. Greene, "Water-soluble vitamins" in Lebenthal (ed.) *Textbook of Gastroenterology and Nutrition in Infancy.* (Raven Press, 1982)p. 591-2.

[29] A.M. Smith et al, "Selenium intakes and status of human milk- and formula-fed infants", *Am. J. Clin. Nutr.* 1982, 35, 521-6.

[30] B.A. Wharton, "Food for the suckling: revolution and development", *Acta Paediatr. Scand.* 1982, suppl. 299, p. 6.

[31] L.K. Dahl; L. Tassinari, "High salt content of Western infant's diet: possible relationship with hypertension in the adult", *Nature*, 1963, 198, 1204-5.

[32] Conversation, Ascot October 1983.

[33] Roy, "Metabolic alkalosis from chloride deficient formula", in Jelliffe and Jelliffe (1982) reference 19.

[34] J. Laughlin et al, "Changing feeding trends as a cause of electrolyte depletion in infants with cystic fibrosis", *Pediatrics* 1981, 68, 2, 203, 206-7.

[35] D.B. Coursin, "Convulsive seizures in infants with pyridoxine-deficient diets", *J. Amer. Med. Ass.* 1954, 154, 406-8.

[36] B. Walker, "Lead content of milk and infant formula", *J. Food Prot.* 1980,43, 3, 178-9.

[37] *Food Chemical News* September 1980 makes good reading.

[38] American Pharmacy Association, *Handbook of Non-Prescription Drugs* (APA, Washinton, 5th edition 1977.) p. 167-8.

[39] L. Salisbury; A. Glover Blackwell *An administrative petition to alleviate domestic infant formula misuse and to provide informed infant feeding choice.* Presented to the US FDA and the Department of Health and Human Services, June 17, 1981.

[40] *Food Chemical News*, Feb. 25, 1985, p. 28-30.

[41] Professor J. Post, Testimony to House of Representatives Oversight and Investigations Sub-committee of the Committee on Energy and Commerce, June 17, 1981. (Serial number 97-73).

[42] J. Braithwaite *Corporate Crime and the Pharmaceutical Industry* (Routledge and Kegan Paul, 1984).

[43] V. Packard *Human Milk and Infant Formula* (Academic Press, 1982) p. 64.

[44] E. Birenbaum et al, "Neonatal hypernatraemic dehydration due to excessively concentrated prepared milk formula", *Clin. Pediatr.* 1981, 627-9. Such mistakes are common: see R.A. Jones; E.M. Belsey "Common mistakes in infant feeding: survey from a London borough", *Br. Med. J.* 1978, 2, 112-4.

[45] C. Sadler, "Mineral water unfit for babies", *Nurs. Mirror* 1983, June 15, p. 13.

[46] *Food Chemical News*, June 17, 1985.

[47] ibid., Nov. 28 1983, p. 29.

[48] ibid.

[49] Discussion with one manufacturer at an international conference, 1984. The product he condemned was one of the most expensive on the market; he asserted that change had resulted from his interventions.

[50] *Food Chemical News*, Sept. 20, 1982; July 11, 1983, p.15; Sept. 12, p.25; Oct. 17, p. 7; Oct. 24, p. 40. See also D.C. Havery; T. Fazio, "Estimation of volatile N-nitrosamines in the rubber nipples of babies' bottles", *Food Chem. Toxic.* 1982, 20, 6, 939-44.

[51] *FDA Consumer*, March 1984, p. 18-9.

[52] N. Solomons, "Mineral interactions in the diet", *Mod. Med Austr.* March 1984, 23-6.

[53] Cf. *ALCA News* (Dec 1996) 7: 3; 34-6.

[54] C.L. Rosen et al, "Hypoxaemia associated with feeding in the pre-term infant and full-term infant", *Am.J. Dis. Child.*, 1984, 138, 7, 623-8.

[55] Lawrence (reference 8, 1985 edition) p. 71-7.

[56] L.M. Janas; M.F. Picciano, "The nucleotide profile of human milk", *Pediatr. Res.* 1982, 16, 8, 659-62.

[57] E.E.Zeigler; S.J. Fomon, "Lactose enhances mineral absorption in infancy", *J. Pediatr. Gastroent. Nutr.* 1983, 2, 2, 288-94.

[58] Gaull (reference 17) p. 55. Some degree of lactose malabsorption is common in breastfed infants; this may have beneficial effects. Lactose is more completely metabolised by the formula-fed because of the 'unnaturally delayed gut transit time' of their food: see Wharton, "Immunological implications of alternatives to mothers' milk", in Wilkinson (reference 11) p. 111.

[59] W.S. Biven; B.N. Heinen, "Production of ethanol from infant food formulas by common yeasts", *J. Appl. Bacteriol.* (1985) 58, 355-7.

[60] A. Aynsley-Green, "Hormones and postnatal adaptation to enteral nutrition", *J. Pediatr. Gastroent. Nutr.* 1983, 2, 418-28.

[61] K. Borch-Johnsen et al, "Relationship between breastfeeding and incidence rates of insulin-dependent diabetes mellitus", *Lancet* 1984, ii, 1083-6. Since repeatedly confirmed in many different populations.

[62] L.C. Read et al "Changes in the growth-promoting activity of human milk during lactation", *Ped. Res.* 1984, 18, 2, 133-8.

[63] L.C. Read et al, "Growth factor concentrations and growth-promoting activity in human milk following premature birth", *J. Dev. Physiol.* 1985, 7, 135-45.

[64] N.F.Butte et al, "Human milk intake and growth in exclusively breastfed infants", *J. Pediatr.* 1984, 104, 187-94.

[65] N. E. Hitchcock et al, "The growth of breast fed and artificially fed infants from birth to twelve months", *Acta Paediatr. Scand.* 1985, 74,240-5.

[66] C.Garza, "The unique values of human milk", Report of the US Surgeon General's workshop on breastfeeding and human lactation, June 1984.

[67] J.A. Lemons et al., "The energy content of infant formulas", *Early Hum. Dev.* 1982, 6, 3, 305-8.

[68] G.J. Ebrahim, *Breastfeeding, the biological option.* (Macmillan 1979) p. 59-60.

[69] D.C. Heiner, "Modern research relating to food allergy and its implications", *Clin. Rev. Allergy* 1984, 2, 1-5.

[70] R.K. Chandra, "Nutrition and immunity", in Lifshitz (reference 15) p. 317-27; *Lancet* 1983, i, 688-91.

[71] Lawrence (reference 8) p. 105-8. See also several papers in the Workshop on Current Issues in Feeding the Normal Infant. *Pediatrics* 1985, 75, 135-215.

[72] Lawrence, chapter 5.

[73] W.A. Walker, "Effect of colostrum on the maturation of intestinal host defences", in

Lebenthal (reference 28) p. 234-5.

[74] J. Bienenstock et al, "A common mucosal immunologic system involving the bronchus, breast and bowel", *Adv. Exp. Med. Biol.* 1978, 107, 53-88; M. Fishaut et al, "Bronchomammary axis in the immune response to respiratory synticial virus", *J. Pediatr.* 1981, 99, 2, 186-91.

[75] A.S. Cunningham, "Breastfeeding and morbidity in industrialised countries: an update" in Jelliffe and Jelliffe (eds.) *Advances in International Maternal and Child Health.* (Oxford University Press, 1981)

[76] J. Soothill, "Immunological aspects of infant feeding", in Soothill, Hayward and Wood (eds.) *Paediatric Immunology.* (Blackwell Scientific Publications, 1983)

[77] A. Høst, S. Husby, O. Østerball, "A prospective Study of Cow's Milk Allergy in Exclusively Breast-Fed Infants", *Acta Paediatr. Scand.* (1988) 77: 663-70.

[78] T. Vukacic, "Intestinal absorption of IgA in the newborn", *J. Pediatr. Gastroent. Nutr.* 1983, 2, 2, 248-51

[79] A.S.Goldman; C.Garza et al, "Immunologic factors in human milk during the first year of lactation", *J. Pediatr.* 1982, 100, 4, 563-7; "Immunologic factors in human milk during the second year of lactation", *Acta Paediatr. Scand.* 1983, 72, 461-2.

[80] See also M.K. Minchin, "Nucleotides", *ALCA Galaxy* (Dec. 1997) 8: 3; pp. 12-14.

[81] A.S. Goldman et al, "Immunologic components of human milk during weaning", *Acta Paed. Scand.* 1983, 72, 133-4.

[82] Packard, reference 43, p.100-2; 164-5.

[83] Edmeades et al, "Infantile gastroenteritis: relationship between cause, clinical course and outcome", *Med. J. Aust.* 1981, 2, 29-32. See also "More about infant diarrhoea", *Br. Med. J.* 1977, 2, 1562.

[84] S.A. Larsen; D.R. Homer, "Relation of breast versus bottle feeding to hospitalisation for gastroenteritis in a middle class US population", *J. Pediatr.* 1978, 92, 417.

[85] H. Patti et al, "Episodes of illness in breastfed and bottlefed infants in Jerusalem", *Isr. J. Med. Sci.* 1984, 20, 5, 395-9.

[86] Macfarlane; V. Miller, "Human milk in the management of protracted diarrhoea of infancy", *Arch. Dis. Child.* 1984, 59, 260-5.

[87] R.I. Glass et al, "Protection against cholera in breastfed children by antibodies in breast milk", *N. Engl. J. Med.* 1983, 308, 1389-92.

[88] D. Tyrrell, "Breastfeeding and virus infections", in Wilkinson (reference).

[89] F.D. Gillin et al, "Killing of giardia lamblia trophozoites by normal human milk", *J. Cell Biochem.* 1983, 23, 1-4, 47-56.

[90] M.V. Khan et al, "Role of breastfeeding in preventing acquisition of roundworm and hookworm in Dhaka slum children", *Indian J. Pediatr.* 1983, 50, 493-5.

[91] M. Kajosaari; U. Saarinen, "Prophylaxis of atopic disease by six months' total solid food elimination. Evaluation of 135 exclusively breastfed infants of atopic families", *Acta Paediatr. Scand.* 1983, 72, 3, 411-4.

[92] S.P.Fallstrom et al, "Influence of breast feeding on the development of cows' milk protein antibodies and the IgE level", *Int. Archs. Allergy Appl. Immun.* 1984, 75, 87-91; S.A. Roberts and J.F. Soothill, "Provocation of allergic response by supplementary feeds of cows' milk", *Arch. Dis. Child.* 1982, 57, 127-30.

[93] A. Lucas et al, "Latent anaphylactic sensitisation of infants of low birth weight to cows' milk proteins", *Br. Med. J.* 1984, 289, 1254-6.

[94] P.D. Buisseret, "Allergy", *Scientific American,* 1982, August.

[95] M. Minchin, *Food for Thought: a parent's guide to food intolerance.* (George Allen & Unwin, Sydney 1985; Oxford University Press, Oxford, 1985); chapter in *The Lactation Consul-*

tant's Guide (Avery Publishing, New Jersey, 1985); talk in *Proceedings*, 20th International Congress of the International Confederation of Midwives, Sydney, September 1984.)

[96] J. Glaser, in F. Speer; R.Dockhorn, *Allergy and Immunology in Childhood* (C.C. Thomas, Illinois, 1973) p. 403.

[97] T.Matsamura, "Food allergy in adults and children", in reference 19, p. 348.

[98] P.J. Kilshaw; A.J. Cant, "The passage of maternal dietary proteins into human breast milk", *Int. Archs. Allergy Appl. Immun.*1984, 75, 8-15; J.W. Gerrard, "Allergy in breastfed babies to foods ingested by the mother", *Clin. Rev. Allergy*, 1984, 2, 143-9.

[99] Packard (reference 43) p. 39.

[100] H.M. Wallace et al, "Comparison of infant mortality in the United States and Sweden", *J. Trop. Pediatr.* (1985) 31: 223-8.

[101] Useful reviews are A.F. Williams et al, "Humnan Milk Banking", *J. Trop. Pediatr.* (1985) 31: 85-9; and Williams and Baum, *Human Milk Banking* (Raven Press, 1984).

[102] "Report of the Task Force on the assessment of the scientific evidence relating to infant-feeding practices and infant health", *Pediatrics* (1984) 74, 4, part 2. The chapter, "Problems with human milk and infant formulas", is not only misleading, but plagiarised from a 1979 report. Attempting to have this publicly noted has proved to be a fascinating exercise, which I shall discuss in the next book I write.

[103] Milk in Hawaii was contaminated with heptachlor sprayed on pastures; in Australia a "market basket" survey found beef so heavily contaminated with DDT that the area was quarantined for a time.

[104] Senn, "The Firemaster Incident", in Jelliffe and Jelliffe (1982) reference 19, p. 133.

[105] Fytianos, K et al, "Preliminary study of organochlorine compounds in milk products, human milk, and vegetables", *Bull. Environ. Contam. Toxicol.* (1985) 34, 504-8.

[106] *The Age*, Melbourne, Feb. 6, 1985, p. 3, and later issues.

[107] In 1980 one U.S. formula company was under investigation after a concerned employee rang the local newspaper and revealed that cans had been sprayed with methyl bromide, aired for 4 hours, then put into the processing line. The company did not make records of quality assurance laboratory tests available to the FDA "as a matter of company policy"; no tests for residues were performed by the company.

[108] C.B.S. Wood; JA. Walker-Smith, *Mackeith's Infant Feeding and Feeding Difficulties.* (Churchill Livingstone, Edinburgh, 1981) p. 106.

[109] reference 68, p. 59-60.

[110] D.L.J. Freed (ed.) *Health Hazards of Milk* (Bailliere Tindall, 1984) ch.10-12.

[111] K. Borch-Johnsen et al, "Relation between breastfeeding and incidence rates of childhood diabetes mellitus", *Lancet* 1984, ii, 1083-6.

[112] S. Auricchio et al, "Does breastfeeding protect against the development of clinical symptoms of coeliac disease in children?" *J. Pediatr. Gastroent. Nutr.* 1983, 2, 428-33.

[113] S.L. Bahna; D.C. Heiner *Allergies to Milk* (Grune and Stratton, 1980) p. 51.

[114] O. Bergstrand; G. Hellers, "Breastfeeding during infancy in patients who later develop Crohn's disease", *Scand. J. Gastroenterol.* 1983, 18, 903-6.

[115] D.A. Campbell et al, "Breastfeeding and maternal donor renal allografts: possibly the original donor-specific transfusion", *Transplantation* 1984, 37, 4, 340-4.

[116] Gaull (reference 17), p. 60.

[117] A.E. Dugdale, "Infant feeding and child health", *Med. J. Aust.* 1981, July 25, p. 107.

[118] L. Hambraeus, "Proprietary milk versus human milk in infant feeding", *Pediatr. Clin. N. Am.* 1977, 24, 1

[119] J. Dobbing in Freed (ed.) reference 109, p. 63. (An amazingly selective chapter which criticises others for being selective!)

[120] C.G. Neumann; E.F.P. Jelliffe (reference 19) p. 547-8.

[121] Le Leiko, "The effects of various diets (cows' milk, soybean, and elemental) on the growth and development of premature and full-term infant", in Lebenthal (ed.) reference 28, p. 285.

[122] C. D. May et al, "Pathogenesis of megablatic anaemia in infancy: an interrelationship between pteroylglutamic acid and ascorbic acid", *Am. J. Dis. Child.* (1950) 80, 191-206.

[123] D.B. Coursin "Convulsive seizures in infants with pyridoxine-deficient diets", *J. Am. Med. Ass.* 1954, 406-8.

[124] D.P. Davies et al, "Blood urea: Normal values in early infancy related to infant feeding practices", *Arch. Dis. Child.* 1973, 48, 563-5.

[125] reference 19, p. 544.

[126] D.L. Phelps, "Vitamin E: where do we stand?", *Pediatrics* 1979, 63, 993-5; M.K. Horwitt, "Vitamin E: a re-examination", *Am. J. Clin. Nutr.* 1976, 29, 569-78.

[127] T. Stapleton et al, "The pathogenesis of idiopathic hypercalcemia in infancy", *Am. J. Clin. Nutr.*1957, 5, 533-42.

[128] L.I. Gardner et al, "Etiologic factors in tetany of the newborn", *Pediatrics* 1950, 5, 228-30.

[129] reference 101, p. 643.

[130] M.K. Hambidge, "The role of zinc and other trace metals in pediatric nutrition", *Pediatr. Clin. N. Am.* 1977, 24, 95-106.

[131] A.E. Hansen et al, "Essential fatty acids in infant nutrition: clinical manifestations of linoleic acid deficiency", *J. Nutr.* 1958, 66, 565-76.

[132] D. Cornfeld; R.E. Cook, "Vitamin A deficiency: unusual manifestations in a 5½ month old baby", *Pediatrics* 1952, 10, 33-9.

[133] R.L. Schreiner et al, "Lack of lactobezoars in infants given predominantly whey protein formulas", *Am. J. Dis. Child.* 1982, 136, 437-9.

[134] reference 107, p. 105-6.

[135] Task Force Report, reference 101, p. 643

[136] *Am. J. Dis. Child,* 1960, 262, 351-3.

[137] C.J. Richardson et al, "Seven year experience with NEC: association with feeding", *Pediatr. Res.* 1982,16:153A. Abstract 446.

[138] Food Chemical News, June 1984

[139] ibid., Jan. 28, 1985.

[140] in H.A. Moss; R. Hess; C.Swift, *Early Intervention Programs for Infants.* (Haworth Press, 1982) p. 106.

[141] *Pediatrics*, 1984, June,p. 876.

[142] *IPA Bulletin*, 1976, 5, 45.

FURTHER READING 1998

I have deliberately chosen not to update all references, for reasons outlined in the introduction. However, at the end of this chapter it may be useful to include a short list of some key papers that strengthen my belief that artificial feeding harms all infants and is acceptable only when it is unavoidable. In addition, a few reviews of the truly astounding qualities of women's milk are included, as knowledge in this field has also advanced.

• M. Hamosh, "Breast-feeding: Unravelling the Mysteries of Mother's Milk", Medscape <http://www.medscape.com> Women's Health 1(9), 1996.

• L.A. Hanson, M. Hahn-Zoric, U. Wiedermann et al, "Early dietary influence on later immunocompetence"; in "Nutrition Reviews 1996", *Pediatr.* 11: S23-S30.

• J.T. May, "Antimicrobial factors and microbial contaminants in human milk: Recent studies", *J. Pediatr. Child Health* (1994) 30: 470-5.

- K.G. Auerbach, et al., "Infant Feeding Comparisons: A Hazard to Infant Health?", *J. Hum. Lact.* (1991) 7: 63-71.
- ILCA Position Paper on the Hazards of Infant Formula (available from ILCA in the US, or ALCA, PO Box 192, Mawson, ACT, 2607. (see Resources pages)
- M. Minchin, "Infant Formula: A Mass, Uncontrolled Trial in Perinatal Care", *Birth* (1987) 14: 1; 27-35.
- M. Walker, "A Fresh Look at the Risks of Artificial Feeding", *J. Hum. Lact.* (1993) 9: 97-107. Gabriellle Palmer also updated my list of defective formula in her 1992 edition of *The Politics of Breastfeeding* (Pan Books), a book well worth reading.
- K.I. Kennedy, "Effects of breastfeeding on women's health", *Int. J. Gynecol. Obstet.* (1994) 47 (suppl): S11-S21.
- M. Beaudry, R. Dufour, S. Marcoux, "Relation between infant feeding and infections during the first six months of life", *J. Pediatr.* (1995) 126: 191-7.
- K.G. Dewey, J. Hernig, L.A. Nommsen-Rivers, "Differences in morbidity between breastfed and formula-fed infants", *J. Pediatr.* (1995) 126: 696-702.
- L.J. Horwood, D.M. Fergusson, "Breastfeeding and later cognitive and academic outcomes", *Pediatrics* (1998) 101: 1. URL: <http://www.pediatrics.org/cgi/content/full/101/1/e9>.
- D.J. Pettitt, M.R. Forman, R.L. Hanson et al, "Breastfeeding and incidence of non-insulin-dependent diabetes mellitus in Pima Indians", *Lancet* (1997) 350: 166-8.
- U. Saarinen, M. Kajosaari, "Breastfeeding as prophylaxis against atopic disease: prospective study until 17 years old", *Lancet* (1995) 346: 1065-9.
- A.C. Wilson , J.S. Forsyth, S.A. Greene et al, "Relation of diet to public health: sever year follow up of cohort of children in Dundee infant feeding study", *BMJ* (1998) 316: 21-5.
- K. Cook, "The implications of breastfeeding on a sexual health practice", *Venereology* (1995) 8: 2; 92-102.

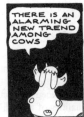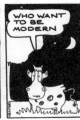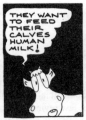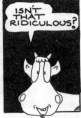

Figure 1   Dumb animals?   **(Cartoon by Brunner, courtesy UNICEF)**

2. WHO IS RESPONSIBLE FOR BREASTFEEDING FAILURE?

In developed countries, greater skill in managing breastfeeding will do more good than 'hot-gospelling' about its benefits. During the last 50 years, the incidence of breastfeeding has fallen in many countries. This fall has happened while doctors and nurses have been urging mothers to breastfeed, which should make us review our educational techniques... Mothers in lower socio-economic groups get poorer support and advice on breastfeeding than middle-class mothers, a situation that the medical and nursing professions could correct. A low incidence of breastfeeding is not inevitable in industrialised countries with a high proportion of women working; in Russia mothers mostly breastfeed. Furthermore, the proportion of mothers breastfeeding can be doubled by appointing a skilled 'lactation nurse' uninvolved in the other duties of a maternity department.

C.B.S. Wood and J.A. Walker-Smith, *Mackeith's Infant Feeding and Feeding Difficulties* (Churchill Livingstone, 6th edn, 1981), p. 98.

The previous chapter should have convinced you that there is no adequate substitute for human milk, and nor is there ever likely to be. The promotion of breastfeeding and human milk banking must be major health goals in developed and developing countries alike.[1] US paediatricians accept that probably 95% of women are physiologically capable of breastfeeding their babies successfully;[2] but where women attempt to breastfeed and fail, they are very often blamed for their failure, subtly or otherwise, the explanations ranging from selfishness to psychological inhibitions.

In an attempt to relieve mothers of the burden of guilt which those judgements impose, professionals everywhere have joined in a conspiracy of silence: we mustn't say too much about the intractable differences between breast and bottle, because those mothers who've tried and failed to breastfeed, or who 'choose' to bottle-feed, will feel guilty. Our whole culture denies the possibility that women who 'fail' in a basic biological role will feel failure in varying degrees; that to mother a child while bottle-feeding is intrinsically more difficult; and that many health and developmental difficulties may be the result of not breastfeeding. Women have largely accepted the burden of responsibility for not breastfeeding, yet most women have very little real responsibility for either breastfeeding failure or bottle-feeding choice.

This situation has not been helped by the way in which breastfeeding has been presented as part of a middle-class lifestyle, presupposing adequate income for a woman not to work, a supportive husband, etc. This is a package that many women cannot identify with. They wish to, or must, work; they are solo parents; or they simply feel ill

45

at ease with sentimental images of mothering, which they recognise as a job worth doing, indeed, but not as their sole job or the only job worth doing. Breastfeeding is a biological act, a way of feeding a child. It is as flexible as any other mode of feeding and has significant advantages for just such groups of women. But because such groups do not fit the romanticised image of mother-devoted-to-child, little has been done to ensure that breastfeeding is practicable for them. That's another issue, and it's time feminists, unionists, politicians and employers did something about it – not to mention childbirth educators and breastfeeding advocates!

Partly as the result of the widespread failure of breastfeeding, many women have developed a defensive/aggressive attitude towards those who, like myself, state plainly that breastfeeding is superior to even the most advanced formula. I am not attempting to criticise the bottlefeeder when I criticise bottle-feeding. Perhaps more than most people, I can understand why bottle-feeding is so 'normal'. But to me it has been ludicrous to see healthworker organisations debating how far they can endorse breastfeeding without upsetting women who bottle-feed.[3] Women will be disturbed to discover what is known about breast and bottle; they will be anxious about what this might mean for their children's long-term health. But if they know all the facts after they have bottle-fed, they will not feel guilty, but instead angry with those people who withheld information or imposed practices contributing to their bottle-feeding. Anxiety and anger are perfectly valid human emotions, appropriate to the situation, and able to be channelled constructively. Those who conceal information, for the sake of sparing some mothers anxiety, are doing greater harm. When 'failed breastfeeders' sit down and discuss their experience in detail, it becomes clear that they failed because others failed them. And the fence-sitters who try to avoid causing guilt (or perhaps dealing with their own sense of it) by concealing truth are failing women everywhere.

Who else fails women? A large part of the responsibility for breastfeeding failure is due, very simply, to professional ignorance. The case histories in Chapter 12 bear witness to this. Stated baldly, that sounds shocking – something we all acknowledge privately but are never so tactless as to state publicly. But until this problem is publicly acknowledged, little will be changed. I am not imputing negligence, or stupidity or malice, or making any other moral judgements. I know that most professionals are hardworking, humane, and dedicated. I am reporting that there is a degree of professional ignorance which is historically quite understandable, but no longer tolerable. In a society where skill and money can produce heart transplants and coronary bypasses, ignorance about breastfeeding is inexcusable.

It's true that nowadays, because of the greater morbidity and mortality of bottle-fed children in both developed and developing countries,[4] most doctors and nurses do urge the mothers to breastfeed and are supportive of mothers who wish to do so. However, words are one thing, deeds another. Of the women leaving hospital with their babies, 85 to 95 per cent should be fully breastfeeding, and where the percentage is lower, I think the hospital staff need to look to their actions. Probably no social institution is as powerful as the hospital in this regard: women are there for the first days of their lactation, and are dependent, at a time when their bodies are adjusting to major changes, on those doctors and nurses. If those mothers are still not breastfeeding at their six-week check-up, the hospital is failing to do all that it can and should – and all that some hospitals do – to promote the health of mother and baby.

So what follows is a checklist for health professionals, to see just how many harmful practices they perform, without critical appraisal or any rationalisation except short-term saving. It's a checklist also for mothers and grandmothers, to see just why they failed to breastfeed successfully or against what odds they succeeded. It's a checklist for childbirth educators involved with local hospitals; where the hospital is in error, you can continue to work for change while also trying to forewarn mothers of the hazards to successful breastfeeding. If you find some hospital staff intractable (and human nature being what it is, this is to be expected) take comfort; there are authoritative texts and international initiatives that can be used to move the laggards along, which will be referred to in this text.

Antenatal period

Hospital (and other) antenatal classes should routinely include:

- Discussion of the nutritional and immunological functions of breastmilk, and the known hazards of bottle-feeding; and an explanation of how infant formulae are devised.
- Explanation of how the breast is constructed and how it works, hence the need for feeding ad libitum (flexible feeding).
- Discussion of ways to collect and store breast milk so that the mother need not feel 'tied down'. Supply of literature on this topic
- Discussion (with fathers and mothers and grandparents) of the common 'old wives' tales' about breastfeeding, and examination of the source of some of the opposition they might still encounter. Discussion of breastfeeding and sexuality is an important facet of this.
- Provision of reliable non-commercial patient-education materials and books to read, such as Stanway's *Breast is Best*; Renfrew, Fisher and Arms's *Bestfeeding*; Cox's *Breastfeeding: I can do that!*, and the MIDIRS *Informed Choice* leaflets.
- Attention to mother's medical history, with special interest in all forms of allergy, food intolerance or hypersensitivity; and practical dietary and nutritional advice, which could lessen the chances of infant sensitisation.[5]
- Advice about smoking and its affect on maternal and child health,[6] preferably given by a non-smoker, because gravel-voiced doctors and nurses who smoke are singularly unconvincing.
- Proper nutritional instruction and oversight, which needs to include strong assurance that this is for her own sake, as the milk will be fine for the baby regardless of her diet (although her own allergens may need to be eliminated or reduced).
- Instruction in simple relaxation techniques.
- Practical advice about coping with housework and a new baby.
- The information that breastfeeding should not hurt, and that squashed nipples are

an early sign that it will hurt if she does not get better help with positioning and attaching the baby.

Of all these important messages, the crucial ones are

- That it matters enormously to her baby and her own health that she breastfeed; and
- Well-positioned and attached babies do not squash nipples and hurt mothers;
- Not all health professionals know how to help with breastfeeding and if difficulties arise, she needs to persevere till she finds one who does.

These classes should utilise as many graphic media as possible, such as the excellent inexpensive slide sets available from TALC (Teaching Aids at Low Cost), P.O. Box 49, St Albans, Herts. AL14AX England. Above all, these classes should involve local breastfeeding mothers, both to familiarise the parents-to-be with the sight of babies feeding and to establish links that could be developed after the new mother returns home.

Hospital (and other) antenatal classes should not include:

- The display of material supplied by commercial interests such as Mead Johnson, Wyeth, Bounty and so on. These state subtly, or crudely, that breastfeeding failure is normal and that bottles are a necessary part of childhood. They also encourage the use of artificial infant foods.
- Demonstration of bottle-feeding techniques. Where this is necessary it should be taught to the individual mother in the postpartum period, after breastfeeding has been attempted. Its indiscriminate demonstration implies that it is normal and approved of by the hospital, and is in any case a poor instructional technique.
- Teaching by educators, whether doctors or nurses, who are not adequately skilled in and enthusiastic about the promotion of breastfeeding. This requires in-service training programmes to be set up, and creation of a general awareness that there is a lot to learn in this area, as in any other area of medicine.

Australia has lagged behind some other Western countries in setting up centres that specialise in the management of breastfeeding problems. This may be due to complacency: our breastfeeding rates compare favourably with other countries, because of a host of confluent sociopolitical factors in our history. (Although when those figures are broken down by parity, class, ethnicity, or geography it becomes very clear that complacency is not warranted.) Even breastfeeding support groups have not yet realised the significance of some recent work in these overseas centres. Hence to educate the professionals is not an easy task. One real difficulty is that in Australia there are few vested interests keen to promote breastfeeding and scores of such interests clamouring for professional attention to their area of concern.

Of course, there are difficulties with antenatal education. Birth itself is the focus of many women's perceptions. Some remember little about other issues. For many women, the child is not real until after the birth, and to concentrate on details of feeding is largely a waste of time. Yet detail is necessary if we are to convey the reality that breast is best and to forewarn women about such disastrous practices as complementary feedings. Orientation is important, and if the mother only retains a clear sense that she wants to breastfeed because it does matter, some good has been done, for in successful breastfeeding the mother's motivation counts for as much as management. The mother who perseveres through difficulties is the mother who has some motivation to do so. In contrast, if the mother believes the manufacturer's slogan, 'Yes, breast is best, but our product is almost as good' – which both parents and professionals have believed in the past – the mother will turn to bottle-feeding in any difficulty. And that message is still being widely broadcast, especially by hospital-based paediatricians who have not updated their knowledge of infant feeding.

However, as learning to breastfeed is a practical skill for which one needs a baby and a (preferably) postpartum breast, much remains to be done during the first days in hospital.

Immediate postpartum period

Most Australian women give birth in hospitals, and hospital policies and practices therefore heavily influence their chances of successful breastfeeding. It is interesting to study the history and trace the reasoning that gave rise to many now-outdated attitudes and practices – they seem less bizarre and irrational once their origins are known – but in this chapter my sole concern is with their impact on lactation.

Drugs to induce or assist labour

These drugs may be necessary but should be avoided wherever possible.
- The use of synthetic hormones to induce labour might make the breast unresponsive to the smaller, physiological doses of oxytocin needed for successful lactation. This happens in dairy animals, according to one dairy physiologist.
- Drugs given in labour may depress the infant's natural reflexes, causing difficulty in feeding.[7] Poor feeding may lead not only to scanty volumes but to decreased production because of lack of nipple stimulation.
- Drugs may also increase the baby's degree of jaundice, leading to phototherapy and additional fluids.

Delayed suckling after birth

The sucking reflex is strongest in the first hour after birth. Thereafter it fades, and if feeding at the breast is delayed for 24 hours the infant may need to be taught what to do, particularly if bottles are given during that time.[8]
- The infant's feeding stimulates the release of oxytocin and prolactin, hastening the production of milk.
- Colostrum is not only important nutritionally and immunologically; it also has a laxative effect. High levels of jaundice are associated with delayed opening of the

bowels. 'Diluting' colostrum by additional fluids may have the same effect; this could be due to increased reabsorption from the bowel, because of delayed transit time (see p. 55).

• It has been documented since 1977 that mothers whose infants feed within the first hour after delivery go on to breastfeed much longer than other mothers.[9]

Restricted feed times (one, three, five minutes, etc.)

• There is no evidence that this reduces the incidence of nipple soreness; a properly positioned baby causes no soreness whatever the length of feed. It has been documented since 1952 that 'demand' or ad libitum feeding actually reduces the incidence of nipple problems.[10]

• There is evidence that restricted feed times cause anxiety and tension. Under stress many normal women find that their milk does not 'let down' in time for the baby to receive any; hence she becomes engorged and the baby goes hungry, and a cycle of lactation failure begins.[11] Studies of milk flow in Oxford mothers revealed a high degree of variability "in respect of the length of nutritive feeding, the initial rate of milk flow, and the final milk intake." The authors concluded that "it is illogical to offer advice regarding the length of a feed on the basis of an arbitrary time schedule... Mothers... should be encouraged to time their feeds according to the responses of their own infants."[12]

• Clocks have no place in successful breastfeeding. They are the antithesis of the idea that the mother-child interaction is unique and variable and that each must learn to be sensitive to the other in a mutual relationship. It would indeed "seem obvious that changing the baby from one breast to the other would be determined by the baby's stopping sucking rather than some arbitrary time limit."[13]

Routine/scheduled feed times

• A schedule is simply not appropriate for the very young infant, who may need to suckle almost constantly at times. Mothers should not ignore their infant's expressed need. Where simple body contact will not settle a young baby, feeding is indicated. It is also less arduous and much quicker than endless walking, back-patting or rocking, or even listening to the baby cry – as well as better for the mother's supply.[14]

• The amount of protein in a mammalian milk seems to correspond to the frequency with which suckling is necessary.[15] Human milk has a low protein content, which is ideal for the young infant, but it is therefore frequently needed. (High-protein diets place great stress on immature kidneys, liver and brain.)

• Scheduled feeds impose a great burden on staff, because all the mothers and babies need help simultaneously! Flexible feeding means that mothers who need help ask for it at different times, and there is less pressure on ward facilities.[16]

• Recent studies have shown that even premature infants benefit from demand feeding.[17] Indeed, Colombian experience has proved this to be a life-saving form of appropriate technology.

• Frequent breastfeeding may be important in the prevention of jaundice.

• Frequent feeding helps to establish a high basal concentration of prolactin, which is important to successful lactation as well as in maintaining infertility after childbirth. This lactational amenorrhoea has been recognised recently as the world's most important contraceptive.[18] After this period of frequent feeding however, many babies settle into a routine of 5-8 feeds per day.

Use of additional fluids

Healthy breastfed babies have very low average intakes in the first two days postpartum. (Day one average: 37ml in feeds of 7ml; day 2 average: 84ml in feeds of 14ml; day 3 average: 266ml in feeds of 38ml.)[19] This is almost certainly because babies have small stomachs and limited kidney capacities, and have to shed fluid as they reduce the blood volume needed in utero. This fits in well with the hormonally-delayed onset of lactation, with the second stage of lactose synthesis beginning roughly 20 hours after birth and milk volumes increasing gradually from then on. Such a neatly tailored arrangement suggests that interventions (such as giving additional fluids) must always be justified, and in fact rarely have been.

1. *Water*

Obviously oral rehydration is indicated if the baby is dehydrated. But water is not the most appropriate rehydrating fluid in true dehydration, which is rare in breastfed infants. (And breast milk is a more effective rehydration fluid than plain water.)[20] The common practice of forcing fluids in the first few days, until mother's milk 'comes in' has been shown to result in increased weight loss, and infants thus fed were less likely to start gaining weight before leaving hospital than entirely breastfed infants.[21] This could be because any additional fluid will depress baby's thirst, decrease the vigour of frequency of feeding, and hence upset the delicate balance of supply and demand. Therefore, even water should be given only when necessary. One recent study found that water supplementation made no difference at all to physiological jaundice in breastfed infants.[22] This could have been expected, as water does not bind bilirubin. In any case, if re-circulation of bilirubin occurs in the breastfed infant, it just may be because it is a powerful and needed anti-oxidant.

2. *5% glucose*

Curiously, very little seems to be written on the effects of supplementation with 5% glucose. I found no investigations of the effect on immature insulin balance or other endocrine mechanisms; no discussion of the possibility of reactive hypoglycaemia (common in adults); no follow-up of children given glucose regularly after birth.[23] After my dealings with food-intolerant families, I suspect such studies are overdue, because where only one child had received 5% glucose he or she was notable as the family's sugar-addict. At present we seem to know very little about what such an unphysiological fluid does to infant bodies – besides, of course, decreasing breast milk intake and thus causing problems. A recent study showed clearly that the routine use of glucose water, theoretically to reduce the risk of jaundice or excessive weight loss, made no difference to either. What it did do was to greatly decrease the number of

mothers still breastfeeding exclusively at three months: 81 per cent of the unsupplemented group, compared with only 53 per cent of those who received glucose water,
were still being fully breastfed. Of the mothers who had discontinued breastfeeding,
38 per cent gave as their reason their baby's preference for the bottle, to which the
infant had been exposed when so young. The neonatologist concluded: "I believe that
routine early neonatal supplementation of breastfeeding with glucose in water should
be discontinued. It usually does not serve any purpose and, more important, it seems to
be a major factor interfering with successful breastfeeding."[24] Calories may be necessary for a child threatened with hypoglycaemia, but is 5% glucose given orally preferable to breast milk? In fact, 5% glucose is more irritating to the lungs and gut than
breast milk would be, which makes nonsense of the old idea that 'if the child aspirates
it won't matter'. Intravenous administration of dextrose seems much more logical
when it is necessary. Perhaps the neat little disposable bottles once so thoughtfully
provided by formula companies seemed more attractive, however unscientific. [It is
interesting to note that in 1998 glucose water bottles seem to have disappeared from
maternity wards, though studies of their consequences still have not been done.] If a
dehydrated child is well enough to take fluid orally, it should be breast milk or oral
rehydration solution. The 1996 monograph, *Hypoglycaemia of the Newborn: a review
of the Evidence*, published by WHO Geneva (WHO/NUT 96.2) should result in
changed practice in many hospitals.

3. *Artificial formulae (usually cows' milk based)*
• There is real risk that even one feed of foreign protein may allow a baby to become
infected by bacterial or viral pathogens. It has been shown that one feed dramatically
alters the flora in the baby's gut, encouraging the growth of pathogens normally suppressed by human milk. This effect has been shown to last for some weeks – normal
gut flora may take that long to be re-established, even under exclusive breastfeeding.[25]
• There is a real risk that one feed of foreign protein will sensitise the baby and set
up a lifelong intolerance to cows' milk.[26] The extent of this problem has been seriously
underestimated in the past, and seems to have worsened with each generation –
perhaps because the sensitised mother gestates an even more sensitive child, perhaps
because whey-dominant formula is more allergenic than casein-dominant, and since
1980 has become the most common formula type in some countries. Studies on allergy
rarely examine the antigenicity of particular types of bovine formula, much less of
individual brands and their composition and market share over time. Yet we have one
UK study showing that infant formula antigenicity varies greatly, between and within
brand name and by physical type (powder/liquid).
• The presence of other foods decreases the availability of nutrients in breast milk by
interfering with enzymes, transfer factors, etc., that make breast milk uniquely well
absorbed. Giving iron-containing foods, for example, can result in iron deficiency.[27]
• The unnecessary use of these fluids simply because they are convenient is the best
advertisement the companies could have. In Sweden in 1984, all infants were given
human milk in hospital, whether they were later to be breast- or bottle-fed. In this way
hospitals state clearly that only human milk is good enough for human babies. Austra-

lian parents of pre-term infants obviously believe that the hospitals' use of formulae (based on cows' milk) proves that they are equivalent to breast milk. Companies know that parents will continue to use products endorsed by the hospital – hence the special deals to get their brand into use.

The very least hospitals could do when using such products is to adhere to the WHO Code's standards.[28] As one well-informed nursing educator said, "If the hospital administration insists on promoting the milk companies in this way, the nurse might suggest to a mother that the bottle(s) of formula be used to make custard, to pour on her own cereal, or into her tea."[29] I couldn't agree more, though the taste might surprise parents!

4. *Human milk supplied by other mothers*

This is usually preferable for newborns, especially milk freshly obtained from a mother who has given birth recently. Many hospitals have maintained excellent milk banks since the 1920s with very few problems.[30] Others routinely employ healthy wetnurses.[31] However, there are real problems with donor breast milk (just as there are for blood and sperm – and even AIDS hasn't closed blood or semen banks!). Care needs to be exercised in screening donor mothers, not only for hygiene, but also for diet, drug intake, smoking, etc. A precise temperature pasteuriser should be available to minimise the risks, and maximise the benefits, of donor milk. Careless handling of human milk greatly affects its composition. We don't have all the answers in this area, but that should lead to more and better research. The fact remains that countries such as Finland have maintained milk banks for 50 years or more with very satisfactory results, and in Norway 80% of hospitals now use donated human milk, a rise of 20% in the last decade: whereas in Australia almost no hospital does![32] Even in the UK milk banking is reviving in the nineties. And here in Australia the Red Cross is investigating milk banking, following an influential ALCA Vic seminar on the subject.

Use of bottles and teats

These are more problematic in the first weeks of lactation, although they can be useful later in situations where scrupulous hygiene is possible.

• Bottles and teats are sources of infection in any community, in Australia especially of thrush, for example. This is not always recognised as the cause of nipple soreness.

• Teats may wrongly condition the suckling reflex in susceptible babies because they require different muscle action and tongue positioning.[33] They do have adverse facial consequences, as the growth of orthodontistry testifies.

• Food flows instantly and continuously (presuming the hole is large enough), thus making the baby reluctant to persevere at the breast until milk is let down. Conversely, where the hole is small and flow is slow, a baby learns to chew more forcefully on the teat, an action which can be painful on a nipple.

• At least some breast refusal is the outcome of complementary feeding before the baby is well educated in breastfeeding. Alternative methods – cups, spoons, syringes, nursing supplementers or eye-droppers – have none of these disadvantages although they are slower. But when mothers (not nurses) are giving these additional feeds, staff time is not an issue.[34] Ideally in the first couple of days, or when milk volumes are tiny, hand expression and teaspoon or syringe feeding are used. Pumps and cups come into their own only as volumes increase.

Use of breast pumps

• Hand expression is a skill that should always be taught, and for many women vastly preferable to pumps. However, breast pumps can be useful in long-term lactation.

• Old-fashioned bulb-type suction hand-pumps are extremely difficult to centre so as to avoid nipple damage, and it is hard to control the degree of vacuum created. Some breast pumps are unpleasant instruments of torture, causing nipple fissures.[35]

• They are also common sources of cross-infection, because the rubber bulb is difficult to clean.[36] All pumps require care with hygiene.

• The Kaneson-type cylindrical pump can be very useful, but nurses and mothers need careful instruction in its use, to avoid nipple damage. The new Avent Isis diaphragm pump is easier to manage one-handed than any other hand pump currently on the market, and some mothers are enthusiastic about its virtues.

• A well-designed electric alternating pressure pump should be standard equipment for maternity hospitals.[37] The well-managed mother of a full-term baby will rarely need to use it except to relieve engorgement or to donate milk, but it is invaluable for mothers whose babies are too small or too drowsy to suck well. A simple foot pump can make this expensive technology accessible in less affluent communities, although hygiene remains a major concern wherever resources are scarce.

Night feeding

• Night feeding minimises or prevents engorgement problems. As breasts become over-full, the levels of inhibitory peptide secreted in the milk, and the pressure that develops in the breast, means that the glandular tissue receives the message to stop synthesis or even suppress lactation. Failure to remove milk has only one significance in nature: the baby has died and the milk is therefore not required. It may take days of frequent suckling to reverse that message and build up an adequate supply.

• Many mothers wake during the night for the first weeks, needing to go to the toilet or to check on the baby. If unsure whether staff will wake her if the baby needs her, a mother sleeps lightly or stays awake. If sure that they will bring the baby to her, she can sleep heavily, wake only to feed and go to the toilet, then sleep again, as the lactation hormones help her to relax and rest.[38]

• Mothers do 'need their rest'. Prolactin levels are highest during sleep, and some Japanese hospitals actually encourage mothers to sleep more for that reason.[39] However, to feed a baby need not involve waking up fully or getting up at all. Mothers need to learn to feed lying down with baby in bed. My third child stayed in the hospital bed with me at night, and we both slept soundly; to reassure the staff (not because it was needed) I used a sling to ensure that she could not fall out.

• Timetabled night feeding is a physiological absurdity. Feed time should be when each individual baby needs feeding. Mothers who would not feel comfortable with their baby beside them ought to know that hospital staff will provide the warm body contact the newborns often need at night. (A baby sling has uses for nurses too!)

Test weighing

Keeping track of baby's weight loss or gain overall is very important. But test weighing as a routine is useless, however useful it may be in research. Using standard ward equipment, the figures are almost always inaccurate, especially for large or small babies.[40] It is harmful, because it creates stress (affecting the results), inhibits or prevents demand feeding and interferes with the synchronisation of the mother-baby feeding relationship. It is even positively hazardous, not only because of the additional cold stress to the infant, but also because the results are often thought to justify giving complementary cows' milk bottles. Nurses are often unaware of the wide variation in human milk composition and secretion and therefore use the very rough and ready nature of the old rule of thumb (2½ oz per lb). A breastfed baby receiving a high fat milk may well need less volume than he or she is 'supposed' to. And anyway, one day's secretion in the first week is a meaningless figure, given women's different responses to the stress of 'performing' for the nurses, and to hospitalisation in general. Many women become profoundly depressed by test-weigh results and some even give up, convinced that they can't breastfeed. Very few realise that if babies needed large volumes immediately after birth, breasts would be making more sooner. Many newborns simply can't handle large volumes of fluid – their kidneys are too small and immature. The average intake on day 1 is just 37ml in total, in feeds of about 7ml – a teaspoon and a half. The incredible survival of newborn babies in the Mexican earthquake makes it quite clear that additional fluids are rarely necessary.

Infant weight loss

A degree of weight loss is normal and may even be beneficial, as shedding the additional fluid reduces the working load of the heart, and may therefore "lessen the risk for the patent ductus".[41] Failure to recognise this fact can lead to supplementation with other fluids, long before such concern is warranted. The length of time an infant takes to regain his or her birth weight will be as variable as all the factors influencing the mother's milk supply and the baby's hydration (such as air-conditioning). Concern about adequate weight gain should be directed towards minimising the stresses and negative influences on mother, as well as monitoring an infant's clinical signs.

Infant jaundice

• Fear of jaundice has often, and unnecessarily, caused breastfeeding failure.[42] Prevention of jaundice should be a concern that informs pregnancy, labour and postpartum care, for many drugs commonly prescribed for women in these periods can contribute to infant jaundice (salicylates, some sedatives, tranquillisers, diazepam, diuretics and antibiotics; oxytocin, steroids, sulpha drugs; even caffeine, in all its myriad forms).[43]

• If a child does become jaundiced, concern to continue breastfeeding should inform the care given. The baby should be removed from bili lights frequently for feeding and care; phototherapy should not be ordered for more than 12 hours at any stretch, as long periods of light therapy flood the bowel with bilirubin that can cause gut damage and lactose intolerance. It has been clearly shown that early, frequent and unsupplemented breastfeeding lowers the incidence of jaundice[44] (possibly because of laxative effects of colostrum, as gut reabsorption in the gut is a major factor,[45] or simply because increased caloric intake lowers bilirubin levels. Cavalier treatment of jaundice has caused much infant distress and early weaning, together with parental perceptions that the child is at serious risk of brain damage and especially vulnerable for long periods.

• Those who wish to maintain out-dated practices of routinely giving water 'to prevent jaundice' should be aware that there is no scientific basis for this.[46] There is no such thing as *breastfeeding* jaundice: it is more accurately called mismanaged-breastfeeding jaundice, or (as it is in adults) starvation jaundice. High rates and levels of jaundice suggest poor breastfeeding care.

• *Breastmilk jaundice,* or more accurately, normal bilirubin levels (elevated relative to deficient formula-fed babies) persisting beyond 10 days post-partum, have gone from being a "disease" in the 1960's to being seen as possibly protective. A search of Lactnet archives will find numerous useful comments by Dr. Larry Gartner, a key AAP committee member with a special interest in jaundice. If definitive diagnosis is needed to exclude haemolysis or some other concern, or if levels rise beyond 350-400mmol, and breastfeeding is interrupted briefly, any alternative feeds given[47] when the baby is not nursing from its mother should be breastmilk. The last thing a jaundiced baby needs is the additional metabolic stress of coping with the excessive protein and mineral loads of artificial formulae, and a dramatic change in gut flora.

Management of infant crying

Hospital attitudes to crying infants will influence the new mother's behaviour. If babies are left to cry, she receives the impression that to ignore a crying baby is appropriate, and so learns to ignore her child rather than respond sensitively and immediately. Babies responded to immediately later cry less than babies who are not. And infant crying is a risk factor for infant abuse. It could be said that hospitals which encourage mothers to ignore their babies' cries are also promoting child abuse. Crying is a signal of need and distress. It distresses mothers, which does not help lactation, because stress hormones may interfere with milk production. It distresses the infant, who may then be too exhausted to suckle well before falling asleep. Babies who are not hungry can readily be soothed by being walked or rocked or held close to a warm body. Baby slings should be standard in all maternity hospitals. But no device compensates for constant access to mother's skin and breasts.

Consistency and accuracy of breastfeeding advice

Mothers need sensitive, skilled help. Only women who are professionally competent and preferably (but not necessarily) have enjoyed breastfeeding a baby are ideally qualified to help a new mother. Nurses who have never breastfed or who chose to bottle-feed and are hostile to 'all this emphasis on breastfeeding' can do enormous harm. So can enthusiastic but ignorant amateurs. This is an area where new research into problems is finally happening; new techniques are being developed. Every hospital needs to appoint one person whose task it is to keep up with lactation research, and who is accepted as the authority on the subject, with a mandate to educate all other staff. Appointing a full-time International Board-Certified Lactation Consultant would be a beginning. (The national professional Association for IBCLCs is the Australian Lactation Consultants Association, the only association whose members all must have passed the highly-regarded International Board Examination; ALCA can provide names of IBCLCs in any locality. See the Resources section on p. 364.) And every hospital should be working to achieve accreditation as a Baby-Friendly Hospital.

The fundamental things that mothers must get right are:

- the logic behind correct positioning of a baby (see Chapter 3)
- comfortable positions – sitting and lying – for feeding,
- recognising the let-down reflex by watching the baby's jaw movements,
- early warning signs of breast and nipple problems, and their treatment (see Chapters 5-6).

Nurses will not be able to help in these areas until their own education has been improved. Far less *detail* about breastfeeding is taught than is needed (and some of what is taught is wrong). As Gunther has said, "Feeding should not hurt the mother at all, and whenever it does the cause should be investigated. Exact diagnosis is made by looking carefully, and this is a part of good practice as in other branches of medicine."[48] To my mind, this is where much more careful research is needed, and the results of the research should be taught in continuing-education courses, compulsory for all who work on maternity wards.

Sleeping pills

- By lowering basal metabolism, sleeping pills slow the production of milk.[49]
- They make it difficult for a mother to feed at night, and perhaps dangerous to handle the baby unassisted or to sleep with the infant in bed.
- Residues in breast milk could affect the baby, either to excite or to sedate. Diazepam (Valium) has been known since 1976 to cause lethargy and impaired suckling in infants.[50] The drug's half-life in babies is much greater than in adults, so the effects are more dramatic.

Tea, coffee, diet drinks

It is almost unthinkable to challenge these socially accepted drinks, but all are pharmacologically active and need to be taken in moderation rather than our usual Western excess.[51] Many women drink 10 or more cups per day, often extremely strong. Newborn infants lack the enzyme needed to metabolise caffeine (and perhaps other compounds) so that it will accumulate in their bodies; its half-life is 4 days. Tea is constipating; it may affect iron absorption[52] by rendering some iron supplements insoluble. (How many women swallow prescribed iron supplements with a cuppa?) Both tea and coffee have been associated with colicky or unsettled infants and poor milk supply; increasingly too with mastitis and fibrocystic breast disease (see p. 157).

Smoking

In theory forbidden in any health institution, smoking by postpartum women still occurs, and nurses who smoke may condone it, or even help write guidelines that suggest reassuringly that some arbitrary number of cigarettes (often 10 per day) is OK. No cigarette smoke is safe for infants. Some babies react very sensitively to amounts others apparently tolerate without harm, although it is clear that smoked over babies will be at greater risk for not only respiratory and gut problems but also allergic disease and cot death. Smoking must be outlawed near infants, and near other nursing mothers, who will excrete nicotine to their babies if exposed.[53] Breastfeeding mothers who smoke should be encouraged to stop, because smoking is associated with changes in milk composition, and many toxic compounds reach the baby through the milk. Being smoked over (by parents, grandparents, friends or relations) will result in shorter, less intelligent, less healthy children. If mothers/fathers cannot quit, they should be encouraged to smoke well away from the baby, outside the house, the car, or any enclosed space shared with the child, and after rather than during feeds.

However, the single most important message to communicate about smoking is this: *if you smoke, you cannot afford to bottle-feed, because it compounds the harms that smoking does to your baby, while breastfeeding reduces that harm. So if you smoke, you must breastfeed. Don't give up breastfeeding because you're worried about what's in your milk.* A full discussion of this will be found in my next book, updating a review article written for the *Journal of Human Lactation* in 1991.[54]

Maternal breastfeeding problems

1. *Engorgement*

Extreme engorgement is now being seen as iatrogenic,[55] as it is rare when babies are fed ad libitum from birth. But some mothers will suffer a degree of engorgement even when fully demand feeding, as milk production can proceed faster than the baby's ability to remove milk. An excess of milk in the breast, combined with the vascular and lymphatic congestion common as the breast switches on to lactation, can create pressures that prevent milk outflow or lymphatic drainage. This leads to a degree of oedema needing assistance for prompt resolution.

The most important thing to remember is that milk can flow out of the breast, while oedema must be resolved by getting lymph back into the circulation. The basic principles for the resolution of oedema can be adopted: rest, ice, compression and elevation. Treatments include the following:

- 'Binders'. These would seem to work on the principle of persuading the breast to slow or stop milk production by mimicking the feedback pressure effect of total distension. They do cause pain to subside more rapidly when lactation is being suppressed.[56] This, however, may not be a recommendation when lactation is to continue, as it may merely indicate greater efficiency at suppressing milk production. Before dismissing the idea of binders as unhelpful, we should listen to the reports of mothers who have found them to increase comfort when applied by skilled midwives willing to adjust them as often as needed: in all other cases of oedema, compression relieved as often as necessary is found to be useful. But unadjusted binders on breasts are as cruel as unadjusted plaster casts put on broken bones before the swelling has reached its maximum. Just as we break open casts that are too tight, if we use binders of any kind, we need to adjust them as needed to deal with breasts still increasing in size. A simple "knickers bra" made from 2 pairs of large underpants can provide comfortable and firm support without compression, and hold ice packs in place. (See the Appendix to this chapter for instructions on making such a bra.)

• Hand expression. This needs to be very gentle to avoid bruising an overdistended gland. Such expression has caused mastitis and bleeding when too vigorous. Nurses often have no idea how exquisitely painful engorged breasts can be. If it hurts, don't do it! The hot jar technique discussed in the mastitis chapter can be used initially. So too can warmth, gentle massage and expression by the mother herself, preferably in a warm bath or under a warm shower, with someone at hand to give the baby to mother to try feeding, then take the baby away again.

• An electric breast pump can be used to 'empty' the breast at the end of the day, after the last feed. Following this, cold packs can be applied for brief periods to reduce the lymphatic congestion in the breasts. Often with this done, the breasts settle down as drainage is possible. Milk expressed can be frozen for later use.

• Borrowing a hungry baby with more vigorous and efficient sucking techniques can also be useful, if one's own baby is too full or sleepy to co-operate.

• Drugs can reduce over-supply, but are problematic (see ch. 4).

Unless this initial engorgement is adequately dealt with, it can progress to obstructive mastitis and even infectious mastitis. Badly managed, this may bring about lactation failure. It can certainly cause a temporary supply problem. Mothers should be taught to look for lumps or painful spots in the breast or under the armpits and to ensure that these clear away with massage during feeds, etc. They should also be taught that much of the fullness of their breasts is vascular and lymphatic congestion, not milk; that when this subsides they may find their supply is just a little low and be prepared to feed more often. Mothers who think that they have been bursting with milk tend to assume that when the congestion resolves they have lost their milk altogether, and some try to 'save it up' by going longer between feeds.

It is worth noting that engorgement is a general term that means overfullness or distension; it is a phase the breast can go through in the weaning process, or preceding mastitis, and the two fronts to work on remain: moving milk and ending oedema.

2. *Nipple soreness*

Again, an iatrogenic problem, usually caused by poor positioning or engorgement, and rarely accurately diagnosed. Sensible treatment is outlined in Chapter 5. Treatments contraindicated by basic logic are still suggested in some hospitals.

3. *Low supply*

• High-protein milk drinks may cause or exacerbate food intolerance problems in mothers and infants. No mother should eat or drink any food in excess or any food that makes her feel ill.[57] Mothers do not need Just for Mum or any such milk-based food – except perhaps in malnourished communities, where such foods are unaffordable and often indigestible anyway!

• Excessive fluid intake is no remedy[58] and may actually suppress milk production. US literature used to urge grossly excessive consumption, yet the only studies done indicate that extra fluid probably suppresses lactation, and that slightly too little is more effective.[59] In general, mothers should drink only as much as they feel they need to, and that should be a low-sugar, low protein, low salt, caffeine free drink. Any deficiency in fluid intake will result in over-strong urine long before it affects milk production; mothers should drink enough to keep their urine pale.

• Encouraging more frequent feeds, whenever baby will suck, usually solves the problem. More complicated cases are discussed in Chapter 4. But in general, mothers simply need reassurance that their supply will be adequate and that such frequent feeding is usually only a temporary thing, with the milk supply building up so that baby soon goes for longer intervals between feeds. The emptier the breast, the faster the rate of milk synthesis between then and the next feed, so expressing after feeds does work.

Paternal and family involvement

For very many reasons – including its beneficial effect on breastfeeding rates – hospitals should be actively encouraging fathers (and other family members, where appropriate) to become involved in the care of the breastfed infant. Fathers need to know the advantages of breastfeeding so that they can bolster the mother's confidence. If they learn the basics of how breastfeeding works, they can help their partner through many difficulties. Other family members, especially grandparents and children, may need help from hospital staff to accept breastfeeding as normal and good for both mother and baby. And too often, siblings' needs for reassurance are overlooked.

Free samples of brand-name products

Many hospitals still give mothers a take-home pack of free, branded sample products. Some of these products can be useful, and it's common sense to accept what may be the only sample of baby products that one can afford. (The exorbitant price of baby goods naturally includes the cost of this promotional gimmick.) However, it seems irresponsible to provide such 'goodies' without explaining why many of these may be unnecessary at home. Naturally parents assume these products are approved of, or even necessary to rearing the child safely. I have known mothers to go on using lotions containing hexachlorophene for months, after seeing this used in hospital. In such cases the child was actually at risk of being harmed by the continuation of what was meant to be a short-term protection against infection; hexachlorophene is now considered unsafe for such use. Hypochlorite bleaches, too, can range from the very expensive (promoted for infant care) to the very cheap, but parents will generally stick to the brand they saw in hospital. No one tells parents that a mother's greatest anti-infective measure is to keep herself healthy and well nourished and exclusively breastfeed her baby; or that sunlight, soap and hot water are better than expensive nappy sterilising solution (which may cause dermatitis, as well). What may be reasonable hygiene for a hospital situation can be excessive and expensive at home. An infant needs to build up immunity to the family bugs. He or she does not need a mother exhausted from trying to keep the house spotless, and from worrying about the cost of all these baby goods.

Indeed, hospital concern about infection has had other bizarre consequences. Staff were once very conscious of themselves as clean, and families as unacceptably grubby. Infection used to be blamed upon visitors. This led to rigid separation of mother and baby, as well as restriction on visitors. More recently it has been realised that it is usually the professionals who carry the most dangerous pathogens in their respiratory tract, while those organisms colonising the mother are the ones to which she has antibodies, so that the breastfed baby is protected against them. The logical corollary is that babies should be handled as little as possible by anyone but family members.

The advertising or supply of free formula among these bundles of 'goodies' has surely ceased since the promulgation of the WHO *International Code of Marketing of Breastmilk Substitutes* (see ch. 10). After all, that Code and subsequent World Health Assembly resolutions pointed out the moral responsibility of those supplying formula to see that parents who needed it had continued access to the product at a price they could afford. (This could mean the hospital continuing to provide infant formula or subsidise it for the whole period it was required.) Everyone accepts that if there is formula on hand, mothers are more likely to give a complementary bottle than to allow the baby to breastfeed more often, as is usual on first going home, particularly among socially disadvantaged mothers. If hospitals are still providing sample formula, or goodies such as magazines advertising formula or bottles and teats, please report them to APMAIF (see ch. 10).

Community liaison

Too many mothers go home, and that's it – they have no further contact with anyone knowledgeable about breastfeeding. They are very vulnerable to all the women (and not a few men) of their acquaintance, who ply them with well-meant advice. Hospitals need to be part of an on-going system of support. Here in Australia the baby health clinics are a useful part of such a system, but they are under enormous pressure to accept unrealistic case loads and certainly cannot do the amount of home visiting that could be required. Step 10 of the Baby-Friendly Hospital Initiative mandates such community support. Of course, every time a mother sees a doctor instead of a maternal and child health nurse the community pays more, but state governments are happy to increase commonwealth costs while saving on their own outlays.

Summary

Hospitals that have modified their routine to eliminate the major obstacles to breastfeeding, all report gratifying results. The percentage of women successfully breastfeeding their infants continues to rise, and in notable cases approaches 100 per cent. But hospitals that continue to employ dogmatic authoritarian staff, addicted to order and routine, or staff without the clinical skills needed to assist mothers, will continue to have less satisfactory rates. Obviously there will be differences between hospitals because of the cultural, socioeconomic and ethnic backgrounds of their patients, but such differences should serve as a stimulus to finding ways of communication with cultural subgroups. Here I would enter a caveat. To improve breastfeeding rates in some hospitals initially is easy. This is a natural system, geared for success in most women, and resistant to all but gross interference of the kind that has been institutionalised as usual. Get the basic protocol right, and the average woman will succeed without too much trouble, particularly when she is motivated, has support and is secure. Next comes the difficult bit. There will be mothers who have problems which require skilled diagnosis and management. Because average advice has helped the average mother, professionals and lay helpers tend to act as though it should work for everyone. It will not. The harder task ahead of us is to learn to recognise and help those mothers – not thrust back at them the blame for their failure, which is really the result of our ignorance. Let's not cheer too soon about what has been achieved, considerable though that is.

Changing all such institutions is a vital prerequisite to promoting breastfeeding more widely in the community. If we concentrate our efforts on telling mothers that 'breast is best', which most already accept, without acting to change institutions and attitudes that make breastfeeding difficult or impossible, we do two things. First, we create additional problems of guilt and anxiety for those who try and fail. Second, we help to create a backlash against the promotion of breastfeeding by women's groups tired of being told yet again they have done the less-than-optimal thing for their children. Feminists and breastfeeding advocates have for so long swallowed the mythology of bottle-feeding convenience – what a joke! – that they have lost sight of the ways in which commercial, medical and social pressures have created an inadequate substitute for women's own product.[60] For these and other reasons, I feel that it behoves those who promote breastfeeding to be working at the process of social change, working to change the conditions and attitudes and ignorances that make bottle-feeding seem an inevitable part of a flexible lifestyle and which cause a rapid fall-off in the number of women breastfeeding after they leave hospital.

After leaving hospital

The care of the newborn has always devolved upon the midwife, and it is right that it should remain her special province. But neglect of the study of lactation... has had two results. In her management of breastfeeding the midwife has worked largely by rule of thumb, and understandably she objects to being asked to alter. In hospitals where much of the day-to-day teaching of pupil midwives is part of the charge-sister's duties, this attitude can seriously impede progress. Another obstacle is the short period of the midwife's supervision and her consequent unawareness that her patient's failures to breastfeed are often the direct result of the management they received in the lying-in period. A higher rate of success cannot be hoped for until she and her auxiliary, the health visitor, are better instructed and work in close contact. This applies also to the medical practitioners with whom they work.

Harold Waller, *The Breasts and Breastfeeding*, (Heinemann Medical, 1958), p. 50

How many mothers leave hospital breastfeeding comfortably, confidently, exclusively? We don't really know. The 1997 APMAIF Report[61] gives a figure (based on the Australian Bureau of Statistics 1997 Survey) of 88% of women initiating 'breastfeeding'. There are very wide differences between hospitals and social groups. 'Breastfeeding' may not have meant exclusive breastfeeding, or feeding without complementary bottles. It may also not mean comfortable breastfeeding. This may be a significant caveat. Under this definition, in 1976 I too was discharged 'breastfeeding', but my son had been given formula for seven of the eight days I was in hospital, and continuing to breastfeed therefore meant having him at the breast virtually day and night as he strove to build up my supply. I also left hospital with extremely painful nipples, which were the direct result of hospital ignorance about positioning and attachment. These too could have meant rapid weaning for another, less-motivated mother. One does not have to be a genius to see many pathways to failure which are the direct outcome of poor hospital practice, however many women leave on day two or day seven 'fully breastfeeding'. Waller recognised this in the 1950s.

But the problems created by hospitals are only part of the reason for the later decline in breastfeeding. And decline it does. By two months, it is 68 per cent; and by six months, perhaps only 47 per cent give even one breastfeed (compared with 90 per cent in Norway, where 98 per cent initiate breastfeeding). Many of these babies at two months will be well on the road to weaning, as other foods and drinks are still introduced too early. In short, breastfeeding at all to four months of age has been managed by only a minority for the past three decades.[62] Figures for breastfeeding exclusively would be much lower. Only a minority of Australia's children receive what is now regarded as optimal nutrition. This makes a mockery of Australian complacency about our high breastfeeding rates. These figures conceal even further problems.

Breastfeeding initiation rates are very low in areas of socioeconomic deprivation.[63] Among those who may well need it most, human milk has been almost totally replaced by artificial substitutes, some of which are grossly unsuitable for young infants. Despite warnings from the National Health and Medical Research Council, the use of substitutes other than infant formula is likely to continue because the so-called 'humanised' formulae are very expensive. (It would be interesting to see a cost analysis[64] of these infant formula. A 'prices justification' enquiry would be useful.)

In this section I want to look at the problems the new mother faces in continuing breastfeeding after leaving hospital. Even the best-informed and most highly motivated mother will have difficulties in any society where artificial feeding has become commonplace, especially a society such as ours where many people have psychological problems related to sexuality.

No one can tell the new parents how it feels to take that tiny bundle home, and wake to the realisation that this seemingly fragile life depends entirely upon them for its care and nourishment. Because we are so unfamiliar with babies, and because we lack an extended family on the spot, that sense of responsibility can be devastating. I have known women who weaned their baby because they couldn't cope with the burden of feeling entirely responsible for the baby's growth; surely a 'scientific' formula would be safer than something they produced and couldn't measure? (In any case, it gives them something external to blame for any difficulties.) When the breastfed infant cries and cannot be pacified, it does give one an intensely personal feeling of failure. ("Just as a biological unit, which is a basic level of functioning, I'm a failure – I can't even feed my child properly, when I seem to be normally equipped to do so.")

But if parents are blessed with a contented thriving child who provides positive feedback to them as parents, they'll still have problems. Bottle feeding has become the normal 'decent' way to feed a child, thanks to commercial influences over successive generations. We give little girls dolls and bottles with disappearing milk; we use teenage breasts to sell cows' milk; we are encouraged to "live on milk";[66] we see advertisements for bottles, even apparently miraculous 'anti-colic bottles',[67] we see bottle-feeding babies advertising nappies and much more; we have a cultural obsession with germicidal products, which are used for everything connected with babies as though their use compensated for the loss of protective factors in breast milk. In our culture, breasts are for sexual display, for titillation. They should (at present) be firm

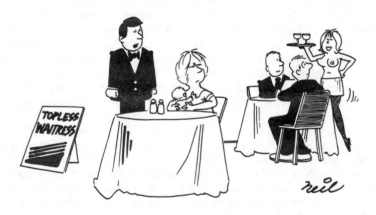

"I'm sorry madam, we don't allow breastfeeding in here."

Figure 2.1 Courtesy of Neil Matterson, from *Is He Biting Again?* (Marion Books, 1984)

and round and high, not soft and low and milk filled. To wear a low-cut evening gown indicates that one is not a prude; to slip a strap aside and to attach a baby, thus covering up a great deal of cleavage, is to shock one's friends. Many women are not able to feed in public at all: one Greek woman wept as she told me how she loved feeding her baby but was only permitted to do so in her bedroom, so she put him on a bottle and he failed to thrive. This sense of modesty, whether natural or culturally induced, means that for women in our society to function there must be reasonably private feeding-rooms provided in public places. Such facilities are scarce, despite NMAA's campaign, so those unable to steel themselves to public feeding must stay home. Rita Whitehead's victory in having the Victorian Equal Opportunities Board rule that she had been discriminated against when a hotelier allegedly abused her and refused her service because she was discreetly breastfeeding, was something of a landmark, although in 1998 the Equal Opportunity Tribunal is having to print posters to inform women that they do indeed have the right to breastfeed in public, after boorish incidents led to ignorant comment from political and community leaders. And what message is conveyed when, at major airports, one sees the sign 'Nursing Mothers' accompanied by a graphic bottle?

Here I would like to enter a strong plea for less emphasis on 'discreet' public feeding. It is not that I want to see every mother baring her bosom to all and sundry, and certainly it is useful for the new and shy mother to know ways of clothing herself so that she is not too obvious when she feeds in public. But that initial sense of embarrassment quickly passes if the mother is feeding flexibly, in response to her baby's needs. Only other people perpetuate it, by their reactions or by their moralising about all public feeding having to be discreet. It was with a sense of shock sometimes that I realised that I was feeding at all, in the middle of an engrossing conversation. (What better way to keep the baby happy so that conversation could continue?) And my awareness that I was feeding usually was prompted by someone else's surprise, approval or disapproval. Such unselfconscious feeding is practiced around the world, wherever cultural hang-ups do not include crazy attitudes to breasts. It seems to me, though, that we acquiesce in that craziness by telling mothers to feed discreetly. Let them feed as they feel comfortable doing. If some bare skin is showing, so what? Hasn't anyone noticed what non-lactating women wear in our society? We will only break down the mindless prejudice against public breastfeeding if enough women do it for it to lose its novelty and shock value.[68] People must be desensitised to the sight of babies at breasts. People who sell special nursing shawls and garments designed to shield onlookers from the appalling prospect of a mother baring her breast to her child really need to think about whether they are part of the problem. Women must be more assertive and refuse to accept that their very basic need to be able to feed their children wherever and whenever the children need feeding should be circumscribed by the neurotic attitudes of others. Those who object are the ones with problems. Let them sort out their problems, not foist them upon others. I refuse to accept that breastfeeding is the sort of activity that properly belongs in the privacy of one's home. There is no analogy with sexual behaviour of other kinds – what society around the world accepts intercourse as a proper subject for public display, yet controls public breastfeeding?

Only bits of 20th century western culture. Most human societies recognise that breast-feeding belongs wherever women belong. Anything less is blatant discrimination.

There is, of course, no need for a woman to be exposed during public feeding; nor am I advocating that most women should blithely bare all. But the present negative attitudes to public feeding do discourage many women, or so restrict their lives that they give up feeding, as the Greek woman mentioned above did. Therefore those of you who don't mind where you feed, and who are not bothered by criticism, go right ahead – with my thanks for your role in liberating other women from such nastiness. As Donelda Ellis rightly said, "Such role modelling of breastfeeding must increase if society's nurturing of feelings of embarrassment, guilt, shame or disgust is to be remedied." Be prepared to reason with the objectors. One of my strongest supporters used to be just such an outraged critic. In the face of my determined rejection of his forcefully expressed outrage and arguments, he thought things through, realised that his responses were simply reflexive, and changed his attitude. Had I given in, he would probably felt confirmed in the rightness of his views.

In some situations, consideration for the feelings of others is reasonable. There is no point in shocking older and less-permissive generations, or cultural groups with different norms of behaviour. Such insensitivity won't win any allies. There are issues of judgement involved in each situation. But sometimes you will receive a pleasant surprise. Once, feeding in a restaurant, I tried to be as inconspicuous as possible to avoid offending an elderly lady at the next table who seemed to be staring at me in disapproval. As she left, she came over to say how pleased she was to see a baby where it belonged – that there was no more beautiful sight in the world! So don't assume that if you are being observed, it is with disapproving eyes. And if you see another mother breastfeeding in public, murmur some encouragement and stop and tell her what that old lady told me. It altered my sense of paranoia to one of pride, and it made my day.

It is artificial feeding that has made public breastfeeding an option rather than an automatic, unnoticed, unremarkable necessity. Our expectations of infant behaviour, too, have been shaped by the bottle, with its "alternating periods of starvation and over-feeding".[69] Born out of the practical needs of 18th-century orphanages, regimes of regular feeding have flourished, so that a baby is 'good' only if it spends most of its time asleep, and feeds at predictable intervals. No matter that we don't function like that, nor do any other animals – babies 'should'. Community ignorance of the normal behaviour of healthy infants creates many needless pressures for new mothers, which only peer-group support and education can dispel. Any breastfeeding promotion campaign which doesn't educate all ages, teenagers to grandmothers, runs the risk of failure or even of fostering a backlash against breastfeeding.

Then there is the cult of fitness and body consciousness. Instead of accepting the bodily changes of pregnancy as normal[70] we retain an idealised image of the non-mature female shape and strive desperately to regain a 26-inch waist within weeks of childbirth. Obstetricians talk about women getting 'back to normal', implying that the appropriate norm for postpartum women is the childless or child-free state, when a new 'normal' is now inevitable. I've known women lose their milk entirely by a combination of drastic diet and exercise. No western woman wants to be really fat, even if one's homeostatic regulators seem to be bent on retaining a prudent surplus. But there are more important considerations than fitting our present unrealistic cultural stereotypes, so well exposed by Greer's comment that "Only in consumer society is the famished female type admired, partly because it is so rare." (Is that why? Are we constantly being manipulated and made to feel inadequate by fashion arbiters whose images are chosen *because* we do not fit them?) Community support groups can serve a positive function simply by bringing together women after childbirth, because in the company of other less-than-'perfect' bodies one feels rather more comfortable than when dealing with the svelte well-groomed career woman. And it is therapeutic to acknowledge one's sense of loss in finding that child-bearing can mean haemorrhoids, stretch marks, painful stitches, stretched ligaments, altered bowel and bladder habits, sciatica, flab, and a host of other minor but depressing realities.[71] Time and hard work may cure some of those ills, but no one enjoys living with them in the present. The woman who accepts them realistically has more chance of continuing to breastfeed physiologically – that is, ad libitum and exclusively for the first five or six months.

Many sensible women quite naturally dislike the experience of breastfeeding because it's painful. I would repeat, emphatically, that feeding should never hurt the mother; as Gunther has said, when it does the basic cause must be found and remedied. There are many and varied practical problems involved in successful breastfeeding. Here I do not wish to discuss them in detail; they are the basis of some subsequent chapters.

Because of our society's distorted sexual fantasies and experiences, some women have profound problems coping with the intimate body contact in breastfeeding. So do some men, watching.[72] While difficulties with intercourse (not uncommon) are seen as reason for professional counselling and help, such an aversion to breastfeeding is not. Yet one could argue that breastfeeding is more important to an infant than intercourse is to a man – I've yet to hear of a man dying for want of coitus with his partner, but death from want of breast-milk[73] is not uncommon. When will we see people with an aversion to breastfeeding being given the special help they need? Not before society acknowledges that it is psychiatrically pathological to be irrationally averse to suckling one's child. Understandable, perhaps; not culpable, certainly; but pathological all the same. Treatment should be given as much for the mother's own sake as the baby's, as it is unlikely that such an aversion does not have its basis in, or consequences for, other areas of the woman's psychosexual functioning. Breastfeeding well-managed can even be therapeutic, a non-threatening way of learning to feel confidence and pleasure in one's own body and a heightening of sensitivity. But up to now, such psychiatric problems have been characterised by extremely poor management, with the bottle as a constant fall-back measure. The availability and 'normality' of bottle-feeding remains the greatest disincentive to any realistic attempts to investigate and solve breastfeeding problems. Why be so 'extreme' as to persevere in the face of difficulties? Both mothers and doctors are often afraid of being thought extreme. Women can suppress very strong feelings about weaning rather than have someone suspect them of social deviance. Is it deviant to enjoy the sensuousness of breastfeeding, to feel grief at the prospect of unexpected weaning, and to be sure that one's own imperfect body can do better than scientists when it comes to feeding babies? So we women sit there quietly when told to wean because of a nipple or breast problem, then go away and agonise over what to do, feeling guilty about whatever decision we make.

Then there are all the other obstacles to continued breastfeeding: physical fatigue in the absence of adequate support networks, coupled with the erroneous belief that it is breastfeeding (not caring for a baby) which is tiring; the many conflicting demands modern women experience; poor nutrition; the isolation of women in many suburbs[74] with physical obstacles that can make taking a baby when shopping almost as difficult as getting around in a wheelchair,[75] the pressure this constant difficulty creates to find a job and childcare so as not to lose totally the sense of oneself as a competent adult;[76] the lack of adequate maternity leave and provision for breastfed babies in the work place,[77] constant pro-bottle propaganda through the visual media and even through books that children bring home from school. Financial difficulties compound these problems, as does a lack of education and assertiveness to find the necessary help. Needless to say, male attitudes and beliefs have a strong influence, too: women are socially conditioned to give the conjugal bond precedence over the maternal bond(s),[69] and if a man dislikes the idea of his partner breastfeeding the baby, she will often defer to his wishes.

And there is the cultural mythology that babies can be 'spoilt' by too much affection and attention; that they must learn 'who's boss', and learn to 'fit in', or run the risk of being maladjusted adults.[78] This is the antithesis of the flexible interpersonal responsiveness that characterises a successful human/breastfeeding relationship, and the profound absorption and delight in the child that can develop when things are going well and the baby provides positive feedback to the parents. People who would never dream of criticising a hairstyle seem to feel free to tell new parents that they are ruining their infant's character by not letting him or her cry for long. Parents are constantly stressed by the conflict between what they are told from various sources, and what their own instincts and reason suggest – which may also be at variance if the parents have not resolved problems from their own childhoods. All such stresses make breastfeeding more difficult. Indeed, considering the postnatal problems, the fact that so many succeed so well at both parenting and breastfeeding can be seen as a tribute to the capacity to cope built into the human species!

All of this implies two things:

- *Many women do require postnatal support for breastfeeding to continue;*
- *National campaigns to promote breastfeeding serve no useful purpose unless they are integrated campaigns, which alter the medical, social, cultural and economic realities which truly discourage breastfeeding.*

So what type of support system would be best promote breastfeeding? A variety of models exist around the world. The more I considered the question, the more I realised that we need to examine these models and evaluate their effectiveness and relevance for Australia. We should not continue as we are, haphazardly, with no long-range planning, whatever the virtues of the systems we have inherited. And I believe that our (now shrinking) system of well-baby clinics has many merits which are being lost in the name of economic rationalism.

One choice is between a separate support system and one integrated with the hospital at which the mother delivered her baby. Many hospitals are aware of the need for some kind of continuity of care. Some hospitals not only provide the standard referral to the Infant Welfare Sister, who will then visit within a few days of the mother's discharge, but also have a team of home visiting nurses, who call within 48 hours of the mother's return home. That, however, is the end of their services unless the mother requires social welfare-type assistance (which is discreetly assessed during pregnancy and at this home visit). There is no further link with these nurses – who are strangers, never before seen by the mother in hospital – so their value is fairly limited as far as breastfeeding is concerned.

More elaborate systems exist. Some hospitals have set up breastfeeding clinics, which serve as teaching centres for professionals as well as providing a comprehensive service for parents. The mother may be seen in pregnancy; during her hospital stay she is helped by staff who have taught rational management procedures and skills at the clinic; and after discharge she has access to 24-hour telephone advice, with regular check-ups at six weeks or more frequently if she needs help. The attitude conveyed by these clinics is very important: it is that while breastfeeding is natural, it is not always easy; that problems do exist but can be overcome by common sense and skilled help; that weaning is not the solution to problems of breastfeeding (indeed, it may be the cause of more serious problems). Because these clinics concentrate on breastfeeding, they are developing a detailed awareness of breastfeeding problems and solutions, which has thus far been almost totally lacking in Western medicine. Until we have a clinic focussed on the actual management of breastfeeding problems, the standard of professional advice will remain poor. This is a matter of basic knowledge, but no one is likely to learn until he or she is aware that there is something to be learnt. When both professional and lay groups keep talking as though we know all we need to know about the management of breastfeeding, progress is impossible. Any random selection of mothers will contain women with problems that do not respond readily to the usual glib generalities. So lactation clinics would help mothers with special needs, train professionals and generally raise the community's awareness of breastfeeding as a specialised subject and as a reputable academic research area. And once there are career possibilities in such research, it can be expected to flourish as other arguably less-important specialities have done. By providing qualified professionals to be integrated into hospital structures as the 'specialist' in breastfeeding, one could reduce the confused and confusing medley of advice still given to new mothers by people who consider that they know as much about breastfeeding as anyone else.

There are dangers in establishing such a specialised clinic with medical/ scientific staffing. The temptation to claim new empires, by going even further into more rarefied and esoteric details, making the management of lactation something only 'experts' can handle, would have to be resisted. A lactation clinic could become the centre for increasing experimentation with hormones and drugs, rather than remaining solidly based on modest, preventive, community health lines. While being convinced of the need to help mothers breastfeed, we must also be prepared to accept that some mothers will not be able to. I would hate to see breastfeeding research going to the expensive technological extremes that infertility research has done, overlooking or ignoring relevant but less spectacular social, nutritional and environmental avenues of research. If we reach the point where most mothers are breastfeeding successfully and enjoying it, the minority may feel cheated if they are physiologically incapable of breastfeeding. Will our society then provide alternative sources of human milk, and help for the mother – or will the mother demand as her 'right' incredibly expensive interventions to enable her to do it herself? Breastfeeding clinics must not become another bastion for the technocrats. The selection of personnel and the involvement of critical lay counsellors would be the key issues in establishing such a centre.

In the last few years many Australian hospitals have begun to offer clinically-based breastfeeding day-stay centres, of the kind I am referring to here, but without the finance or detailed technical assistance that would allow research to be done. One promising example of the sort of mutual collaboration which I had in mind in 1984 is New Zealand's Cry-SOS clinics.[79] Begun by academics, based in a university department, they combined a substantial educational programme with realistic parental consultation and continued academic scrutiny. A really professional breastfeeding clinic could develop along similar lines. And it seems Western Australia could be the first state to set up such a clinic. Dr. Peter Hartmann has recently secured funding to develop a clinic which will utilise scientific research methods as well as basic breastfeeding knowledge to assist women.

A third variety of care integrated with hospitals has been provided by UK research teams who recruited mothers for study while in hospital, then continued to visit them fortnightly after discharge.[80] In Britain, the regular pattern of postnatal care is referral to the local area health authority which provides clinics and health visitors (who go to people's homes more often than here in Australia) and in some areas community midwives. Attendance at clinics is voluntary, and patchy as here in Australia. The health visitor is welcomed by those who are not threatened by her often-unconscious middle-class values; she is sometimes evaded by those who are threatened or who feel her sudden unannounced arrival leaves them at a colossal disadvantage. (Personally, I'd hate to have an official visitor turn up just as I was yelling at the kids and the house was a shambles. If she were a maiden lady, I'd feel that she could never understand, because I didn't until I had my own children. Mind you, she might well understand, seeing so many other mothers, but the new mother finds that hard to believe.) By contrast, the researchers who visited mothers did so at regular intervals, by appointment, and were available by phone during the day, at least. They were well informed, but their information may have mattered less than their presence, with its implicit medical approval of continued breastfeeding. They were predictable; they came to the house; a mother with doubts could air her questions at a specific time in an unofficial and non-judgmental forum, to someone without any coercive powers. Does this suggest that a pattern of regular home visiting could be helpful to at-risk mothers, especially in the first few months of establishing lactation? Does it say something about who should visit? I agree with those who argue strongly for such a system, which new mothers particularly would benefit from. This could readily be integrated into existing Australian patterns, but would cost more than the pittance presently provided for postnatatal care.

Separate systems of breastfeeding support have been alluded to. Here in Australia, the nationalistic and racist concerns of the early twentieth century, and the worsening rates of maternal and child morbidity and mortality, led to the establishment of infant welfare clinics, later named maternal and child health centres. These are staffed by triple-certificated nurses, and theoretically are subject to the authority of the State Health Department, but they are also partly run by local government which employs the nurse. This can lead to enormous variations in the role and scope of the infant welfare clinic. One, in an area where the council is more aware, may serve all sorts of community health functions, providing social groups for new mothers, educational lectures, and a local 'drop-in centre'. Another may seem like an old-style hospital, with rigid emphasis on doing it by the (always outdated) book. Mothers may be so terrified of the sister's opinions that they lie to her, telling her what she wants to hear rather than what is actually happening. In such places (which I would like to believe are rare), the support value of the clinic is zero. It would seem like a good idea for such systems to build in a mechanism for reporting anomalies. Of course, no system is perfect, because no group of people ever are, and it must be conceded that health departments do make efforts to keep clinic sisters fully up to date. But I am not aware that governments consult parents on such issues, and parents rarely volunteer this information except to one another. Until these services are more responsive to the needs of the consumer, they will not realise their full potential for community education and development – including breastfeeding support and education, but much more besides. In 1983 I hoped to see this grassroots development burgeoning as the basic unit of community infant health care, dealing with the usual problems and concerns, but with the backing of a professional referral centre, the specialised breastfeeding clinic, for dealing with the difficult cases. In 1998 I am distressed to report that slash and burn economic vandalism and doctrinaire free-market policies are making this system much less available to mothers on their own terms. The most valuable aspect of the clinics, the fact that mothers themselves determined when and how often they went, has already been lost in many municipalities.

Such a system of infant health clinics, supported by government funds, never existed in America. There the paediatrician gained control of the healthy baby very early in the century, largely due to his control of formula feeding – an unrealised liaison which has probably coloured American paediatrics ever since.[81] It is paediatricians and doctors who have been the architects of the re-shaping of the MCH service in Victoria: it is not surprising that such persons also gave talks on the opportunities this re-shaping would provide for doctors. As of course it has: many mothers are now seeing doctors over issues they would once have asked the MCH nurse about. This is not a gain: the specialised MCH nurse usually has vastly more knowledge about normal babies than most generalist medical practitioners could ever have, and most MCH nurses and midwives have been educating themselves further about infant feeding, aware of their need to know. Doctors in Australia have almost no education about infant feeding, and are heavily reliant on the infant formula companies for information and, of course, free samples and supplies. It is obvious in 1998 that companies are targetting doctors more than ever and providing them with materials and samples that are now supported by advertising: in Mead Johnson's case., even television advertising which carefully avoids naming the product (so as to be able to claim not to advertise formula) but tells parents that there is a new option (not "treatment") for reflux (i.e., their new formula) which their (white-coated male) doctor or some (white-coated female) non-doctor health professional can provide. Medical ignorance about the clinical management of breastfeeding is not exposed once the child is on the bottle: the sicknesses the child then has are all "normal" and doctor can prescribe and treat as usual. Once again industry pushes Australia down the American path to illness. The community pays more for this shift to doctor care, but it shifts costs from state and local government to the commonwealth.

At present there is a growing awareness of past inadequacies of paediatricians in relation to breastfeeding. This has led to a renewed interest in the subject by doctors, and La Leche League International's seminars on breastfeeding for physicians are an apt response to that interest. It has also led to the emergence of a new group of breastfeeding consultants,[82] usually nurses who have breastfed children, who have set up private-enterprise clinics. (The nurse-practitioner is better accepted in the US than here, perhaps partly because of the high cost of an unequal access to medical care.) Major clinics include Dr. Audrey Naylor's in San Diego, the Lactation Institute and Kittie Frantz's UCLA clinic in Los Angeles, both attached to university programmes. Other lactation consultants work in conjunction with obstetricians and paediatricians. And academic programmes in universities, to train nurses and child health workers, are also beginning. Obviously such programmes will be cost effective if they help mothers to breastfeed longer, and they are being developed in some US county hospitals serving poor populations. But these are only very small beginnings, despite the active support of the U.S. Surgeon General for such proposals.[83]

The major burden of providing support for breastfeeding mothers continues to fall on the informal networks of family, neighbours and friends, and the numerous self-help parent groups which have become a feature of Western society. These are mainly feminine networks, and most have not benefited from substantial education about infant and maternal health and diet; some (rare) doctors actually argue that such education is undesirable or useless. On the whole it would seem that such networks, particularly the organised ones, are the natural avenue for increased community health education and participation. International health agencies have done a great deal to promote this idea. The advantages are obvious: making use of a volunteer network reduces costs and in some ways increases market penetration. Help is close by when needed, in a way that paid professionals cannot hope to match, and in a language other mothers can comprehend.

But there are hazards.[84] The unpaid volunteer is a creature of her own time and place. She may be totally unable to relate well to mothers who do not share her background and its inbuilt assumptions. She may convey many negative attitudes and much inadequate, even inaccurate, information, because it is unrealistic to expect volunteers to have up-to-the-minute knowledge. This would not matter so much if the volunteer frankly acknowledged the limits of her information, but many voluntary groups, having created some form of education system, then operate as though that knowledge were definitive, normative for everybody – when, as I have earlier said, breastfeeding is a highly individual process, and there may be good reasons why the rules are not working (other than the insulting assertion that "the mother can't really have wanted to breastfeed"). Clearly, volunteer networks need close liaison with interested and caring professionals, particularly those engaged in research. And if such groups are to bear the burden of promoting breastfeeding, it is reasonable to expect that they will be funded by health authorities or other agencies. I am tired of hearing voluntary groups criticised for not being as fully professional as highly paid and educated people who do not hold down two major jobs! I consider that NMAA Counsellors should be paid, in fact.

It seems almost frivolous to discuss the details of various types of postnatal support when decision-makers do not consider any such support a priority. I'd therefore like to ask you why you think health authorities are so slow to meet this obvious need, and what you think can be done about it. Jenny Phillips' *Mothers Matter Too*, Penelope Leach's *Who Cares?*, and Joyce Nicholson's *The Heartache of Motherhood*, make concrete suggestions and plead for saner social policies on mothering. The issue is a complex one. To help support breastfeeding mothers is to opt for a social organisation that makes ad libitum breastfeeding possible, and this involves a great many changes, large and small, physical, psychological and political. Anyone concerned to promote breastfeeding is inevitably involved in politics. One cannot stand aloof. To sign a petition may be 'political'. Not to sign it is also political, and can be interpreted as meaning that you oppose it, when you may in fact agree but simply not want to be 'political'. In a democracy the key to change is political pressure, and those who don't play that game can only lose.

If government departments or voluntary groups confine themselves to informing mothers about breastfeeding but do nothing about changing hospital practices, solving breastfeeding problems or providing postnatal support, and so on, they condemn mothers to failure with the added burden of knowledge that substitutes are inferior, which makes women feel worse. If women are to continue to be condemned to breastfeeding failure by social policies and practices beyond their control, at least they should be told that these are the reason for their failure. Justified anger is preferable to undeserved guilt and inadequacy, if one is concerned about mental health.

To summarise all the foregoing: Obviously there are dozens of reasons why women who would like to breastfeed are instead giving formulae and solids to their babies. It is important in each particular case to know what those reasons were. From a practical point of view, this enables steps to be taken to ensure that the woman's next attempt does not fail for the same reasons. And from a psychological point of view, it ensures that she does not blame herself for what is not her fault. Such self-blame can have a profound effect on the individual's perception of herself, as well as her relationship with her children, and thus is a concern for all of us attempting to create a healthier, saner society.[85]

Appendices

The knickers bra

1. Purchase 2 pairs of large (size 20+) female full cotton briefs and half-a-dozen or more large safety pins.
2. Fold each brief down the middle, so that you can put your hand through both leg holes at once.
3. Sit the briefs side by side with the holes at the top.
4. Pin them together. This forms the central back seam of a vest-like garment.
5. Put your arms through the legholes, pull the unpinned edges to the front and pin them in a position which is comfortable and supportive, adjusting front and back as necessary. If needed, thermal packs or cabbage leaves can be inserted – cabbage against the skin, cold/warm packs between the two layers of material.

Figure 2.2 Making a knickers bra

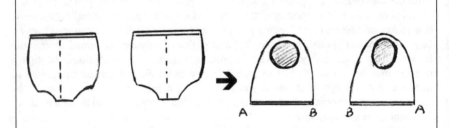

Fold the knickers so that the leg holes are next to each other, and place the two pairs side by side.

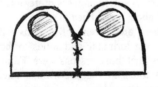

Attach them along one edge.

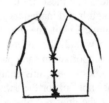

Put your arms through the holes and pin the knickers together at the front.

Teaching the young

What do dolls teach our children about reproduction and breastfeeding? Very negative and inaccurate things, indeed. That sort of propaganda is built into children's play from the time they are tiny. Let's counterbalance it a bit with some physiological learning about babies, bodies and breasts.

First of all, make your own breastfeeding doll. Here you will see how to adapt any cloth-bodied doll for older children who can handle press-studs: simply sew two studs to the doll's front, and find smaller dolls whose mouths can clip onto these 'nipples'. The idea, I might add, was my daughter Elizabeth's in 1982, just before she was three. The usual bottles and dolls were about, and she was playing near me, so I said abstractedly, "Why don't you give dolly a bottle?" She looked at me as if I were half-witted, and said, "Because bottles aren't good for babies, Mum. They need boobies." For her third birthday she got this.

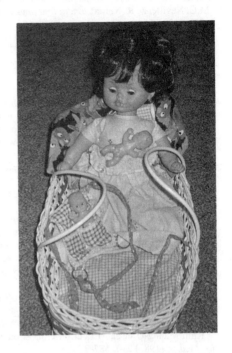

Figure 2.3 A breastfeeding doll

NOTES

CHAPTER 2: WHO IS RESPONSIBLE FOR BREASTFEEDING FAILURE?

[1] Some national and international campaigns are described in S. Freir, A. Eidelman, *Human Milk, its Biological and Social Value* (Excerpt Medica, 1980). (The two year Canadian programme (first year aimed at educating health professionals, second year the public), is described in A.S. Myres, *J. Can. Ass.* (April 1981) 42: 2; 130-141.

[2] American Academy of Pediatrics, Committee on Nutrition: Breast-Feeding. *Pediatrics* (1978) 62: 4; 591-601.

[3] cf. The National Childbirth Trust (U.K.) magazine, *New Generation*, (1983) 2: 2; 36-37.

[4] cf. Cunningham, A. S., "Breastfeeding and morbidity in industrialised countries: an update", in D. Jelliffe, E. S. P. Jelliffe, *Advances in International Maternal and Child Health*, v. i. (Oxford University Press, 1981), and Chapter 1 of this book.

[5] cf. M. Minchin *Food for Thought: a parent's guide to food intolerance* (George Allen & Unwin, Sydney, 1985).

[6] ibid. See also P. Fried, *Pregnancy and Lifestyle Habits* (Beaufort Books, N.Y. 1983), ch. 5.

[7] J.T. Wilson, *Drugs in Breast Milk* (ADIS Press Australasia, Balgowlah, 1981) p. 84. J. Goldfarb, E. Tibbetts, *Breastfeeding Handbook* (Enslow Publishers, 1980) p. 89.

[8] M.C. Neville, M.R. Neifert, *Lactation: physiology, nutrition, and breastfeeding* (Plenum Press, 1983), p. 285-6.

[9] P. de Chateau, B. Wiberg, "Long-term effect on mother-infant behaviour of extra contact in the first hour postpartum", *Acta Paed. Scand.* (1977) 66: 145-51. See also R. Saadeh, J. Akré, "Ten steps to successful breastfeeding: a summary of the rationale and scientific evidence", *Birth* (1996) 23: 154-60.

[10] R. S. Illingworth, *Lancet* (1952) i, 683.

[11] M. J. Houston, "Breastfeeding", *Nursing Mirror*, 1983. Feb 9, (Supplement). 80% of mothers allowed to feed flexibly were still feeding at 6 weeks, whereas only 57% of mothers who had begun with restricted feed times were still feeding at 6 weeks. *Lancet* (1981) i, 392-3.

[12] Howie, P. M., Houston, M. J. et al, "How long should a breast feed last?" *Early Human Development* (1981) 5, 71-77.

[13] Ellis, D. J., "Needs of the breastfeeding dyad: how nurses can assist", *Austr. J. Adv. Nursing,* 1983, 1, (1), 40.

[14] Salariya, E. M. et al, "Duration of breastfeeding after early initiation and frequent feeding", *Lancet* (1978) ii, 1141-3.

[15] Jelliffe & Jelliffe, *Human Milk in the Modern World.* (O. U. P. 1979) ch. 3.

[16] Cruse, P., Yudkin, P. & Baum, J. D., "Establishing demand feeding in hospital", *Arch. Dis. Child.* 76-78. cf. Fisher, C., "Mythology in Midwifery – or 'Making Breastfeeding Scientific and Exact'", *Midwives Chronicle*, May 1982, for the origins and illogic of such practices.

[17] Collinge, J. M. et al, "Demand vs scheduled feedings for premature infants", *J.O.G.N. Nursing* (1982) ii, 1141-3.

[18] Potts, M. et al. (ed.) "Breastfeeding and fertility", *J. Biosoc. Sci.* (1985) Supplement 9.

[19] M.J. Houston et al, "Factors affecting the duration of breastfeeding: Measurement of breastmilk intake in the first year of life", *Early Hum. Dev.* (1983) 8: 49-54.

[20] Khin-Maung-U et al, "Effect on clinical outcome of breastfeeding during acute diarrhoea", *Br. Med. J.* (1985) 290: 587-9.

[21] Lawrence, R., *Breastfeeding, a guide for the medical profession.* (C. V. Mosby & Co., 1980) p. 176. See also Houston, M. J. et al., "The effect of extra fluid intake by breastfed babies in hospital on the duration of breastfeeding", *J. Reprod. Infant. Psych.* (1984) i, 42-48, for a general discussion of the effects of fluid intake in a U. K. situation.

[22] de Carvalho, M. et al., "Effects of water supplementation on jaundice in breastfed infants", *Arch. Dis. Child,* (1981) 56, (7), 568-9.

[23] The new link between bottlefeeding and childhood diabetes might give further food for thought – cf. K. Sikaris, "The association of diabetes and infant feeding method" (review), *ALCA News* (Dec. 1997) 8: 3; 11-13. See also A.L. Drash, M.S. Kramer, J. Swanson, J.N. Udall, "Infant feeding practices and their possible relationship to the etiology of diabetes mellitus", *Pediatrics* (1994) 95: 752-4.

[24] Herram, A. J., "Supplemented versus unsupplemented breastfeeding", *P-N* 1984, May, June, p. 70-71.

[25] Articles by Bullen and Soothill in Wilkinson, A. W. (ed.), *The Immunology of Infant Feeding*, Plenum Press, N.Y. 1981

[26] This whole area is comprehensively reviewed in Minchin, *Food for thought*, op. cit. That sensitisation may occur during the vulnerable neonatal immunodeficient state is acknowledged in the Joint Report of the Royal College of Physicians/British Nutrition Foundation, Food Intolerance and Food Aversion. (*J. Roy. Coll. Physicians of London*), 1984, 18 (2) p. 13.

[27] Lawrence, op. cit., p. 64.

[28] World Health Organisation, *International Code on the Marketing of Breastmilk Substitutes*, (1981); see further ch. 10.

[29] Ellis D. J., "Needs of the breastfeeding dyad: how nurses can assist", *Aust. J. Adv. Nursing*, (1983) i, (1), 39.

[30] Ikonen, R.S. et al, "Bacteriological quality control in a human milk bank", *Klin. Pediatr.* (1982) 194 (5) 295-7.

[31] Clavano, N., "The results of a change in hospital practices", *Assignment Children* (UNICEF) (1981) 55/56, 139-65.

[32] Baum, J.D., Fisher, C. et al. *A Guide to Human Milk Banking* (Oxford 1980). Available from Vickers Medical Publications, Basingstoke, Hampshire, RG249NP, England.

[33] Helsing, E., & King, F. S., *Breastfeeding in practice: a manual for health workers*. (O.J.P. 1982) p. 46.

[34] cf. Avery, J. L. & Fleiss, P. M., *Induced Lactation* (available from NMAA or from 80206. U. S. A.). See also *Pediatrics* (1980) 65: 2; 236-242. Supplyline, the NMAA version of a milk supplementing device, is available very cheaply; see p. 366. Do-it-yourself supplementers are illustrated in *New Generation*, (1983) 2, (3), p. 17. Of course any supplement, given by bottle, spoon or dropper, will interfere equally with milk production – cf. Illingworth, R. S., Barlow, J., Complementary feeds – by spoon or bottle? *Arch. Dis. Child*, (1954) 29, 422-3. Supplyline at least supplies breast stimulation.

[35] Lawrence, op. cit., p. 122. In 1958, in "A cineradiographic study of breastfeeding", *Brit. J. Radiol.*, xxxi, 363, 156-162, Ardan condemned such pumps as inefficient and potentially dangerous. Milk is not extracted by suction - cf. p. 99.

[36] Liebhaber, M. et al, "Comparison of bacterial contamination with two methods of human milk collection", *J. Pediatr.*, (1978) 92, 236.

[37] A number of excellent models are now available. In Australia, consult NMAA.

[38] cf. Bourne, M. A., "Sleep and the Newborn", in *NCT News*, 1983,2,2, p. 16-17.

[39] Talk by Dr Masao Takeuchi, "Effect of low calorie diet on quality/quantity of breast milk", at the LLLI Physicians Seminar, 1983. (Available from LLLI, p. 331.)

[40] Whitfield, M.F. et. al, "Validity of routine test weighing as a measure of intake of breastfed infants", *Arch. Dis. Child.*, (1981) 56, 12, 919-911. Houston, M. J. et. al., "Factors affecting the duration of breastfeeding: Measurement of breast milk intake in the first week of life", *Early Hum. Dev.*, (1983) 8, 49-54. Although accurate electronic scales provide a good estimate of intake, test weighing was not advocated as a routine because it creates anxiety.

[41] Friis-Hansen, B., "Water – the major nutrient", *Acta. Paed. Scand.* (Suppl), 1982, 299, 11-6.

[42] Both because of the weaning unnecessarily prescribed, the poor management of lactation accompanying temporary interruptions, and perhaps even because of the brief separation of mother and child. cf. Elander, G., Linberg, T., "Short mother-infant separation during the first week of life influences the durations of breastfeeding", *Acta Paed. Scand.*, (1984) 73, 237-240.

[43] For good discussions of this, cf. Lauwers & Woessner, op. cit., p. 301-9. see also Cogan, R. and Hinz, "The Etiology of "Physiological" Neonatal Jaundice: The role of Interventions", *ICEA Review*, (1983) 7, 1. An excellent discussion paper loooking at evidence connecting induction, intravenous hydration, epidurals, and early feeding.

[44] de. Carvalho, M. et al, "Frequency of breastfeeding and serum bilirubin concentration", *Am. J. Dis. Child*, (1982) 136, (8), 737-8.

[45] Articles on relationship between passage of meconium (stimulated by colostrum, delayed by other feeds) and jaundice are abstracted in Cogan, R. and Hinz., op. cit.

[46] Drew, J. H., "Infant Feeding and Jaundice", *Keeping Abreast, Journal of Human Nurturing*, 1978, Jan, March, pp. 53-7.

[47] Guthrie, R. A., "Breast milk and jaundice", ibid., pp. 47-53. As far back as 1978, this medical school taught that in the rare cases of true breastmilk jaundice, interrupting breastfeeding for just 12-24 hours a week was enough to keep bilirubin at a safe level. Of course this pre-dated work on exclusive, frequent, breastfeeding from birth.

[48] A detailed review of the scientific literature and wide-ranging discussion on this subject can be found on the tape of the 1984 LLLI Physicians' Seminar talk by Dr. Lawrence Gartner. See also Gartner, L.M., "Neonatal jaundice" (review), *Pediatr. Rev.* (1994) 15: 422-432; Gartner, L.M., "On the question of the relationship between breastfeeding and jaundice in the first five days of life" (review) *Semin. Perinatol.* (1994) 18: 502-9; A. Nicoll, et al, "Supplementary feeding and jaundice in newborns", *Acta Paed. Scand.*, 1982, 71, (5), 759-761; Kuhr, M; Paeth, N., "Feeding practices and early neonatal jaundice", *J. Pediatr. Gastroenterol. Nutr.*, (1982) 1: 4; 485-8.

[49] Gunther, M., *Infant Feeding*, (Methuen, 1970), p. 80

[50] Applebaum, R.M., "The modern management of successful breastfeeding", *Ped. Clin. N. Am.*, (1977) 24, (1), 37-47.

[51] Mirkin, B.L. (ed), *Perinatal Pharmacology and Therapeutics*, (Academic Press, N.Y. 1976)

[52] Morris, M.B. et al, Caffeine and the fetus: is trouble brewing? *Am. J. Obstet. Gynecol.* 1981, 140,6; *Br. Med. J.* 1981, 282, 1474

[53] *Br. Med. J.* 1981, 282, 1474.

[54] Fully documented in Minchin, op cit., where I discuss the hazards of smoking for babies and their families; see also Lyon, J., "Effects of smoking on breastfeeding", *Arch. Dis. Child.* (1983) 58, 224-6.

[55] M.K. Minchin, "Smoking and breastfeeding: an overview", *J. Hum. Lact.* (1991) 7: 183-8.

[56] Applebaum, op. cit., p. 218. For a good discussion of engorgement, see Neifert. M.R., "Routine Management of Breastfeeding" in Neville, M.C.& Neifert, M.R. op. cit., p. 283-4

[57] Brooten, D.A. et al, "A comparison of four treatments to prevent and control pain and engorgement in non-nursing mothers", *Nurs. Res.* (1983) 32, 4, 225-9.

[58] Discussed and documented in Minchin, op. cit. Since then the significance of pregnancy food-aversions and nausea in relation to infant sensitivities has been raised by U.K. researchers. cf. Baylis, J. M. et al, "Persistent nausea and food aversions in pregnancy: a possible association with cows' milk allergy in infants", *Clin. Allergy* (1983) 13, 3, 263-9.

[59] Dearlove, J.C. & B.M., "Prolactin, fluid balance and lactation:, *Br. J Obst. & Gynecol.* 1981, 88, 6, 652-4.

[60] Gunther, op.cit., p.77, 79. Vartan, C. K., "Inhibition of lactation with oestrogen", *Br. Med. J.* (1969) 1, 50.

[61] Kitzinger, S., "Stealing a woman's choice", *New Internationalist* no. 108, Feb. 1982, p. 14-15.

[62] Advisory Panel on the Marketing in Australia of Infant Formula, Annual Report 1996-7, p. 3

[63] Lumley, J., "Breastfeeding in Inner City Melbourne", talk given to NMAA Seminar, Oct. 15, 1983. (Available from NMAA, P.O.Box 231, Nunawading, 3131.)

[64] Williams, H., "Nutrition in the first year of life in a multi-ethnic poor socio-economic municipality in Melbourne", *Aust. Paed. J.* 1983. This is a universal phenomenon at present.

[65] Increasingly such hard questions must be asked. The way in which Australian supplies of essential infant formulae were disrupted in 1983 because of arbitrary price increases shows that societies may be held to ransom by commercial forces. Despite the public outcry, no effort was made to hold the companies accountable – no journalist investigated the basis for charging up to $20 for a small tin of a product now being made on a large scale. (Jelliffe (1982) reported that 'hypo-allergenic products' accounted for 20% of formula sales in 1979. cf. only a 2% a decade earlier. Sales in 1979 were worth $100 million.) Instead the government was seen as the villain, risking infant lives.

[66] The 1983/4 Australian advertising slogan for cows' milk is "Live on milk", and as usual it features semi-naked teenage breasts. Interestingly, in 1974, U.S. milk producers were forced to drop the slogan "Everybody needs milk" as charges were laid this was false, misleading, and deceptive advertising. cf. Oski, F.A., *Don't Drink Your Milk!* (Wyden Books, 1977, Mollica Press, 1983).

[67] The Maja anti-colic bottle has been widely advertised in women's magazines. It is expensive, and quite useless in those cases of colic due to the contents of the bottle (alien milks) rather than its mode of delivery. But it continues to be sold without any protests from enraged parents.

[68] Brack, D. C., "Social forces, feminism, and breastfeeding", *Nursing Outlook* (1975) 8, 556-61.

[69] Bullen C.L., & Willis A.T., "Resistance of the breastfed infant to gastroenteritis", *BMJ* 1971, 3, 338-343.

[70] cf. Greer, G., *Sex and Destiny*, (Secker & Warburg, 1984) ch. 1 for a stimulating discussion of these questions.

[71] Lennane, John & Jean, *Hard Labour* (Penguin 1979) covers some of the grimmer realities. I found this very helpful after too much saccharine positive propaganda!

[72] Kitzinger, S., *Woman's Experience of Sex* (Collins Australia, 1984), p. 225-230.

[73] Neumann, C.G., & Jelliffe, E.F.P., "Effects of Infant Feeding" in Jelliffe & Jelliffe (ed.), *Adverse Effects of Foods* (Plenum Press, 1982), cf. p. 543-50.

[74] See Phillips, J., *Mothers Matter Too* (Thomas Nelson, 1985).

[75] Leach, P., *Who Cares?* (Penguin, 1979) for a description of such obstacles.

[76] Kamerman, S., *Maternity Leaves and Benefits* (Columbia University, 1981); Clearinghouse on Maternal and Infant Nutrition, Government Legislation and Policies, on Pregnancy, Maternity and Infant Feeding, and Marketing of Breastmilk Substitutes. Report no. 1 (June 1983).

[77] UNICEF Manila have produced a neat leaflet urging employers to provide such facilities, and have had some success. It is interesting to note that since 1919 the International Labor Organisation has had a convention obliging signatories to provide such facilities, and two paid nursing breaks, for breastfeeding mothers.

[78] Cook, P.S., "Child-rearing, culture, and mental health", *Med. J. Austr.* (1978) Special supplement, August 12.

[79] Write to Dr John Kirkland, Education Department, Massey University, Palmerston North, New Zealand,for details. See also his book, *Crying and Babies – helping families cope.* (Croom Helm, 1985).

[80] Houston M. J. et al, "Do breastfeeding mothers get the home support they need?", *Health Bulletin* (1981) 39, (3), 166-172. Houston, M. J., "Breast-feeding success or failure", *J. Adv. Nursing* (1981) 6, 447-54. "Home support for the breast-feeding mother" in Houston (ed.) *Maternal and Infant Health Care* (Churchill Livingstone, 1984) ch. 3. Hart, H. et al, "Community influence on breast feeding", *Child Care Health Dev.* (1980) 6, 3, 175-87.

[81] Apple, R.D., "'To be used only under the direction of a physician.' Commercial infant feeding and medical practice,1870-1940", *Bull. Hist. Med.* 1980, 54, (3), 402-17.

[82] The professional certified Lactation Consultant Program set up in the United States. For more details, write to JoAnne Scott, 3400 Charleson St, Annandale, VA 22003. Tel. (703) 560 1039.

[83] *Report of the Surgeon General's Workshop on Breastfeeding and Human Lactation.* US Dept. of Health & Human Services, 1984.

[84] cf. Lauwers, J. & Woessner, C., op. cit., part 1. *W.H.O. Women and Breastfeeding* (Geneva 1982), p. 23. Meacher, M. *Self-help groups for parents under stress.* Available free from Mental Health Foundations, 8 Hallam Street, London, WIN6DH. England.

[85] If you find this hard to believe, read some of the accounts in Chapter 12, particularly case histories 3, 4, 7 and 10.

REASSURANCE SCIENCE CAN OFFER...
OR PERHAPS YOU FIND IT DISTURBING??

Establishing a maximal level for protein recognizes that excessive protein not only offers no advantage, but because of increased renal solute load *[and potential adverse neurological impacts due in part to high loads of neurotransmitters, rarely mentioned in public by industry]* may be deleterious. Milk-based infant formulas contain approximately 2.3g protein per 100kcal. The standard also states that the protein must have a protein-efficiency ratio (PER) at least 70% that of casein. Interestingly, the PER reflects the protein quality for a growing rat. *[Since laboratory-fed rats, along with pigs and other animals, have been used in the research which has developed many of the still-unquestioned standards in human infant nutrition.]* In PER studies with human milk, rats did not grow optimally, *[although of course infants do]* providing some doubts about the utility of PER studies for evaluation of protein for human infants.... *[Isn't that reassuring to hear?]* p.306

There is a paucity of information on the safety of foods and food additives as they occur in infant formulas. *[And we have been feeding them for a century.. Do parents know this fact, still true a decade later, is accepted without comment by scientists?]* Newborns of a species like swine, which are physiologically similar to human newborns and could be used routinely for nutritional studies from the day of birth, offer many advantages towards understanding the effects of early nutrition on growth and development in humans. *[especially on cognitive development and learning disabilities, no doubt?]* ...Because piglets grow at a faster rate than human infants *[why not use blue whales or elephants, given this logic?]* they have more stringent dietary requirements *[they need more protein to grow more lean muscle mass faster, so they can be turned into bacon more profitably, but outside Hollywood no one ever heard of a talking pig. It is just conceivable that what is optimal for a pig is disastrous for a human.]* Therefore a diet that supports healthy growth in the piglet will probably be more than adequate nutritionally for the human infant. *[And even if we were convinced by this rivetting piece of logic, is a "more than adequate diet" harmful, perhaps?..]*

Snippets from the Proceedings of the *AOAC Topical Conference on Production, Regulation and Analysis of Infant Formula*, May 1985, Virginia Beach, Virginia. (Association of Official Analytical Chemists, 1111 N. 19th St., Arlington, VA. 22208 USA) No ISBN or publisher given)

MANAGEMENT

The decline in breastfeeding and increase in the number of bottle-fed babies has influenced the educational emphasis on a method of infant feeding. This is noticeable in the nursing literature. The lack of information, and sometimes misinformation, on the part of health professionals, particularly nurses, has led to an increase in failure rate in breastfeeding mothers.

S. Solberg, in *Maternal and Infant Health Care*,
ed. M.J. Houston (Churchill Livingstone, 1984), p. 39

In the next few chapters I want to look again at some areas of practical breastfeeding management. From clinical experience, as well as from basic reasoning, I found in 1983 (and still find in 1998) a good deal to criticise in the way that many professionals manage the initiation of breastfeeding and its problems. There are honourable exceptions: many of the ideas in this section were culled from the world medical and nursing literature. Nevertheless, what amazes me is how little notice has been taken of advances in breastfeeding management. Gunther and Newton wrote on nipple problems in the 1950s, yet the vast majority of health professionals have still never heard of their findings. This is despite the growth of lactation consultancy and world-wide movements such as the WHO/UNICEF Baby Friendly Hospital Initiative.

It seems to me that neglect of breastfeeding problems reflects the male dominance of medicine and scientific research. What is simply a female problem is of little real interest because we have such good substitutes nowadays, a refrain common since the 1940s at least. Consider what might happen if the only male organ of equivalent sensitivity to the female nipple were regularly to crack and bleed, causing intense agony, during normal physiological use. Would men be advised to give up sexual activity involving their penises now that artificial means of conception, and alternative pleasure techniques, are socially acceptable? Would men be reassured that artificial substitutes for vaginal intercourse were just as good, and that their partners were not missing out on anything important? Would relationship counsellors tell men they had a low pain threshold if they complained, prescribe sunlight, fresh air and lanolin as solutions with no further enquiry, or urge men to stop searching for solutions to this agonising problem? Would solutions discovered in the 1950s be ignored for 40 years? I think not. Rather, I'd expect advances in management of such a devastating problem to be routine medical practice within months, and the original researchers to be feted world-wide.

Difficulties in breastfeeding are real problems, when millions die or are damaged for want of breast milk, and millions more are born into poverty as a result of the loss of lactational amenorrhoea, the world's most powerful contraceptive. Breastfeeding problems are objectively far more important to the world than western infertility or impotence problems, which have created vast medical empires. One might therefore expect a fully scientific approach to the solution of these problems: a scientific approach combining detailed observation with rational and cautious investigation and management. The premises of this approach would be that that difficulties exist, that solutions are possible with careful investigation, and that ignoring that problem and giving a bottle is not a solution but failure. A scientist would rarely advance unprovable and destructive hypotheses such a "tense mother" of a "difficult baby". By these criteria, not many scientists have been writing about breastfeeding.

I wrote in 1984 that "things are looking up. In the past decade there has been a substantial improvement in nursing education and the emergence of a significant group of women who combine practical skills with an ability to do valuable clinical research. Midwives, in particular, seem to be taking on responsibility and seeking to define themselves as true professionals, independent practitioners, rather than doctors' helpers. At the same time, women are ceasing to be 'patients' (what a descriptive title!) and asserting themselves as consumers. Both processes are being encouraged by many men, medical and lay, particularly those who have been involved patients themselves. So I am hopeful that the next decade will bring a great deal of change and great improvement in the management of breastfeeding." In 1998 I feel that my hopes have been partly realised with the development of the accrediting body, the International Board of Lactation Consultant Examiners, and professional associations for IBCLCs such as ALCA, the Australian Lactation Consultants Association; greater scientific interest evidenced in the growth of the International Society for Research into Human Milk and Lactation, the initiatives taken by the World Health Organisation and UNICEF, and a great growth in professional education for healthworkers. Thanks to scientists like Peter Hartmann, Malcolm Peaker and Mike Woolridge we have reliable equipment that would allow us to distinguish between the mother who cannot make more milk and the mother who can; we understand more of the complex inhibitory systems that regulate milk production; and the ultrasound studies of infant suckling I called for in 1984 have confirmed Gunther's understanding of infant suckling as accurate. Much better books are now available: *Bestfeeding: a guide for new mothers*, by Renfrew, Fisher and Arms, was the very first book for mothers in which all the pictures were accurate as well as the text; Henschel and Inch's *Breastfeeding: a guide for midwives,* and Sandra Lang's *Breastfeeding the Premature Infant* are both a quantum leap ahead of previous midwifery texts; Lawrence's pioneering text for doctors has been expanded and improved. For WHO Geneva to publish James Akre's *Infant Feeding: the Physiological Basis* was unthinkable in 1984; the book has had enormous impact where it has been circulated (but there is no money for a revision and update). Both priorities and practice still need to improve.

That improvement will not occur until we accept that we still have a lot to learn. Many practices in breastfeeding management are still wrong; we still cannot help many women. We must get rid of the language of certainty and the confidence that standard advice is enough. I read things like, "There's nothing new in dealing with these management problems. All of the suggested measures are simple. There is nothing difficult, not even contentious any more, in dealing with most of them. The answers to most breastfeeding management problems are easy, but they are not getting to everybody. The real problems are psychosomatic." When I do, I would like to scream with frustration and rage. *We do not have all the answers. In many cases, even in 1998, we are still not asking the right questions. And we certainly have not developed all the investigative techniques we need to search for the answers.* The time for psychosomatic explanations is when there is evidence to support them and all other avenues are exhausted. We are nowhere near that point.

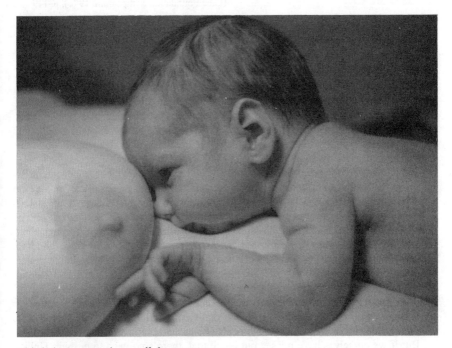

This baby may not know all the answers,
but she knows where to look...

LEARNING TO BREASTFEED

Success or lack of success in the early giving of the breast is probably the strongest influence in the reinforcing or abandoning of breastfeeding.

Mavis Gunther, in *Breastfeeding and the Mother*
(Ciba Foundation Symposium, 1976), p. 149

In mammals, learning to breastfeed is part of a life-long process beginning at birth. Some of the knowledge is instinctive, but much of it is socially acquired – learned from observation of other animals, sharing of babies, and so on. It is well recognised by zoo keepers that animals are likely to have difficulty suckling their young if they have spent all their lives in an unnatural environment where suckling is not visible, where the immature female does not learn to handle and care for the younger members of the group. In 1984 there was the televised spectacle of a heavily clad human mother nursing discreetly in the probably vain hope that a pregnant gorilla will recognise that a baby is fed thus. (But perhaps the human mother stripped off when the television cameras went away.)

We humans are mammals too, and some of our difficulties with breastfeeding arise from our unnatural environment. Unlike humans in traditional societies, we live in small nuclear families and have very few children. In grandma's day, many sisters acted as little mothers to younger children, so babies were much more a part of everyday life. Women began bearing children early and often went on right through their reproductive years. Very few followed the present pattern of two or three children close together in age, then an end to childbearing unless divorce and a second marriage supervene. It's easier to breastfeed if breastfeeding is taken for granted as a natural part of life, rather than being a rare sight which affronts some people; it's easier, too, if handling and carrying babies has become second nature, rather than being a source of great awkwardness and unease. This means that as our children grow, we should give them opportunities to care for other women's babies, and see them being breastfed.

But if we ourselves have missed out on all that, there's no need to despair. Unlike other animals, we can organise ourselves to make up for that deficit. Pregnant women are well advised to attend meetings of the Nursing Mothers' Association of Australia (NMAA) or similar groups. And we can read, although learning from books is usually more difficult than absorbing experience unconsciously. Furthermore, elaborate teaching systems have been set up to teach us how to breastfeed, both before and after leaving hospital. The defects in the hospital teaching process have been mentioned in the previous chapter. Now let us look in more detail at what women have been taught, the actual mechanics of getting a baby to suckle. Books have influenced both mothers and nurses alike.

In 1984 a typical description of how the first-time mother should put her baby to the breast read something like this:

> With your first and middle fingers supporting the nipple from just outside the areola, touch the nipple against your baby's cheek and, as he instinctively turns his head towards it, slip it into his mouth. You may have to repeat this a couple of times if the nipple slips out of his mouth.[1]

The pictures that accompanied such descriptions usually showed a baby lying flat on his back in the mother's arms, cheek near the nipple or head turning sideways to grasp the nipple. Before you read any further, pick up a glass of water, turn your head sideways over your shoulder, and try to swallow your drink. Difficult? Consider how much more difficult for a newborn, who first has to milk the breast before there is anything to swallow. Of course the nipple slips out of the baby's mouth, usually despite the baby's best efforts to keep it in by suction alone, which exerts very substantial pressure and can damage the nipple.[2]

Such descriptions were commonplace, repeated in one book after another, without the authors examining what actually happens when a baby successfully latches on to the breast. There was no excuse for this, when Dr Mavis Gunther has been saying differently since the 1950s. In 1970, her book *Infant Feeding* described in great detail the physiology of "a good latch".[3] This was largely overlooked by those who should have recognised its significance until I discovered it in 1976 and popularised it in the first edition of this book. Even after many years of preaching the importance of what Gunther said, while many midwives and counsellors are aware of it, others are not. And when healthworkers do not understand exactly what babies do when they feed, facilitating breastfeeding is often reduced to an arbitrary set of rules and steps, or cute techniques, none of which will work for all mothers.

So just what do babies do when they feed from either breast or bottle? Is it what is so frequently illustrated in breastfeeding books and in advertisements for rubber nipples? If Gunther was right – and her experience of some 40,000 babies suggested that she might be – then the answer to that question is a firm 'no'. What she said, and what I shall develop in this chapter, is easily tested by those with access to a breastfed baby. What is more, since it was written in 1984 it has been proven accurate by Woolridge's ultrasound studies, although its subtleties are still not understood by many, perhaps especially in America, where Gunther's work was unknown.

Gunther pointed out that it is the action of the baby's tongue and jaw, milking the breast, which "not only obtains the milk but... provides the principal stimulus for the milk flow mechanism and the maintenance of lactation." So the baby must get a good mouthful to enable this milking action to take place. Babies' heads need to be at a comfortable angle when feeding, an angle that ensures both that the nipple is well back in the mouth, stimulating the palate, and that the baby can suckle comfortably and

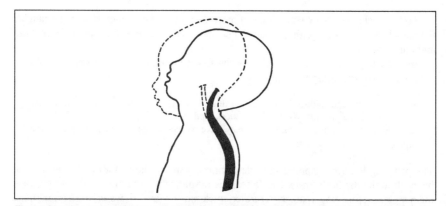

Figure 3.1 When breastfeeding, the baby's head should be tilted slightly back, with the chin against the breast and a good mouthful of breast tissue grasped between his tongue and palate. The dotted outline shows the normal, non-feeding position. modified from *Infant Feeding*, Mavis Gunther (Methuen, 1970), p.40. Reproduced with permission. Methuen.

swallow the milk ejected into his mouth by the breast. *This comfortable feeding angle can only be achieved when the chin is pressed firmly against the breast.* Because newborn babies have limited neck movement and head control, to be at this angle, the baby's body must be held close to the mother's. If blankets or clothes or careless positioning make him too far away, he has to crane his neck forward (or someone else will tip it forward for him) which means that his chin moves away from the breast and his gums cannot milk the ducts but are likely to damage the nipple; as well, his nose is likely to be buried against the mother's breast. Only suction on the nipple itself keeps the nipple in his mouth, and it is this pressure that is responsible for the flattened stripe of positional soreness (see p. 130).

Figure 3.1 shows how the position of the mouth, and the angle at which it will receive the nipple, depends on the movement of the whole head and neck. The baby can feed easily only if the closeness of his chest to the mother's makes him put his head up. The baby can feed and breathe easily if his head is supported at this angle and is not flexed on his neck. In contrast, the common practice of holding his head in against the breast causes him distress and may result in persistent 'fighting at the breast' as the baby struggles to reach the angle at which he can breathe and feed. If he is not being held close against his mother, the nipple will tend to slip out as he pulls back, particularly if her breast tissue is not yet fully protractile, or stretchy, as it does become while she is lactating.

To imagine for yourself what this would be like, get an almost-inflated beach ball. See how your nostrils are clear of it when your chin is against the ball. Then ask someone to push the back of your head forward, flexing your neck. As your nose goes in (and you don't have the flat nose of the newborn), your chin moves away. To see how difficult it would be to swallow at such an angle, try drinking a glass of water with your chin against your chest. Are you surprised that babies fight and get frustrated when well-meaning hands grab their heads and push them forward?

In summary, this is the way a baby should be held in the cradle hold (across the chest) position: The baby should be on its side, chest tucked close to the mother's chest, head supported on the mother's forearm but free to move, mouth directly opposite the nipple, body supported by the arm the mother is using to rest the head. Depending on the length of the mother's breasts, pillows may be needed under the mother's forearm and infant's body to raise the baby to the right level without causing strain on the mother's shoulders or allowing the baby's neck to be twisted or flexed by its body falling away from the breast. The baby's lips may be touched with the nipple if he has not already opened his mouth. When his mouth is wide open and centred over the nipple, he should be brought against the breast so that he gets a good mouthful, his mouth covering a substantial part of the areola, both below and above. The baby's mouth should remain wide open against the breast (see Chapter 12, Figure 12.4), although in fact the baby is brought in so close that his lips are not immediately visible: the curve of the breast meets the curve of the baby's cheek. Visible or pursed lips (see the baby in figure 12.2) are much more appropriate to bottle-feeding and probably mean that the baby is exerting suction on the nipple. Baby's lower lip should be turned out, not rolled back over his gums; the tongue should be under the nipple and visible if the lower lip is gently moved down. The mother's arm should be close to her side, with shoulder and elbow in an straight line, or the baby's head would be wide of the breasts. The breast should not be held between "first and middle fingers" in a scissors hold, but rather between thumb on top and four fingers beneath if necessary. Using the scissors hold very often distorts the shape of the breast that the baby latches on to; it may therefore cause suction to be exerted on the nipple; and the bottom finger may obstruct the baby's chin.

Correct and incorrect positioning are graphically illustrated in a film funded by Nestlé, in which Dr Felicity Savage-King and Sr Chloe Fisher feature[4] and in one I made for the Adelaide Women's and Children's Hospital, called *Latching On: the Key to Successful Breastfeeding*. More recent and clearer depictions can be found in the Royal College of Midwives (UK) video *Helping Mothers to Breastfeed*, and the NMAA Tasmania Branch video featuring Sue Cox has been found helpful by many mothers, although it contains minor details not everyone endorses.

Since 1984 most editions of breastfeeding books have been corrected to reflect some of what is said above, and numerous cheap pamphlets are now available. But as far as I am concerned the one book for mothers which unequivocally gets positioning right in every picture is Renfrew, Fisher and Arms, *Bestfeeding*. Many others, even by reputable authors, do not. There is no substitute for experience here, and good diagrams and films cannot convey what is best taught by skilled instructors.

Of course it should be said immediately, before this all seems to become too complicated, that most mothers and babies manage to find their own ways of feeding comfortably and efficiently. Once breasts have become fully protractile under the influence of hormones and suckling, mothers can feed one-handed, sitting, standing or lying, in every possible position. As babies get bigger too, they exercise more control over their own heads and rapidly adjust to novel postures, using their hands to position the breast if need be. *In stressing the importance of positioning we are talking about the initiation of breastfeeding in the first-time mother, who is quite likely to have problems unless she learns, consciously, or unconsciously, how to hold her baby.* The logic of positioning and the angle of the baby's head on his neck needs to be demonstrated in both sitting and lying positions, while the mother is in hospital. I am amazed by women who assert that they never manage to learn to breastfeed lying down until the baby was much older. It is in those first few exhausting months of new motherhood that the ability to lie down and doze off while feeding can be an absolute lifesaver. After all, those hormones make you drowsy,[5] so why not relax and enjoy a catnap?

As well, it should be said that *babies, and breasts, are individual and constantly changing.* Very large soft pendulous breasts will need to be treated differently from small firm breasts; huge nipples from flat ones; and so on. I have seen nipples that point in different directions, so to centre the baby's mouth around the nipple will require a change of angle of the baby's whole body in relation to his mother's – but not of the baby's head on his neck or the angle of the nipple itself. Large breasts usually need support while feeding, for two reasons; firstly, to reduce the effort the baby would otherwise need to make simply to keep the weight of the breast from pulling the nipple out of the mouth; and secondly, to improve drainage within the breast. If the breast constantly slips out of or even just forward in the baby's mouth during feeding, the baby gets frustrated, the nipple is often damaged, and the breast will not be properly emptied. Figure 3.2 shows how the position of the hand can alter the angle at which the baby receives the breast-nipple teat: for some mothers this would be helpful, for some harmful. . *Bestfeeding* illustrates the use of a broad band of soft material as a sling for the breast, to free the mother's hands and keep them from obstructing the baby's mouthful. Making a flatter breast shape can help some babies latch on: bit only if the flatter "biscuit" shape is aligned with the direction of the baby's mouth. If you have breasts to experiment with, try doing all these things watching your breasts in the mirror, so as to see how different actions affect the whole breast, including the nipple. Visualise a baby grasping the breast and the consequences of the changes you make to the shape of the breast in the mouth.

The main stimulus for the baby to begin sucking is the contact of the mother's nipple with the roof of his mouth,[6] so if any technique is associated with suckling difficulties for a particular baby, it might be because the nipple no longer touches the roof of the baby's mouth, and therefore the technique of thumb above, four fingers below, might be preferable.

The mother's own posture is important. The mother in case history 2 (see Chapter 12) was 'taught' to feed her baby sitting on the side of her bed, legs dangling down, without support for arms, back or feet. Many women sit uncomfortably hunched over the baby, without support for their back or arms. When strain is felt, the mother may lean back on to her pillows, without lifting the baby as she does so. The result is that the breast and nipple is pulled forward in the baby's mouth, and he exerts fierce suction to try to keep hold of it. Positional soreness strikes again! Once a baby has got

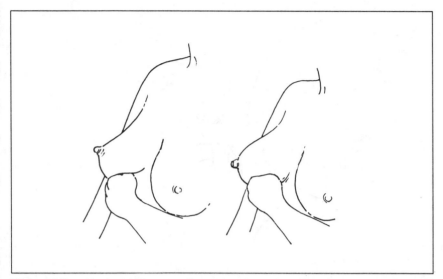

Figure 3.2 How hand positions can affect the angle at which the nipple enters the baby's mouth.

a good mouthful, he needs to keep it; he certainly cannot unless the mother realises that the whole baby must move with her whole body.

The clothes the mother is wearing may make correct position difficult. As Gunther said, "The mother's part – her holding and positioning of the baby – would be almost automatically successful in... conditions where mother and baby were naked: the newly born slippery infant could only be so held to the breast that his whole trunk was against her chest. In this position the lower jaw (the principal moving part in the feeding process) comes automatically against the breast and the baby can instinctively take the breast... I am not arguing for nakedness but for the concept that the baby's body should be just about as close as it would be without clothes."[7] Clothes may also obstruct drainage of milk from the breast. It is common for women to discover that night-dresses don't open far enough for relaxed feeding, or that 'trapdoor' bras seem to get in the way. It's false economy to put up with such problems. Make the opening bigger or use T-shirt or pyjama tops and bottoms (more practical in many ways.) Get a comfortable fully opening bra (or wear none if you're so inclined and your breasts are not too heavy).

Similarly, a baby bundled up hospital-fashion, with its hands and layers of clothes between its chest and the mother's chest, may make correct positioning difficult. Unwrap the baby, put his bottom arm around mother's ribs, his top hand free to pat the breast, then cover him loosely to keep warm. Most babies like their hands free to explore; some actually get very frustrated by being tied up tight, although they may need to be swaddled to sleep so that their arm movements don't wake them. (One

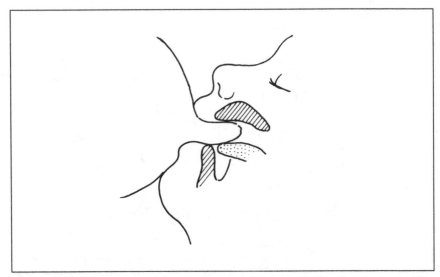

Figure 3.3 The usual depiction of what happens during breastfeeding. Incorrect unless the baby is tongue-tied.

small word of warning: a baby who discovers that twiddling the other nipple hastens let-down should be persuaded to twiddle or pat other areas of the breast before the habit becomes so well established as to be a social or physical liability.)

Once lactation counsellors, professionals or amateurs, understand the basic rationale of positioning, they can very often see instantly why a mother is having difficulties. But they must see the mother feeding to assess the problem. Experienced counsellors know that one visit can be worth a dozen phone calls. Mothers usually recognise when the baby is 'on right', after which they have learnt what productive suckling feels like. 'It's not hurting - what did you do?' is the usual response to getting a good latch, as Chloe Fisher puts it. Because this is pre-eminently a practical skill, it needs to be learned firsthand. Health professional education still has a long way to go in this area. The following figures may help make a few more points clear, so I am retaining them in this edition.

Figure 3.3 was said to show what occurs during feeding. What it illustrates is the problems a tongue-tied baby would have. Fisher[8] criticised this, correctly, because of the tongue position and also because the top lip was further away from the nipple than the bottom lip. Correcting this to its reverse – i.e. the bottom lip further from the nipple, which means the chin driving more closely into the breast – improved many cases of nipple soreness. Fisher then offered this next figure as showing the correct position:

In Figure 3.4, the baby's oral structures are approximately right. Certainly the tongue will project at least that far over the gums. (Where the tongue cannot be seen

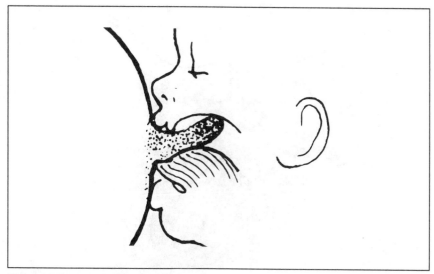

Figure 3.4 Fisher (1983) after Ardran (1958).

when the bottom lip is gently moved aside, the baby's cheeks will usually be sucked in as he sucks on his own tongue.[9] The tongue was not down as he took the breast into his mouth, and now lies above the nipple, so break suction, take the baby off the breast and start again!) However, in this diagram the breast is all wrong, and therefore the baby's chin, instead of driving against the underside of the breast, is not even touching it. If breasts were this shape, as they can be when engorged, the baby would have great difficulty drawing the nipple and areola into his mouth.

Figure 3.4 was taken from a cineradiographic study[10] of breast- and bottle-feeding done in the 1950s. The author, Ardran, did valuable work in reviewing what was then known about the process of feeding itself. But he did not realise that in posing a breastfeeding baby so that clear pictures resulted, he was in fact distorting the normal position for a newborn to feed in, and so altering the mechanics of feeding. An experienced breastfeeding mother, with protractile breast and nipples, and an experienced breastfeeding baby could successfully feed in this or any other position, particularly if the baby was used to different types of objects to suck (dummies, bottles, fist, toys). The baby simply alters what it does to keep the nipple in and the milk flowing. An attentive mother can watch and feel this happening by moving the baby around into different positions while he is still attached to the breast; it is sometimes also noticeable if you put a finger into a baby's mouth. (The rhythm of the breastfed baby's suck feels different from that of a bottle-fed infant.) Therefore in studies like this we need to know a good deal about both mother and baby's experience before deciding on the relevance of the conclusions for feeding *inexperienced newborns at inexperienced breasts*, which is where problems originate.

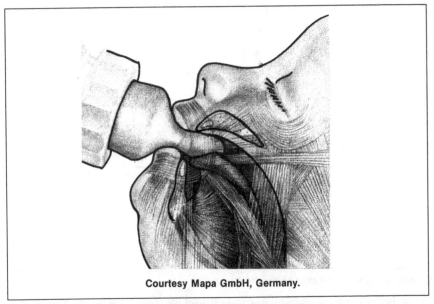

Courtesy Mapa GmbH, Germany.

Figure 3.5 Cross-section of a baby's mouth when bottle-feeding.

Figure 3.5 illustrates what one manufacturing firm claims to occur during feeding from their teat. That may well be. However, this is not, as they claim, what happens during breastfeeding. The tongue is back behind the gums, and the baby's mouth is barely open, simply circling the small diameter of the neck of the teat. The tip and front of the tongue may be exercised, but there would be none of the coordinated undulating movement, from front to back, of the whole tongue which one can feel in the breastfeeding baby. To say, as advertisements do, that a small-holed teat provides a 'workout similar to breastfeeding' is to ignore the reality of the milk flow reflex, which sends milk gushing into the baby's mouth initially and later during the feed. It must be very tiring for a baby to have to extract every drop by means of tongue thrusting and chewing motions – no wonder that so many mothers widen teat holes despite the 'glossopathic dangers' (see p. 205). It should also be obvious that any baby nursing a breast in this manner would be abrading the nipple surface, particularly on the underside, and compressing it as well. (See Fig. 3.6 for the characteristic facial appearance.)

This is probably what happens in what has been described as the nipple-confused baby. Frantz described it as follows: "Since liquid flows easily from the bottle nipple [if the hole is big enough] infants frequently position the tongue at the tip of the rubber nipple, thrusting forward and slightly upwards to slow down the flow to keep from gagging. The jaws do not need to compress the nipple to extract the fluid, so there is little chewing movement of the jaw. When an infant tries to suckle the breast the same way, he fails to extract milk from the breast effectively, or to stimulate the letdown.

This is called nipple confusion and often results in a frustrated infant who begins to prefer the bottle."[11]

It would be less confusing if Americans called bottle teats teats and not nipples!. Certainly the description of what an infant does while bottle-feeding matches the illustration a manufacturer of orthodontic teats provides. But feeding at the breast is not more 'difficult' or tiring – reasons often given for small babies not breastfeeding – some babies merely have to make a few active movements at the breast, then they can lie back and try to keep up with the flow it actively ejects. That the actions required are *different*, I have no doubt. That they require co-ordination which can be quite complex seems likely. That they are difficult for babies already imprinted to an unnatural way of feeding also seems likely. The solution then would be to ensure that no baby was given unnatural objects to suck before he or she had experienced breastfeeding and turned instinctive into learned behaviour.

It was interesting in 1984 to talk about nipple confusion with nurses in Los Angeles and Philadelphia. In Los Angeles, such problems were commonplace; in Philadelphia, rarely seen. Both groups tended to think the other wrong to over- or underemphasise this problem. Yet the Los Angeles counsellors were seeing women only after birth, when problems had developed; the Philadelphia mothers, educated during pregnancy about early causes of breastfeeding difficulty, probably had fewer such problems because their postpartum management was so much better. Nipple confusion was just as contentious in 1996, with a few eminent names in breastfeeding decrying the existence of such a problem altogether, despite the consensus of their colleagues. But this 1996 battle seemed to me a battle of semantics rather than substance. Obviously *not all babies get confused by being given dummies or teats to suck on*, or breastfeeding would be extinct in western cultures. No one ever suggested that all babies were adversely affected by early bottle feeding. Equally obviously, *there are just too many clear-cut cases of young babies imprinting on a teat and being very difficult to breastfeed thereafter, to consider such a problem non-existent*. It is what we do to treat the problem that has become contentious. Tincture of time? Suck re-training?[12] We know too little about the issue and the suggested remedies for dogmatism. But we can all agree that these babies above all need skilful positioning, and lots of patience, and lots of support to the parents.

To return to 'orthodontic' teats. How did they become accepted as simulating the shape of the breast during feeding? Possibly on the basis of studies like Ardran's cine-radiographic study. In 1983 I wrote to a number of manufacturers for further information on this, and got nothing valuable in reply. NUK claims their teat was designed after taking a plaster cast from the breast and nipple of a mother who had just fed. (!!) Technically this would be either impossible or inaccurate. Ardran states the obvious: that once the baby releases the vacuum in his mouth, the breast-nipple teat immediately begins to shorten and thicken, rapidly returning to its non-feeding shape. Any nipple that remained flattened and compressed would be one so badly positioned that all circulation had been disrupted. Hence this is not a model one wants to reproduce.

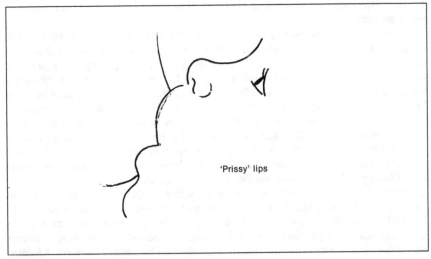

'Prissy' lips

Figure 3.6 Baby bottle-sucking the breast.

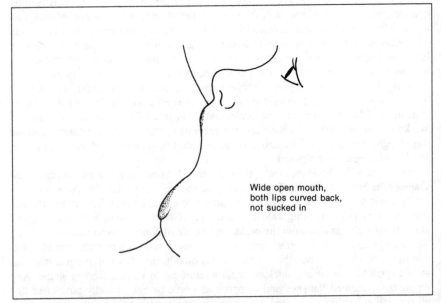

Wide open mouth,
both lips curved back,
not sucked in

Figure 3.7 Baby actively suckling the breast.

Despite the many ultrasound studies (not all of well-positioned breastfeeding babies) since I called for them in 1984, there are still unanswered questions about what goes on inside a baby's mouth while breastfeeding. It is perfectly clear, however, that Figure 3.5 is inaccurate. A breastfed baby has a great mouthful of breast to manage, so the mouth is agape, not prissily pursued. Compare Figures 3.6 and 3.7. In the latter, the baby's tongue draws the areolar tissue into the mouth and shapes it into a teat. The tongue then stays extended under that teat and extracts milk by an undulating motion. This undulation is coordinated with the jaw movements in different rhythms which depend on the rate of milk flow. An older baby at the breast will be able to stop and smile at mother, even laugh, without letting go of the teat he has formed of breast tissue; by then the nipple and areolar tissue will be so flexible that the baby's mouth will not need to be so wide open. But one never sees a properly positioned baby with those round pursed lips as shown in Figure 3.6. Indeed, the well-positioned baby is unlikely to have lips showing at all, but rather the breastfeeding image is "two curves meeting at the mouth": the curve of the mother's gently rounded breast and the curve of the baby's fat cheek. Observing badly positioned breastfed babies and generalising from them may explain the origin of such diagrams, just as it explains the prevalence and duration of nipple soreness.

Orthodontic teats have had their champions among breastfeeding counsellors. Rice called orthodontic pacifiers "mother and baby's friend" and urged training baby early to them by stroking baby's palate to stimulate sucking; she also advocated using an orthodontic nipple over mother's nipple when baby has a short tongue, mother has "not prominent nipple", or mother has too large a nipple. I simply could not see in 1984 how such practices would not cause major difficulties, as there is no physiological basis for them that I can see. It therefore did not surprise to read Rice's account of a mother whose baby had been fed only with an NUK teat who had difficulty getting him to take the breast. If the baby was "imprinted to the proper thrust of the tongue for breastfeeding" and the NUK truly simulated the shape of the breast, "some jelly to entice" would not be necessary, unless the mother's breast was oddly shaped. Nor was I surprised when in 1990 Denise Drane and I reviewed all the research literature about teats and found indications that the long-term use of orthodontic teats may lead to more facial deformity than plain longer ones. This was part of an investigation by the Trades Practices Commission set in train by Queensland lactation consultant Robyn Noble's complaint to the watchdog agency that NUK advertising was false and misleading. In Australia NUK are no longer able to claim that their product mimics breastfeeding, or is closer to breastfeeding than other teats, and so on, thanks to the TPC and the reviews it commissioned. Where else in the world has NUK stopped making a claim that is demonstrably false and misleading? This issue of teats will be fully discussed in my next book.

Rice frequently mentions the baby's receding chin, suggesting that it is breastfeeding which creates a more normal facial feature. I am not aware of any excessive preponderance of receding chins among bottlefed babies, though such feeding probably does adversely affect facial development in other ways (see ch. 9).

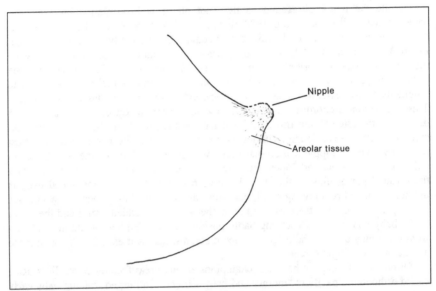

Figure 3.8 Post-partum breast, showing changing curve.

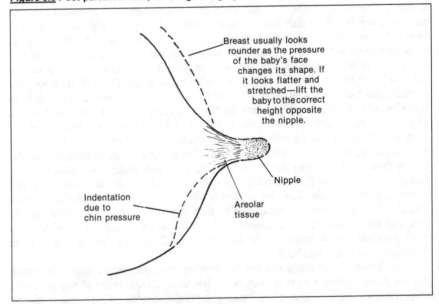

Breast usually looks rounder as the pressure of the baby's face changes its shape. If it looks flatter and stretched—lift the baby to the correct height opposite the nipple.

Nipple

Indentation due to chin pressure

Areolar tissue

Figure 3.9 Breast during feeding – dotted line.

Reflecting on the infant face has made me see how beautifully adapted it is to breastfeeding. A very prominent chin could come between baby and breast, preventing the gums from reaching far enough on to the breast to milk the sinuses. In California an experienced LLLI leader has commented that the snub nose, also so characteristic of babies, prevents problems with breathing while feeding. Only women with very large or soft breasts need be concerned to watch that their breasts does not obstruct baby's breathing. Are these coincidences, or useful adaptations favouring survival? This led to some further reflections.

Western women all recognise, and often bewail, the changing shape of our breasts during life. The cultural ideal at present is the firm, conical, virgin breast symmetrical above and below the nipple – as in the 1950s illustration, Figure 3.4. Yet as soon as we become pregnant, our breasts begin to change. The terms in which we describe that change are almost always pejorative – they sag, or droop, or drop – see Figure 3.8. After thinking about this question of babies, breasts and breastfeeding, I have concluded that the alteration in the normal 'virgin' shape is yet another useful adaptation designed precisely to assist in successful breastfeeding. Look at Figure 3.8. The effect of that 'sag' is to present the underside of the breast further forward to the baby. This facilitates a better mouthful and better milking of the breast by ensuring that the baby's gums compress the sinuses and glandular tissues (rather than having the gums simply pick up elastic areola skin and tissue, and land on the base of the nipple itself). A baby's mouth, going straight on to that breast centred on the nipple, must do what Fisher tells her mothers: get more of the underside in.[13] Exaggerate that advice, and of course the baby could be chomping down on the upper surface of the base of the nipple. This is less likely than the reverse, however, because the mother can see whether the baby has some of the upper areola in his mouth. In fact, Fisher argues that it is often the mother's concern to get the visible, upper areola in, which causes her to position the baby so that the lower areola surface is not in, and the breast therefore cannot be milked efficiently. This accords with my experience, and seems reasonable.

So what happens if we take the baby from Figure 3.4. and put him on a more realistic breast such as in Figure 3.9. Everything is where it ought to be: the chin drives firmly against the breast; the nipple stimulates the palate, which is thought to be the basic nursing stimulus; the baby's head is slightly further back, allowing him to breathe and swallow readily; his nostrils are clear of the breast. Trace off an outline of this baby; try putting him to the breast at different angles, and see where his gums will compress, where the nipple is relation to the tongue, and so on.

Now, every breast is different, so generalities like the description above are true only for the 'average' breast, neither 'too big' or 'too small', with nipples projecting at roughly this angle. But if we understand what goes on here, we may also be able to look at different breasts and see the potential problems they may pose for successful feeding. We should be able to look at a mother's breasts, and then at how she holds the baby for feeding, and correct most cases of painful nipples and inefficient feeding. We may be able to work out why some babies obviously prefer one breast, or why some mothers have problems with fissures only on one nipple. The way mothers use their

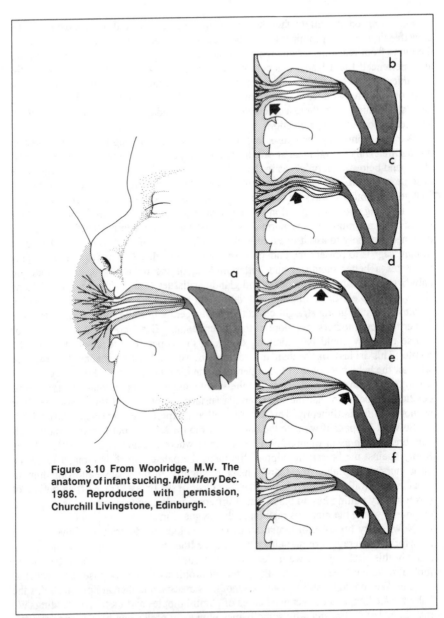

Figure 3.10 From Woolridge, M.W. The anatomy of infant sucking. *Midwifery* Dec. 1986. Reproduced with permission, Churchill Livingstone, Edinburgh.

<u>Figure 3.10</u> Baby at breast; <u>Figure 3.11</u> Anatomy of infant suckling

bodies may come to be seen as a contributory factors; experienced nurses often comment that if a woman is right-handed, it will be her right nipple that is most sore. (Is the arm not held as close to her body?) There must be some basis for this. We can see from such diagrams why it is so difficult to milk an engorged breast; perhaps we should draw a profile of difficult breasts and analyse their effect on feeding? Meanwhile, instead of bewailing our droopy boobs, let's take pride in them as yet another example of our bodies' capacity to do things right, so that we can nurture our children.

The suckling patterns of breastfed and bottle-fed babies

The term 'sucking' has been used to describe what babies do; and 'suckling' is what their mothers do. This is a widely used distinction, but not one I am happy with. Sucking is a very precise term, covering an action that is only part of what babies do while feeding, and not even the most important part (which is the vigorous milking action of the jaw and tongue.). Babies do not suck milk from the breast as we suck liquid from a straw. Some mothers think they do, and some breast pumps are designed as if the stronger the suction exerted on the nipple the more milk will be extracted. In fact, the only purpose of suction is to relax the muscle sphincter which prevents milk outflow when the ejection reflex occurs, and to hold the teat (breast or bottle) securely in the mouth. In the bottle-fed baby, suction does help to extract milk, but this is tediously slow, and many mothers widen the teat hole to the point where gravity causes the milk to flow through the hole readily. Ardran's work makes it clear that in breast- and bottle-feeding milk is squeezed out of the teat by the rhythmic compression exerted by jaw movements and tongue action. (As well, it is actively ejected by the breast.)

So what term should we use for what baby does? I try to avoid 'sucking' except where appropriate, and have resorted to 'feeding' or 'nursing' on most occasions. 'Milking the breast' or the baby's 'milking action' probably smack too much of the dairy to be acceptable to mammals supersensitive to their difference from other species, rather than proud of what all mammals have in common, a unique ability to nurture their young. I wish 'suckling' were able to be used more of the baby, as it is a term that conveys a precise meaning without being limited to one particular action. In some situations it seems to be simply unavoidable, e.g. suckling pattern. 'Feeding pattern' could include frequency and intervals in the day. 'Suckling pattern' means the pattern of movements during feeding.

Just how similar is the feeding action of the breastfed baby and that of the bottle-fed baby? It will be clear from comments earlier in this chapter that I think there are major differences in the way babies use their oral and facial muscles; and the orthodontic teat makers agree, even if they are wrong on details. But what of the frequency of jaw movements, length of feed, and so on? These are called the "temporal dynamics of feeding" by NUK,[14] the major orthodontic teat makers, and they are very clear that there is no difference whatever when their product is used (see Figure 3.12). We'll come back to that shortly.

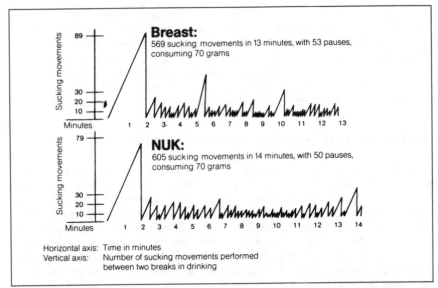

Horizontal axis: Time in minutes
Vertical axis: Number of sucking movements performed
                  between two breaks in drinking

Figure 3.12 Temporal dynamics of feeding according to a major manufacturer of teats. (Courtesy Mapa GmbH, Germany)

In all of the very detailed discussion of these diagrams, great emphasis is placed on the nipple hole being correct. "The relatively small nipple opening requires strong suction so that the infant is not overwhelmed by a large quantity of milk in a short time..."[14] All benefits of "strenuous feeding"[14] are lost if the baby gets milk too quickly, it seems. If this is so, why is there no warning to mothers not to enlarge the hole, as very many do when feeding is taking the recommended "14 minutes for 70ml"? (28 minutes to bottle-feed the baby who takes 140ml; 35 minutes to get 175ml down). These seem to me to be extraordinarily long feeds, when the larger, more efficient, older breastfed baby has often taken his fill in 3-4 minutes. Is it the length of time, or the number of suckling/jaw movements, or the number of swallows, or an arbitrarily fixed amount in the bottle, which determines how long the bottle-fed baby should be allowed to feed? And if the idea is to insist that the baby feeds 'strenuously' to the point of being tired and falling to sleep[14] after a feed, why are babies with cardiac defects, who tire easily, sometimes taken off the breast and given these small-holed, tiring teats to struggle with, rather than a nice soft breast which ejects the milk for them? Is it nipple confusion which results from their earlier exposure to bottles in the special-nursery, their loss of the inborn feeding reflex, which ensures that these babies have problems with breastfeeding so that the strenuous bottle seems easier? Are those bottle fed babies with hypoxaemia during feeding[15] in fact struggling with inappropriate teats and small holes? I don't know, but I wish someone would look at these possibilities. And clearly, instructions in the use of particular teats need to be

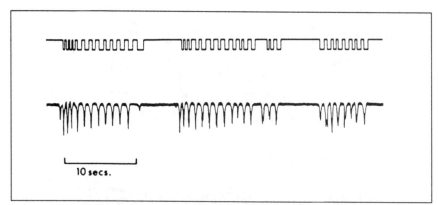

Figure 3.13 A sample of the suckling record. The sucks have been recorded independently (1) manually by direct observation (upper trace), and (2) by intra-oral pressure recorded via a naso-gastric tube (lower trace). (Drewett & Woolridge, 1979)

more detailed; similarly a great deal of rethinking is in order about the products we put into babies' mouths. Now research indicates that premature babies lying by themselves in incubators benefit from being given something to suck[16] (they rest more, sleep more, do not startle as much, and therefore grow better) we need to re-examine this subject from an independent, not commercially motivated, perspective. (That evaluation should include babies receiving Kangaroo Care.)

This re-examination of teats is now beginning, and results do not agree with the claims of the teat manufacturers, as illustrated in Figure 3.12. But then, Figure 3.12 is not very clear. Was this 13 minutes on one breast? If so, why ? If not, at what time was the baby switched to the second breast? (A change in suckling pattern should be evident.) How was a 'pause' defined? It looks as though the mother had severe difficulty with initial let-down and then a very unusual flow rate. Oxford researchers have produced a diagram of what looks much more like a normal suckling pattern, Figure 3.13.[17]

Here it should be said that each baby may have his or her own unique suckling pattern. All three of my children, feeding from the same breasts, had a characteristic pattern which they adapted to meet the changing circumstances such as exercise-induced undersupply or pain-inhibited ejection reflex, and which varied also with their need: after a long sleep, with an empty stomach, the initial attack would be much more energetic; if the breast was required for comfort sucking, the rhythm would be gentler, less impatient, accepting milk flow as a bonus rather than demanding it instantly. During the three months of intense nipple pain, in the virtual absence of an efficient ejection reflex, Philip's feeding was much more continuous and uniform (three or four chomps per swallow) than it became when I solved the problem (initial rapid chomps changing to suck-swallow rhythm). In the evenings, when I had a perennial problem, I had to devise all sorts of games to keep Philip working away at the breast to stimulate the let-down of milk. He tended to come off, look at me in disgust, and yell loudly as though protesting would help me produce. All three babies learned early on that the

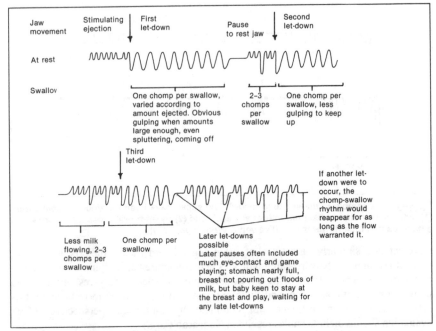

Figure 3.14 An 'average' suckling pattern.

right breast, which had been (unnecessarily) operated on years before, was less efficient, and they would not accept it first when hungry. None of their patterns resembled Figure 3.12, but rather were like Figure 3.14. Observing many breastfed babies since, I think this is a fairly normal pattern. Mothers with oversupply and hairtrigger ejection reflexes would see a pattern more like 3.15.

Mothers with incorrectly positioned babies, or poor supply, might observe the suckling pattern shown in figure 3.16. This pattern of several chomps per swallow can occur late in the feed, as the contented baby stays at the breast to doze, swallowing whenever he or she has a mouthful. It is an indicator of problems only if at the beginning of the feed the baby cannot establish a more equal chomp/swallow ratio, with obviously good milk flow. But the difference between a hungry, frustrated baby and a contented child reluctant to leave the breast is usually obvious.

Many mothers do not realise that a pattern of feed-pause-feed is the normal one. Here again, the image of bottle-feeding may be responsible. According to one advertisement, with Maja, "the baby gets an uninterrupted and soothing feed, and there are no upsetting breaks due to vacuum build-up." Breastfed babies pausing are not upset, but often are taking time to learn and explore, while hanging on to their comfort object, the breast. Watch an older baby in particular, grinning up at mother, or the younger one fascinated by a button, or patting (sometimes pinching!) the breast, or

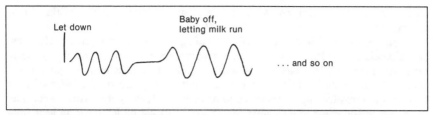

Figure 3.15 Baby's suckling pattern when mother has oversupply or hair-trigger reflexes.

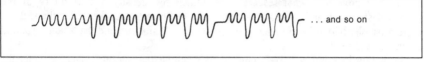

Figure 3.16 Baby's suckling pattern when incorrectly positioned or mother has poor supply.

grabbing for the other nipple. Imagine if we tried to eat our food in one continuous burst of chewing. Naturally babies pause; they should not be prodded to continue without reason.

The bottle-fed babies I have observed did not take more than five minutes to finish a full bottle of milk. When my expressed breast milk was fed to my children, they were very angry if the milk did not flow rapidly, and of course we widened the teat holes. (Doesn't everyone?) As the greater part of breastfed baby's intake occurs in the first five minutes of the feed, this is reasonable for the bottle-fed baby, whose feed is uniform in composition, and who might just as well suck on as empty pacifier as struggle hungrily to obtain food from a slow-flowing teat, perhaps falling asleep before taking the amount needed.

The breastfed baby is another matter. While the greater part by volume is taken in the next few minutes, the generally higher fat content of milk obtained in smaller quantities later in the feed may be important for the baby's growth and satiety. Therefore it is indeed "recommended that mothers should be told of the highly individual nature of breastfeeding and should be encouraged to time their feeds according to the responses of their infants",[18] who may fall asleep utterly satiated after a few minutes or who may feed contentedly for 20 minutes. It must emphasised that the initial pattern established in hospital may not last. The mother whose baby goes on feeding for half an hour may find that at two months the baby is off the breast in three minutes, ready to play. In scientific studies of the frequency of feeding, very many babies were feeding only 5-8 times or less per day, even though in the first week they fed 10-20 times. Needs change as babies do. This is another of the great advantages of breast-feeding as opposed to bottle-feeding: women can meet all these varying needs without calculation other than whether she can spare the time to sit/lie down and feed. It is "impractical to recommend a policy regarding the length of a breastfeed which would be appropriate for all mothers."[18] Which makes it difficult, surely, to claim that 13 minutes breastfeeding is exactly the same as 14 minutes using an orthodontic teat? And that this is necessary to avoid the "glossopathic danger"?

I don't doubt for a moment that "NUK suckling requires an even greater effort than breast suckling", but I'd like some independent scientist to show me that this is necessarily an advantage. Of course, NUK and the orthodontic teats may still be the best choice for the bottlefed infant – but to claim that they are on the basis of their closeness to breastfeeding seems to me to be dubious. Readers are invited to consider the evidence and come to their own conclusions. I would be interested to hear from manufacturers who make differently shaped teats, to know how they arrived at the shape they now sell, what research determined the density and elasticity of the rubber/plastic used, and so on, as Ardran[19] showed clearly that the stiffer the teat the more difficulty babies had in compressing it to squirt milk out, and that shape, size and so on affected feeding.

With this in mind, I was fascinated to examine the various advertisements for several very different teats, in an edition of American Baby, a magazine sent free to childbirth educators for distribution to pregnant mothers. The Playtex "Natural Action" nipple is "Most like Mother". Both terms are registered trademarks. It is "designed to imitate the natural action and shape of mother's breast. Soft and flexible, the unique shape fits into baby's mouth comfortably... placing the formula at the front of the mouth where proper digestion begins." (In breastfeeding milk is ejected at the back of the mouth, and comes complete with digestive enzymes.) The Playtex teat is totally unlike the NUK shape and totally unlike any breast I ever saw, in that the stiff rubber repeatedly rebounds out of the baby's mouth. As well, Binky Pacifiers discuss their various products, all very different shapes, stating that any of them will promote "the healthy oral development an orthodontic nipple will." Whom do you believe? Let's have a moratorium on advertising literature which makes claims that not using their teat, or not using their teat properly, could result in mental or social deficiencies! (See the glossopathy tree, ch. 9.) Even I, with my low opinion of bottlefeeding, find that, shall I say, hard to swallow.

To put such claims into historical perspective, I cannot resist drawing your attention to earlier commercial advertising claims about bottles and teats, via an illustration (fig. 3.17) of a Maws 'murder bottle.' With the benefit of hindsight, the faults of these long tubes, impossible to clean, are obvious: though not perhaps to the manufacturers who are creating such internal tubes for bottles and selling them around the world in 1998 (fig. 3.18) as useful to allow babies to feed themselves when they cannot yet even hold the bottle at the correct angle. How many babies will die before a second ban? And (this is the frightening thought) will people in 50 years time find all other current advertising claims just as absurd, and we as stupid as the parents who used long-tube bottles and the health professionals who recommended them?? Use your common sense, and think of chemical plasticisers, hygiene and the risks of scalding and choking as you look at the photos on p.388: which of these do you think should be available in any country that cares about children?

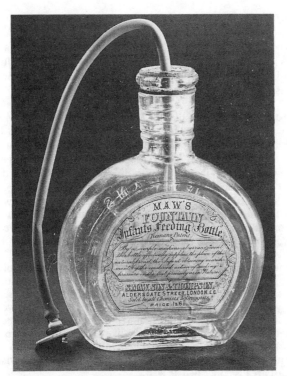

Figure 3.17 A nineteenth-century 'murder bottle' with insert tube, from the Sovereign Hill Historical Park's collection. It claims to act 'precisely as in Nature'.

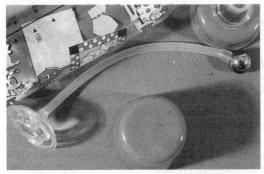

Weighted metal ball with hole for milk to be sucked through fine silicone tubing to teat. Sold in 1997, as a new device to allow babies to self-feed before they can hold the bottle themselves. Impossible to clean

Figure 3.18 'Murder bottles' reinvented, 1997: fine tube with metal ball on end to facilitate infant self-feeding. (Photo: James Maher Photography)

UK addendum re positioning

Simple instructions incorporating all these ideas about position and attachment are possible. Below is a copy of instructions given to mothers at the John Radcliffe Hospital, Oxford. My thanks to Chloe Fisher and the Oxford Breast-feeding Research Group for permission to utilise them. [Interpolated comments are mine.]

Place your baby on a pillow so that his bottom rests on your lap. Move your arm along his back and support his shoulders with your hand. Your fingers should gently cradle the back of his head. [This confuses some babies. An alternative is to support the baby's head on your forearm or in the crook of your elbow, making sure your arm is moved across your body so that the baby is directly opposite, and at the same level as, your nipple.] Your baby's head should not be held rigidly, but should be free to move, and his chin should be positioned so that it is tilted slightly upward, pointing at your nipple. Leaning slightly forward, turn your baby toward you as you move him close to you. (Remember that babies are more mobile than breasts!) Let his mouth touch your nipple. This activates his rooting reflex, causing his mouth to open. Wait until it is wide open. Now he is ready to latch on.

It's important to remember to aim his *lower lip* well down the areola (the darker area surrounding the nipple). Your baby's tongue will then be under the nipple and areola and he can move his top lip into position and will begin to nurse. Proper nursing action lets your baby squeeze the milk ducts which are located well behind the nipple, instead of sucking the nipple where much less milk can flow into his mouth.

Once you know what a proper latch feels like you will be able to achieve it at each feeding. *Recognise a proper latch.* You generally won't be able to see any of the areola when your baby is nursing. If the areola is large, some may be visible; if small, some of the breast area is concealed as well.

If he's suckling properly your baby's jaws will be moving, causing his whole head to move. If you watch carefully you'll notice that his ears may wiggle while he's nursing. There shouldn't be any hollow in his cheeks – if there is, he's not latched on properly. [Or is pre-term and lacks fat pads in his cheeks. Nor should the baby be making loud clicking tongue noises, although swallowing can sometimes be noisy.]

Watch his sucking patterns carefully: regular, even, short sucking [for more than the first few minutes of stimulating the let-down of milk] means a poor latch. A true sucking motion is irregular: a few rapid sucks, a pause, then slower, longer drawing sucks. This pattern will be repeated throughout feeding. Pauses are part of the normal feeding pattern, they do not mean that your baby is going to sleep and needs waking up.

Your baby should seem relaxed and contented while nursing. A baby who is wriggling and seems restless isn't sucking properly. If he sucks contentedly for a few minutes he may break the pattern and wriggle slightly. You may want to sit him up for a moment and let him burp and then latch him on again. Watching his movements carefully lets you tune in to his particular needs.

If you feel that the latch is wrong, put your finger into the side of your baby's mouth, letting in air to break the suction, and begin carefully again. [With some babies who hold on as hard as they can, and some mothers with sensitive nipples, it is best to put your finger right between the gums. Keep one little fingernail cut right back so as to avoid hurting the baby accidentally.]

Your baby should be allowed to nurse for as long as he wants to on the first breast. If he's properly latched on he will automatically stop when he is ready, and push the nipple out of his mouth. Change to the other breast and let him continue. He may only suck for a few minutes on the second side or not at all. It's when your baby isn't sucking effectively that feedings go on for hours. Do not judge your baby by any other baby, some babies take all they need in five minutes, some take half an hour or more, all babies are different. Remember to begin with the second breast next feed.

As to *when* to teach this business of getting the baby to feed successfully, here is a comment from another experienced midwife, Mary Renfrew.

I'd like to add something about the importance of the first feed, and its usefulness as a teaching time before any bad habits can be formed. Here is my recipe for success:

1. Let the baby feed/nuzzle the nipple at delivery if the mother wishes, although my experience is that in the first excitement and busy-ness, babies and mothers don't feed well. It may work if the mother is experienced, and usually what happens then is a comfortable and slippery nuzzle.

2. Complete any necessary stitching and the baby's initial check. Make mother and baby warm and comfortable-shower or wash, clean clothes, comfortable bed for mother – and the departure of everybody except parents, baby and midwife. Then in peace and quiet, about 45 minutes after delivery, you have an open book to make breastfeeding successful.

3. Explain baby's behaviour and needs; usually the baby is awake and alert at this stage. Look at breasts and nipples and baby's mouth, and explain positioning and its importance. The mother should just hold the baby at this point – unwrap him or her, play with fingers and toes, get the feel of the baby – and talk about her feelings about breastfeeding. Briefly explain supply and demand; anxiety and its effect on let-down. All this is a five-minute chat.

4. Help to position mother and baby, explaining as you do. Usually mother is lying down or at least semi-recumbent, and on one side, because of a sore bottom. When the baby is positioned and sucking well, you have an ideal opportunity (and trust of the parents) to talk about one or two potential problems. Not too much, overloading them with information, but enough to convey the warning that problems can happen, and, if they do, she should get help quickly. It's also an ideal opportunity – and there are so few – to talk to father about breastfeeding.

5. Then you can leave them alone, being in the room to answer questions but writing up case notes or doing something unobtrusive. You can help the baby to change to the other breast, using all the baby's behaviour as a teaching experience. (Parents are very receptive.)

6. All of this takes 15-20 minutes maximum, at a time when it's a good idea to be around anyway, to check the uterus and bleeding, and so on. To try to teach feeding at delivery time is to court disaster. We would be replacing one set of rules dictating feeding at four hours with another set of rules dictating feeding at delivery. Too

much is going on for such a first feed by such an inexperienced mother to have the best chance of success.

Even if there are complications with delivery (retained placenta, caesarian section, etc.), the first feed is still important. It may be delayed slightly, but should proceed in the same peaceful low-key manner.

NOTES
CHAPTER 3: LEARNING TO BREASTFEED

[1] Llewellyn Jones, D., *Breastfeeding: how to succeed*, (Faber & Faber, 1983), p. 45.

[2] Gunther, M., *Infant Feeding*, (Methuen, 1970), p. 81.

[3] ibid., p. 38-9.

[4] Write to Nestlé, Technical Assistance Dept. CH-1800. Vevey, Switzerland if you have any trouble locating this. The title is "Helping with Breastfeeding".

[5] Bourne, M. A., "Sleep and the Newborn", *New Generation* 1983, 2 (2), 16-17.

[6] Gunther, M. *Proc. Roy. Soc. Med.* (1958) 51, 305

[7] Gunther, M. in *Breastfeeding and the Mother* (CIBA Foundations symposium 45, Excerpta Medica 1976), p. 155

[8] Fisher, C., Positions of Success, *New Generation* (1983) 3, 20-21.

[9] Rice, Ilene, *Heartstart* (self-published, available from 2392 Nancy Place, St. Paul, MN. 55113, U.S.A.), P.59.

[10] Ardran, C. M. et al, "A cineradiographic study of breastfeeding", *Br. J. Radiol.* (1958) 31, 363, 156-62.)

[11] Frantz, K., "Slow weight gain", in Riordan, J., *A Practical Guide to Breastfeeding* (C. V. Mosby & Co., 1983) p. 218.

[12] Marmet C, Shell E. "Teaching neonates to suck correctly", *MCN* 1984; 9: 410-7.

[13] Fisher, "A proper latch – instructions given to mothers at the John Radcliffe Hospital, Oxford." See also Positions of Success, op. cit.

[14] Literature supplied by Mapa GmbH (the German manufactures of NUK) Postfach 12 60, D 2730, Zeven, West Germany.

[15] Rosen, C.L., et al, "Hypoxemia associated with feeding in the pre-term infant and full term infant", *Am.J.Dis.Child.* (1984) 138, 7, 623-8. If a breastfed baby had such problems, feeding position should be investigated first.

[16] Bernmarm,J.C., et al, "Non-nutritive sucking during gavage feeding enhances growth and maturation in premature infants", *Pediatrics* (1983) 71, 1, 41-5. Kessen, W.; Leutzenodff, A.M., "The effect of non-nutritive suckling on movement in the human newborn", *J. Comp. Physiol. Psychol.* (1963) 56, 69-72. Field, T. et al, "Non-nutritive sucking during tube feedings: effects on preterm neonates in an intensive care unit", *Pediatr.* 1982, 70, 381-4.

[17] Drewett, R.F.; Woolridge,M., "Suckling patterns of human babies on the breast", *Early Hum. Dev.* (1979)3/4, 315-20, see also Bowen-Jones, A.; Thompson, C.; Brewett, R.F., "Milk Flow and sucking rates during breast-feeding", *Develop. Med. Child Neurol.* (1982) 24, 626-33. Lucas, A.; Lucas, P.J.; Baum, J.D., "Differences in the pattern of milk intake between breast and bottle-fed infants", *Early Hum. Dev.* 1981, 5,2, 195-9.

[18] Howie, P W.; Houston, M.J. et al, "How long should a breast feed last?" *Early Hum. Dev.* (1981) 5, 71-7.

[19] Ardran, G.M. et al, "A cineradiographic study of bottle feeding", *Br. J. Radiol.* (1958) 31, 361, 11-22. This and the previous study by these authors are essential reading on this subject.

TOO LITTLE MILK?

Weight is not everything. A baby who has fed on unsuitable starchy food will grow fat and heavy, but he will not be healthy. Baby is not to be fattened like a Christmas turkey or a prize porker. What is wanted is firm flesh, sound bones, and skin of a good colour. If you get weight without this there is something wrong. Many fat babies, even some who have won prizes at baby shows, have been fed on starchy artificial foods and have rickety bones under their pale, podgy skins.

- Glaxo Baby Book, (1919 edition), p.37

One of the most common reasons for a mother weaning her baby is the belief that she has too little milk, or poor-quality milk, and cannot satisfy her baby. This is sometimes represented as being merely a 'socially acceptable'[1] excuse for discontinuing, rather than being a real (i.e., physiological) problem. Those who make such pronouncements usually also believe that simple measures such as more frequent feeding are all that is needed to increase the amount of milk a mother makes and a baby takes. Are they right?

I had to feed almost constantly in order to satisfy my first child – until I resolved the cause of my problems: poor positioning and attachment. My second child was easier, but I still had to have her attached to the breast, almost like a limpet, throughout the evening, which, with a two-year-old as well, became more of a problem, and towards five months I was hard put to satisfy her. My third child made me stop and try lateral thinking to solve the "six o'clock starvation syndrome", as I dubbed it. Clearly I was not impressed by simplistic advice about demand always creating supply – I should have been awash with milk if that always worked. Because I had such difficulties, I was more sensitive to other women who reported similar problems. Rather than deciding that if more frequent feeding did not work, the mother 'didn't really want to',[2] I came to accept that this was a real and a major problem, relating to the ability of a mother to synthesise milk in harmony with her baby's ability to consume it. (What I could not accept were cultural pseudo-explanations advanced by formula companies to explain this phenomenon.)

Sometimes, of course, the problem is not physiological but psychological, a failure of belief. We women seem all too ready to believe that the quantity or quality of our homemade product is somehow less satisfactory than that made to a 'scientific' formula, whose manufacturer asserts that the mixture contains all that baby needs. Without discussing why we are so under-confident or whether our faith in science is fully justified, at this stage, let it be repeated that, firstly:

109

- *The milk we make is, almost without exception, a better product than any laboratory can ever devise.*

and secondly:

- *Almost every woman is physically capable of feeding her child fully for at least six months – and most women can feed more than one child, and for much longer.*

So problems of quality and quantity should be rare, in theory. Yet it remains true that most women who wean early believe their milk is inadequate in quantity or quality. How can we tell just what the problem is? Let's look first at the quantity.

Quantity of milk supply

How can one tell whether a breastfed baby who is exclusively breastfed is getting enough milk?

- If the baby's weight gain is good, he or she is getting enough over the day (though perhaps not at certain feeds).
- If the baby is contented and sleeps well, despite smaller weight gains, he or she is probably getting enough. The baby may still wake at night, but babies vary greatly in this, whether breast- or bottle-fed.
- There are some babies who are meant to be slow gainers. Where there is a family history of small stature or slow growth, this is more likely than for the child of a family of six-footers. A normally slow-gaining child should, however, be a contented, alert child with no sign of abnormal health or behaviour, and growth should be reasonably consistent over the first year. The importance of monitoring child growth cannot be overemphasised, even if the interpretation of that growth has changed markedly during this century.
- Six to eight wet cloth nappies in 24 hours is a sign that a baby is getting enough milk, provided he or she is not being given other fluids or solids. Strong-smelling yellow urine indicates that the baby does need more fluid, either water or breast milk. Scanty, strong urine is one of the early warning signs of dehydration, which is rare but possible in hot weather or when the baby becomes overheated. Bowel motions are harder to interpret. A child may have several in a day, or one in several days, and still be healthy. However, the baby with frequent fluid stools is losing a lot of water with each and so should be offered the breast more frequently, or even in very rare instances offered water (preferably the breast if the baby's weight gains are average or less, although some overfed lactose-overloaded babies do better if their mother temporarily reduces the frequency of feeds, spacing them to intervals of 3-4 hours, or ensures that they feed well at and "finish the first breast first".
- The baby's general clinical signs can be assessed by any professional. Good skin tone, clear bright eyes, alertness, normal fontanelles (these sink in when dehydration occurs), all suggest a healthy adequately-fed baby.

If a baby meets these criteria, it is very unlikely that he or she is having difficulty obtaining enough milk from mother. Yet there are times when mothers of just such babies suspect that they are starving their children and therefore offer second-rate supplements.

When do women commonly suspect low-supply problems?

• When breasts that were engorged or full seem to be soft and 'empty', in hospital or on arriving home. This simply means that the breasts have settled down to efficient production. There is no supply problem at all.[3]

• When the newborn baby needs more feeds than he was having in hospital. This may indeed indicate that a return to home and its activity and responsibilities has caused a minor drop in supply; or it may indicate that the baby is growing more alert and responsive and can use more milk. Sometimes simple temperature changes cause an increased appetite: much of baby's food goes to keep him warm, and his temperature controls are very immature. If he is either too hot (losing energy and fluid to sweat) or too cool (spending energy to keep warm), he will need more food. The simple solution is to feed ad libitum – i.e. whenever and for as long as the baby seems to indicate a need – and supply will probably increase. It's interesting to note here that in very hot weather milk may become more watery, helping to protect baby against dehydration. (Its low electrolyte content makes dehydration less likely than in the bottlefed infant, in any case.)

• When the baby can't be pacified by anything but suckling at the breast all evening – the 'six o'clock starvation syndrome'. It is a fact that some women, like me, seem to 'run dry' by late afternoon or evening. Some find that a nap after lunch makes all the difference here. Others have found an even more certain solution: at the first feed or two of the day, they allow baby to feed on one breast while expressing the other into a breast pump. Collecting, say, 50ml each morning and giving this after an evening feed, many mothers have reported that the previously wakeful constant suckler, suddenly began to sleep soundly. Because the breasts are making this milk daily, there is no decrease in overall supply. Baby may sleep a little less before the second or third morning feed, until the breasts have begun to make the extra, and he should be allowed to suckle freely on the second (expressed) breast. Daytime feeds should also be allowed to go on until baby is content: if the stimulus of constant evening suckling is suddenly withdrawn, supply could drop unless that stimulation is being given at other times; similarly the mother could run the risk of becoming pregnant if night feeds (and ovarian suppression) are abruptly discontinued.

• When the older baby suddenly needs more frequent feeds. Increases in feeding frequency are commonly reported at six weeks, three months and six months, but can occur at any time because no two babies grow at exactly the same rate. In this case baby is saying either that supply is a tad inadequate at the moment, or that he needs more comfort all of a sudden. But the baby's demand for more frequent feeds is both symptom and cure. Allow him to suckle freely, and supply will quickly build up to his needs – usually.

• When the baby stops feeding after two or three minutes. If he seems contented, he may well have already got all the milk he needs, believe it or not. Babies become very

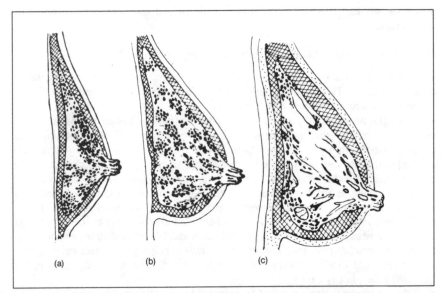

Figure 4.1 Three breasts. (a) Small breast with plenty of glandular tissue. (b) Average breast with plenty of glandular tissue. (c) Large breast with little glandular tissue, much fat.

expert at emptying the breast, and the let-down reflex may be equally efficient. When baby's weight gain is good, don't worry about how long a feed takes.[4] However, if his weight gain is poor, or he is obviously miserable, leaving the breast after a couple of minutes may have another meaning (see p. 123).

• If the breasts decrease in size and rarely feel firm or full. By itself, this may simply mean that they are well adapted to milk production. Can you imagine a tiny Cambodian woman being able to nurse her own and five other babies? One such case has been reported in respectable public journalism. Size is no guide to efficiency. Large breasts may be filled with fat and connective tissue, not glandular tissue (see Figure 4.1). However, it is true that storage capacity of the breast may help determine the pattern of feeding needed to fully nourish the baby: just as a car with a small fuel tank can drive as far as one with a larger tank, but will need re-filling more often. The same is true of babies' stomachs, of course! And rates of milk synthesis can rapidly adjust to ensure that the small-storage-mother can make enough milk, just as rates of stomach emptying can mean changes in baby's intake.

• When 'test weighings' reveal very little milk. Even when carried out over a full 24-hour period, these can be misleading and even wrong[5] unless administered by people who know how to interpret the results obtained by using very accurate equipment. To judge milk volume by a single test feed is utterly unscientific[6] – the mother is usually under stress, so the yield is naturally less, apart from many other considerations. The baby takes different quantities at each feed, and the relative amounts of fat vary

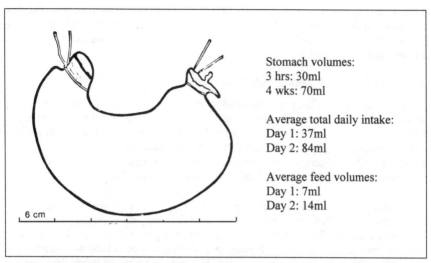

Stomach volumes:
3 hrs: 30ml
4 wks: 70ml

Average total daily intake:
Day 1: 37ml
Day 2: 84ml

Average feed volumes:
Day 1: 7ml
Day 2: 14ml

6 cm

Figure 4.2 Outline of the stomach of a newly-born infant, actual size. Attributed to Holt by Jellet (1922) (Diagram courtesy of JoAnne Scott, Washington.)

widely. A high-fat, volume feed may be quite adequate for baby but may not be "sufficient" by weight, just as 100gm. of a chocolate bar will provide more fuel than 100gm of carrots. What's more, it's quite clear that the old formula whereby baby's needs were assessed (21/2 oz/lb/day) is due for revision anyway.[7] Breastmilk is so different from formula, so much better utilised by the body, that babies need less of it, much less than was previously thought. Exclusively breastfed, thriving babies have been shown to be receiving as little as 71±17 kcal/kg/day, where the old belief was that they required around 115 kcal/kg/day. Mothers are sometimes encouraged to hand express after such test-weighings and are dismayed when they get very little milk. Do remember that what is expressed is never any indication of what baby can obtain.

• When a baby is grizzling and constantly wanting to feed. This can be because the child is in pain and wants comfort, as with teething in some babies, or with colic in others, or it can indicate some suddenly increased need for milk because of other factors not readily suspected. (See case history 1 in Chapter 12. This child fell asleep immediately after drinking a bottle of boiled water – he was thirsty because slightly dehydrated.) A baby who is constantly feeding, day and night, is as wearing a problem as one who fails to gain weight adequately, and his constant suckling can be misinterpreted, especially by isolated mothers without access to scales.

In the majority of cases, a seemingly poor milk supply is due to unphysiological ideas how babies 'ought' to be fed. Anxiety about not having enough milk can by itself produce the problem in some people, so that expressing and storing the early oversupply can be a great psychological boost. One very useful diagram to show the new mother is Figure 4.2, an illustration of the actual size of an infant's stomach at birth. Even though it rapidly expands after birth, it does not take litres to fill this container. Little and often is the rule. Many Australian mothers are daily producing half a litre or more of milk by day three[8] after birth, so it is obvious that they will be having oversupply problems for a time.

When the baby isn't getting sufficient

Having disposed of the problems of an imagined poor supply, let's now look at that minority of cases where the problem is indeed real. There will be times in some women's experience of breastfeeding when they do not produce enough milk or their babies are not getting enough of what they have. The result will be:

- A baby who is discontented, unable to sleep long, always wanting to feed. (There are other reasons for this, such as food intolerance or overfeeding.)

or:

- A lethargic baby, without energy to suckle long, with either scanty urine, or very infrequent stools. (This, too, may be the result of physiological problems in the infant.)

Such babies should be carefully checked over for signs of illness. The key indicator to a genuine and continuing supply problem is that both types of baby will gain weight only slowly, if at all. Growth rate *by itself* is a poor indicator of infant development and is useless in trying to assess milk supply problems. Growth must be assessed in the context of infant behaviour, including activity and excretion. One miserable wakeful child may not gain weight at all, but if he has profuse loose stools the problem may be intolerance of something in mother's milk, or infection, or both. Another baby may have profuse loose stools due to maternal oversupply and continue to gain weight well. No one factor can be diagnostic, and only careful investigation of both mother and baby will give a clue to the cause. The slapdash attitude is: "She isn't growing fast enough, give her a bottle or some solids." This is extremely poor practice, especially when we don't know precisely how fast the baby should be growing, either individually or against present tables, and when bottle or solids can lead to malnutrition. Obesity, too, is a form of malnutrition.

As well, such an attitude is positively risky. The baby who is not thriving at the breast may be suffering from conditions that will worsen dramatically on any second-rate diet, such as problems with metabolising an adequate intake. Obviously, we must do everything we can to identify the cause of the poor growth and remedy it, being careful to "first, do no harm", such as unnecessarily disrupting the infant's gut flora and reducing the bio-availability of nutrients in breast milk (that is, giving a bottle).

Causes of an insufficient quantity of breast milk can be found in both mother and baby. The most common causes lie in the breastfeeding experience itself.

- Scheduled limited time or infrequent feeding. There are still some mothers who truly believe that babies need to feed only for 10 minutes each side (or less) every four hours, and these women cannot accept that the pattern may change over a day from intervals of four hours to half an hour. After the regularity of feeds at some hospitals, this is hardly surprising. But the fact is that babies are people, like us, who want to eat when they feel hungry. And, like us, they all have their own body rhythms. Similarly, suckling times are variable.

- Poor positioning of baby at the breast. This was discussed in Chapter 3. Unless the baby's body is comfortably close to the mother's body, with his head slightly back so that his chin touches the breast, he will not be able to feed and breathe easily. If feeding is an exhausting struggle to stay on the breast and to get enough air, he'll give up too soon. (See also ineffective suckling.)
- Feeding from one breast only. This does seem to reduce the stimulation needed to maintain an adequate supply, although women can succeed in breastfeeding and never use both breasts.[9] However, in most cases, the baby should determine what he takes – so offer him the second after he has left the first. Massage or gentle stroking of the breast from the armpit towards the nipple as baby feeds may also help. Curiously enough, voluntary one-breast feeding may prove to help some babies; those with frequent fluid stools and abdominal discomfort, whose mothers have a bountiful supply and forceful let-down. Overfeeding, if it leads to lactose overload and intolerance, may also cause poor weight gain.

What about hormones? Successful lactation depends on the production, release, and action of body hormones. Many factors can upset the proper balance of these hormones:

- retained placental material,[10] or the administration of progesterone immediately after birth;
- pain from stitches, nipple or breast problems, inhibiting milk flow;
- extreme blood loss sufficient to damage the pituitary;
- over-tiredness, which is common no matter how baby is fed;[11]
- breast surgery damaging nerves in the nipple;[12] or destroying drainage outlets by severing ducts;
- emotional stress in some women;
- oral contraceptives and other drugs;[13] Danish researchers argue that the change to progestogens and IUDs, and away from high-dose combined contraceptives may be partly responsible for the resurgence in breastfeeding: a causal connexion?[14] In Australia, only the mini-pill is recommended in lactation (and that can cause problems in a minority.)
- hypothyroidism or other hormone deficiency, such as severe antepartum oestrogen deficiency, with low prolactin levels postpartum; or decreased prolactin levels due to smoking;[15]
- menstrual problems;[16]
- supervening pregnancy.[17]

These factors can influence both the amount of milk made (production) and the amount that flows from the breast to the baby (ejection). There may be a role for hormonal drugs, for analgesia, for positive relaxation techniques in managing some of these problems, but those interventions are relatively familiar and I shall not go into them in detail. I would comment, however, that in cases of poor weight gain Frantz considered problems of milk ejection to be very rare and relatively minor. So do I. So does Dr. Michael Woolridge in the UK.

Maternal diet, too, can affect the quantity of milk available. The general prescription of a balanced and varied diet, and avoidance of 'junk' foods, is fairly common. But mothers may be more at risk from an excess of 'healthy' food. The use of B vitamin supplements, or consumption of large quantities of brewers' yeast, has become very common; yet it has been shown that B_6 inhibits lactation,[12] and some babies begin to refuse the breast after the mother consumes large quantities, possibly because of taste differences. Over-the-counter premenstrual tension (PMT) medications usually contain high doses of vitamin B_6. These are being widely promoted and used. Frantz noted in conversation (June 1984) that problems were already being seen among mothers using them. Mothers were often told to drink large volumes of fluid, particularly in America, but this, too, may actually help to suppress lactation (see p. 60). Fluid intake generally is related to urinary rather than mammary output.

The mother's genetic endowment may be involved. In any mammalian species this will be the case. While it is very rare, there will always be a few women who are genuinely unable to produce enough milk for their baby. For some mothers, metoclopramide may be useful,[18] although this should be approached with caution (see case history in Chapter 12). Sulpiride too[19] could be assessed for its clinical usefulness. But drugs affecting hormone levels will be useful only if hormone levels are the basic problem, and they may not be. Neifert has documented some women who had very little glandular tissue in apparently average breasts.[20] It has been known for years that breast size provides few clues to the internal structure of the breast[21] (See Figure 4.2). I am somewhat concerned that these problems could be caused or accentuated by the extraordinary infiltration of hormonal drugs into our food supply, or via administration to women or their mothers, but know of no studies relating to this. However, even women with such problems can usually provide a little breast milk if they would like to nurse for a time, and the baby may happily accept the breast as a pacifier, while receiving nourishment from a bottle. These are women who should have a priority claim upon human milk banks, and access to skilled and sensitive counselling to enable them to accept these bodily defects in a matter-of-fact way, and not to interpret the baby's likely rejection of their breasts as rejection of them as mothers.

Many mothers presume that genetic factors are responsible for their poor milk supply. When they have difficulties they leap to the conclusion that this 'runs in the family', just because their mother and aunt and sister all failed to breastfeed successfully. It is more likely that they too were victims of poor management of their breastfeeding problems. Poor management is not a new phenomenon – remember that it's only a generation ago that women were told that they must feed four-hourly or ruin their child's character for life![22] And each woman within any kinship network who has failed at breastfeeding can have many subtle effects on other women. The anxiety produced by knowledge that they failed may contribute to the new mother's tension; the advice they give, based on their experience, may be inappropriate or damaging; the fact that they give advice which is not consistent with other trusted sources is another source of tension. So breastfeeding failure in the family can contribute to poor supply problems without there being any predetermined genetic component at all.

There is some evidence that a few women tend to produce less milk as they grow

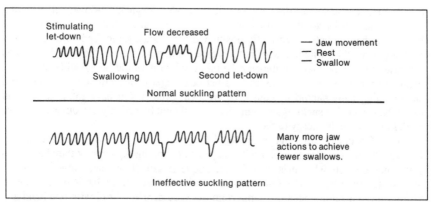

Figure 4.3 Suckling patterns: normal, and ineffective.

older.[23] However, this must be kept in perspective. Thousands of older mothers, and even grandmothers, have successfully breastfed twins. For the genetic poor milker, age may be a further problem, but for most women it's not. One case I know of personally: a woman was having her second baby at 40. The child was premature, and it was decided to transport him from the country to a regional hospital, without mother. There he was given cows' milk formula. Later transferred back on a very hot day, he became slightly dehydrated so was given Lactogen. He became extremely constipated and eventually spent almost two weeks in hospital. Staff attitudes to the mother expressing her milk or feeding the baby were very negative, and she was unable to express very much. But she wanted to feed, despite her fears about her age. Within a week of the baby being at home he was fully breastfed and never looked back. He was breastfed for much longer than her first child, born a decade previously. Every lactation counsellor could tell of similar cases.

Then there is the baby who is simply a poor feeder. Downs' syndrome babies, or babies who were premature, ill, jaundiced, heavily sedated or neurologically impaired at birth sometimes are unable to feed vigorously, or imprint the wrong type of suckling pattern in the first crucial days of learning how to feed. They are what Kittie Frantz describes as "ineffective sucklers".[24] The term "flutter suckle" is now widely used in America to describe what seems like babies' initial rapid-jaw motion: a chew-chew-chew pattern, which stimulates the let down of milk. Good feeders then switch to a chew-swallow pattern, but these ineffective sucklers rapidly revert to the chew-chew-chew motion. I attempt to illustrate this in Figure 4.3. To me, this suggests not only poor suckling habits, but also poor positioning of the baby, because the correctly positioned baby will stimulate a flow of milk that will force him to "suckle right or drown", as Frantz put it (in relation to a nursing supplementer).[25] Frantz advocates the use of a "burp and switch" technique: allow baby to feed for three to five minutes on one side, then burp and switch to the other side, for as long as the baby can be persuaded to stay awake and keep trying. This is said to take advantage of the fact that baby's first few sucks are the strongest; it stimulates frequent let-downs of milk and doesn't allow baby to doze off. However, it could also work by increasing the likelihood that the baby is correctly positioned for at least some feeds. In a normally suckling baby, this switching does not increase the total volume of the feed, but it does increase the volume taken in the first 10 minutes,[4] so it would be valuable for babies unable to summon the energy to feed for periods longer than 10 minutes. Feeding of a slow-gaining baby should of course be frequent even if you have to wake baby at times. Non-nutritive suckling on dummies, etc., should be actively discouraged – these babies need all their energy to feed.

Some US doctors in 1984 encouraged the use of the Valsalva technique: gently jack-knifing the baby so that blood is pumped to the brain. Apparently they have consulted neurologists who insist that the technique is safe (Lawrence, however, warns against this as risky[24]). The following description is taken from Jan Riordan's book. "Hold him in a supine position, supporting the shoulders and head with one hand and the legs with the other. Then bring his knees toward his head as far as possible, trying to touch the infant's nose. Repeat several times to increase his circulation and stimulate his alertness." Riordan illustrates this procedure,[26] as does Danner, who calls a modifed version the "dolls eyes technique".

In extreme cases, the use of a supplemental nursing system (to supply expressed breast milk while baby feeds at the breast) may work wonders. The Rolls-Royce of these is Medela's version, the SNS, although it is startling to see that opaque materials and impressed numbers make this needlessly hard to clean. Cheap versions can be made with a feeding tube and container of breastmilk. If the baby dozes, keep him at the breast and express milk into his mouth; he learns to swallow and suck as he sleeps.

Reasons why a baby is not receiving sufficient quantities of milk may also include genetic or developmental problems in the baby: physical abnormalities of the oral structures, such as cleft palate, a very high palatal arch, and so on. Some poor-gaining babies may be neurologically impaired. These are well described by Lawrence[27]. It is all too easy to blame the breast and urge a change. It would seem that neuro-muscular therapists have assisted some babies, though this must be seen as experimental until proper studies are published.[28] Tongue-tie can also prevent the breast being adequately milked by the tongue. It's therefore a possibility worth eliminating by a careful medical examination, and remedying by snipping the frenulum. Quite a number of doctors are once again doing this, and mothers report immediate differences in the suckling, and in weight gains thereafter.

The Dancer hand position (see figure 4.4) may help a baby suck more effectively because he needs less energy to hold his jaw steady (in order to compress the areola). Sarah Danner has described this as follows: "Simply slide the hand which is supporting your breast forward, so that the breast is supported by three fingers rather than four. Such support is still necessary to keep the weight of your breast from pressing on your baby's chin and mouth. Bend your index finger slightly so that it gently holds the other cheek. Your thumb and index finger form a U, and his chin sits in the bottom of the U." Later, as muscle tone improves, chin support alone using the index finger may be adequate. This idea arose from working with handicapped older children who had similar problems with efficient eating because of lack of jaw stability, and it has worked successfully for many mothers.

Other infant problems, such as illness, may cause slow weight gains[29] that are interpreted as indicating low milk supply. If a baby has to use nutrients in fighting off infection, he or she cannot use it to grow adequately. For this reason it's worth avoiding exposure to serious infections, even though the baby would be substantially protected by breast milk. Infectious challenge, or even the immune response after vaccination or the stress of painful surgery, often accounts for a week of slower growth, or even weight loss. But a healthy child will bounce back from that, and the baby's capacity for 'catch-up' growth usually means that over a month or more his weight gain remains in proportion. Hence mothers shouldn't worry about a one- or two-week dip in weight gain: it does not necessarily indicate dwindling supply, only that baby had to use food for purposes other than growth.

Allergic disease is not uncommon in babies. When this takes the form of nasal congestion, it can directly interfere with feeding. Babies who cannot breathe through the nose cannot breastfeed adequately. Nasal decongestant drops and eucalyptus rubs are available but may be dangerous for young babies, as they cause a rebound reaction after continuous use in which the breathing problem is even worse[30] and potentially fatal. A clean twist of wet cotton wool can help to clear the nose. In such cases, allow the baby to feed from both breasts with the least-blocked nostril uppermost, i.e. switch from a 'cradle-hold' breast-feeding position to a 'twin' position, with baby's legs going under the arm; support the baby's body on pillows so that the arm doesn't get tired. And of course, do all you can to identify the cause of the nasal allergy. (Nasal congestion caused by a respiratory infection will have the same effect.)

Food intolerances and allergies can also contribute to growth problems that are interpreted as indicating a poor supply. Checking the frequency, consistency and volume of a breastfed baby's stools is an essential aspect of diagnosis.

Experts continually stress the need for careful observation and testing for other physical illness while helping the mother with breastfeeding problems. "We found an infant with cystic fibrosis, many urinary tract infections, congenital heart disease, a brain tumour, etc. We learned that a baby who is not gaining at the breast may also be a baby who fails to thrive on the bottle... We feel every baby who is 'failure to thrive' deserves to have illness ruled out before he is switched off the breast."[25] Even simple defects such as a deviated septum in the nose, or a slight misalignment in the neck or jaw (not uncommon) may make for difficulties with breastfeeding. It would be wonderful to think that all breastfed babies were subject to such careful examination before any suggestion of weaning was made. Unfortunately the use of a formula is often the first suggestion, and the mother is deemed odd if she shows reluctance to substitute an inferior product for her own milk. Any signs of lactose intolerance often result in instant weaning – yet lactose intolerance is only rarely a primary disorder and is more frequently a consequence – often of intolerance to the proteins the child is likely to be prescribed (cow's milk and soy) or other foods in the mother's milk.

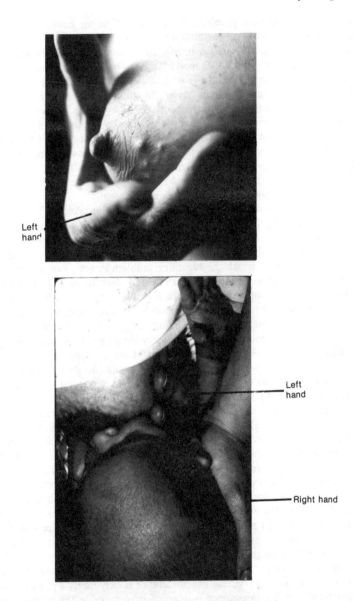

Figure 4.4 The Dancer hand position, which helps a baby to suck without using energy to hold the jaw steady. The mother's thumb and forefinger form a U, and the baby's chin sits in the bottom of the U. Baby and breast must be very close together.

So much for problems of quantity and availability of mother's milk. Can the problem ever be one, not of how much and whether baby can get it, but rather of quality of human milk? Yes, indeed, although nothing like as often as is suspected!

Quality of milk supply

Mother's milk isn't, and isn't meant to be, a totally standardised product. What each mother produces does vary, within a wide range that is normal and adequate for her children's growth. Even severely malnourished women have been shown to produce milk that is not significantly different in quality from that of well-nourished mothers: if anything, it has slightly more fat, even when malnutrition is severe.[31] So there is simply no such thing as milk that is 'too watery' or 'too weak for baby to grow on'. Some of us are surprised when we first see mature human milk, for although colostrum may be creamy, our milk thereafter is a pale translucent blue, compared with the thick opaque milk of the cow. If milk is let stand, a thin layer of fat will collect at the top, just as it does in bottled non-homogenised cows' milk. When a baby suckles the breast, he receives differing amounts of fat at different feeds. A test analysis of the milk from one feed says nothing at all about the overall composition of a baby's diet.

However, if a baby's growth and development is poor and you're certain that it is not a problem of quantity, there are a few possibilities to explore in this area of quality, or composition.

Certain ingredients in maternal diet are reflected in milk, principally the types of fat and the water-soluble vitamins B and C, and these are important in the child's growth.

- Fats and oils: No researcher has yet come to any definite conclusion as to what the ideal balance of saturated and polyunsaturated fats in the mother's diet should be.[32] Yet fats in the diet are key components of enzymes, cellular membranes, the brain, the central nervous system, and the immune system, and may be important in the pathogenesis of some atopic disease states.[33] That being so, it seems sensible for mothers to include in their diet both kinds of fats: small quantities of animal fats, and less saturated vegetable oils, nuts and seeds. The average western fat intake is excessive, and nutritionists urge us not to use fatty spreads and dressings or, if we must, to use polyunsaturated margarines and oils. Yet margarines are a black sludge at one stage in manufacture, and contain colours, anti-oxidants, stabilisers, emulsifiers. In 1984 I suggested a simple way to improve the balance of polyunsaturates in spreads, while still supporting the dairy farmers, was to blend butter with an equal amount of cold pressed (chemical-free) sunflower or other oil. The resulting mix is easy to spread, free of colours, flavours and preservatives (so keep it in the fridge), and much more palatable. Such mixes have since become commercially available, but making your own is still possible. What is important is to increase one's intake of the long-chain polyunsaturates found in fish, in brains, in evening primrose and blackcurrant seed oils. Formulas contain almost none of these (and when they are added they may not work), yet they are crucial to the development of the central nervous system after birth. Getting rid of excess saturated fat in the mother's diet can also result in changes in infant stool habits and growth, and an end to recurrent mastitis in rare cases.

• Vitamin B complex and vitamin C vary according to maternal diet, and the need for both is greater in lactation and infancy. Check the maternal diet for adequacy in both (but do not overdose without specific reason and medical advice). B_{12} deficiency has caused failure to thrive in the children of a few vegetarian mothers;[34] and we have already seen that vitamin B_6 excess suppresses lactation. Extremes are dangerous.

• In a rare case, zinc deficiency in a baby, leading to failure to thrive, came about because of the absence of zinc from the mother's milk, a consequence of some defect in the transfer process.[35] The discovery that some women have sub-optimal levels of zinc in their milk may be due to the routine use of iron supplements, which interfere with zinc absorption in pregnancy and lactation. They should be prescribed only when needed.

• Iron deficiency in the mother may lead to low antibody levels in her milk; by permitting infection to develop more readily this could contribute to slow growth. Poor nutrition has the same effect.[36]

• Recent research[37] has detected the presence of various human growth factors in breast milk. Levels are high in pre-term milk, very high in colostrum and persist throughout lactation. Similar bovine growth factors are found in bovine colostrum, but not cows' milk or formulae based on cows' milk. This may help to explain why the children of severely malnourished (but not starving) mothers thrive while exclusively breastfed. Researchers have long been puzzled about how such mothers on extremely poor diets produce such healthy children. Theoretically, they cannot supply the calories that are theoretically necessary – but there they are, bonny breastfed babies until weaning begins. Perhaps some mothers' milk will be found to contain abnormally low levels of these growth factors or of some other component that stimulates growth or increases bioavailability of nutrients. Such studies are in the future.

• Data from slightly malnourished mothers have been used to support the contention that overnourished Western mothers should be able to sustain lactation more readily. However, there may prove to be differences between the malnutrition of scarcity (when too little food is available, but it is food to which the body is well adapted) and the malnutrition of affluence (when too little fresh food is eaten in conjunction with too much high-fat, high-protein, carbohydrate-rich snack food and the consumption of chemicals such as caffeine, nicotine, etc.). Rats put on diets similar to the latter have many difficulties, ranging from decreased fertility to increased abortion and defect in offspring and greater difficulty with lactation.[38] Theoretically again, the human mother is not greatly affected by such a diet – or I can find no scientist to state this possibility publicly. Yet avocados in excess are said to dry up goats! And for some weeks we lived with a young single mother whose diet included packets of chocolate biscuits, cans of soft drinks, and so on, as well as cigarettes. Her baby's bottom was very sore, and the baby was often very unsettled despite good care from both of us. (However, the baby thrived beautifully despite the constant loose stools; and I realised very often

lk imbalance is impossible: if a baby fails to empty one breast, at the next feed
k will begin with a higher fat content. In other words, it should not be possible
e too much or too little foremilk. This has apparently been demonstrated in
s in Western Australia, and Mike Woolridge years ago showed that fat
ntrations in milk varied greatly within a feed, and not necessarily in a direct
ase from start to finish.

et a few women with oversupply problems and slow-gaining babies have im-
ed baby's weight gain by allowing baby to suckle on one breast only at each feed
day or so, which seemed to reduce their supply until it was more in balance with
y's needs. I find it interesting that experienced breastfeeding counsellors and mid-
es, agree that some women with over-supply problems can improve weight gains
h one-breast feeding for a very short time usually.[40] If the baby's stomach is small,
d the mother has excessive milk, it is possible that large feeds of lactose-rich milk
uld result in severe colic because of the baby's inability to digest all the lactose.
is commonly occurs when the mother is determining the length of the feed at each
east by changing sides every five or ten minutes. The solution may be to increase the
fficiency of feeds while decreasing the volume of milk taken all at once, or increasing
he baby's total fat intake. What that means in practice is allowing the baby to feed
ntil she comes off the first breast, then offering the second breast only if the baby is
clearly ready for more. Then, if the baby wants to feed again in the next couple of
hours, the 'emptier' breast is offered (unless the baby insists on more volume, of
course). We have come to realise that the best option is to allow the baby to determine
this as well as the other aspects of breastfeeding: and often the result is one day of one-
sided feeding (the mother needs to express enough to prevent discomfort and mastitis)
followed by a return to two-breast feeding as the supply drops in response to the
decreased stimulation. Lactose-overload, by causing diarrhoea, can severely reduce
baby's weight gains. Properly managed, it rarely involves taking the child off the
breast. Even when it does, breastmilk can be either diluted to reduce the lactose load,
and/or fortified with additional fat from a second batch of expressed breastmilk that
has been allowed to stand and then skimmed.

Not relevant to this problem of poor weight gains, but perhaps indicating that such
distortions of milk composition might be possible, is the obverse of this problem:
women with obvious undersupply problems whose babies are gaining weight very
rapidly. In one well-documented case, a baby who was constantly at the breast gained
250-450 g each week, despite his mother's severe nipple pain (a consequence of
incorrect positioning). After three months of agony, and inhibition of let-down reflex,
the mother solved her nipple problems. Immediately she began to experience the let-
down reflex, her breasts began to feel full of milk, and her baby began to go two to
three hours between feeds; his weight gain dropped to 175-250 g each week. This
mother now considers that her child was thirsty (therefore constantly at the breast)
although receiving enough milk with high fat levels (hence the enormous weight gain).
He was a very vigorous, barracuda-type sucker – perhaps such babies are capable, like
some breast pumps, of removing excessive mammary lipids not usually available for
nursing?[41]

how important breastfeeding can be as a gob-stopper.)

● Too many oligosaccharides? (complex carbohydrates) (hindm
maintains that some lactating women produce too many of thes the mi
rates in their milk.[39] Because the baby cannot digest them, they ca to ha
causes inadequate weight gain. He did not recommend weanin studie
whether maternal diet might affect the levels of such carbohydr conce
becomes another wait-and-see area of research. incre

● Some drugs can affect infant growth, and this is well discuss prov
Riordan, and other authors. Social drugs – alcohol, cigarettes, mari for
and many medications, will be present in milk in quantities suffici bab
baby; poor growth can be one such effect. Over-the-counter medicatio wi
investigated. Many medications for cold-sufferers, for example, cont wi
ines. A mother who cuts back smoking may see improved weight gain w an
● Good (i.e. nutritious) foods that the mother eats may also affect infan co
baby is to be sensitive to them. This is a highly individual matter, so lac T
should not avoid good foods on the basis of another person's experience. b
are reacting to substances in mother's milk often come eagerly to the b e
minute or two later pull away and scream loudly. (This may be the baby's
a too-sudden rush of milk, which makes baby splutter and choke, but tha
such behaviour is obvious.) Some babies learn to refuse milk altogether on
mother's allergen load is very high. This seems more common in the days be
struation, when prostaglandin levels (which affect gut function) may be elevat
are also sometimes very 'sicky' babies, constantly possetting or even projectil
ing their feeds. Naturally this affects their weight gain, as does the frequent s
that often accompanies colic. One thing should be emphasised: if a baby is resp
to what is in mother's milk, she will almost certainly have a great deal of t
coping with artificial substitutes. So don't consider weaning; instead, investigat
possible problem substances and eliminate those from the maternal diet and env
ment as a first step. Simply keeping a detailed no-cheating diary of maternal
infant behaviour and the baby's stool pattern for a week can identify many problems

The relative balance of components in human milk

Theoretically, and almost certainly in the majority of mothers, human milk is a
fluid of remarkably predictable and stable composition. Yet it sometimes seems that a
few women with massive milk supplies are temporarily producing milk with too little
fat for good growth. If the baby has a large enough stomach, he or she may quickly
take in enough to feel full and stop feeding, yet without adequate fat intake, the baby's
weight gain will be poor. When the mother's oversupply is reduced, the fat content is
more appropriate for the baby's needs.

This has been described in terms of foremilk and hindmilk, terms which have
become quite unhelpful. Some understood that the milk "at the back of the breast" was
fat-rich and tried emptying the breast to get to it. Others talked as though the breast
made two different products, one good and one inferior. Theoretically foremilk-

There are three distinct problems being discussed in this chapter. The first is the question of real or imagined under-supply of short duration; the second, the slow-gaining breastfed baby; and the third, the genuine case of failure to thrive. Only in this latter case is there any immediate cause for concern, and perhaps for immediate supplementation with other foods, before careful investigation of the basis of the problem (despite the risks of supplementing before discovering the nature of the problem). In most cases of low supply or of slow-gaining babies, the problem lies in the breastfeeding process itself and is readily solved.

Many problems can be purely the result of the inaccurate information purveyed in commercially inspired literature, with its talk of "when breastfeeding fails or is insufficient" and talk of the need for rest and relaxation. Breastfeeding is a natural process. While it can go wrong, and is influenced by many variables, such an essential survival process is unlikely to fail easily. The role of stress in the mother, for instance, has been much emphasised in Western literature. This may date from Truby King's "do not let anyone speak to you or worry you in any way while you are feeding baby. Just the effort of conversation sometimes lessens the flow of milk."[42] It is still present, though in a more moderate form, in modern texts. Yet around the world women succeed at breastfeeding in the direst of circumstances. In war, breastfeeding rates rise. Physical factors such as inadequate suckling stimulus (due to mother or infant problems) or physical fatigue are more likely to be significant than such psychological ones, in average women. Our constant insistence on total relaxation as a necessary precondition for success may prove to be both inaccurate and counterproductive. By setting unrealistic standards, we create destructive anxiety, and a negative feedback cycle begins. The belief that the stress of Philip's hospitalisation and surgery might reduce my ability to feed my two-month-old Elizabeth added significantly to my anxiety levels in 1979. Needless to say, I had plenty of milk because my activity was reduced, and had to feed frequently when we returned home to normal workloads. So much for psychological stress!

So the first task in assessing a slow-gaining breastfed baby is to assess the breastfeeding process itself. Useful protocols for the management of this problem are now available;[43] organised history taking such as is provided via the Lactation Institute's forms is strongly recommended.

There have been, and will be, mothers who are unable to breastfeed despite the best help possible and their desire to do so. Until the day when human milk is available for their babies, they must use formula. That is what formula is designed for. They should do so with our support and encouragement, and with detailed advice about, and help with, the many difficulties and problems of artificial feeding. Remember what was said about the interaction between infection and nutrition (see p. 24). If any baby starves because of some obsession with exclusive breastfeeding, the immunological benefits of breast milk will be outweighed by the damage to the baby's immune system because of malnutrition. Now that breastfeeding has become the 'in' thing once again, we don't want to create a class of social pariahs. We breastfeeding mothers have been through all that ourselves. Would we really want to make another woman feel that she should feed her baby only in her bedroom, this time because she's bottle-feeding? We can't know how it came about or what grief it may cause her, so let's accept and support her as just another mother trying to do her best for her child, as most of us do most of the time. We will be less likely to sit in judgement on other women if we know more about the complex nature of breastfeeding problems and the difficulties many mothers, no less caring than us, experience in their sometimes heroic efforts to succeed. And if we talk to bottle-feeding mothers in friendly accepting ways, we may be able to let them know that their problem was simply mismanaged, as many are, thus encouraging them to learn more and perhaps try again. And avoiding the angry backlash silly statements always cause.

NOTES
CHAPTER 4: TOO LITTLE MILK?

[1] Walker,G., "Midwives and breastfeeding – what more can they possibly do?" Proceedings, ICM 20th International Congress, Sydney, September 1984.

[2] Said to me on innumerable occasions, although the literature makes it clear that women are not breastfeeding as long as they want to: see Ellis, D.J.; Hewett, R., "Breastfeeding: motivation and outcome", *J. Biosoc. Sci.* 1984, 16, 81-8

[3] Minchin, M., *About Breast and Nipple Problems* (NMAA, 1981).

[4] Howie, P. W.; Houston, M J., "How long should a breast feed last?" *Early Hum. Dev*, 1981, 5, 71-7.

[5] Whitfield et al, "Validity of test weighing as a measure of the intake of breastfed infants", *Arch. Dis. Child.* (1981) 56, 919-21; Hartmann, P E; Saint, L., "Measurement of milk yield in women", *J. Pediatr. Gastroent. Nutr.* 1984, 3, 270-4.

[6] A valid research tool, test weighing is a harmful routine procedure.

[7] Butte, N F. et al, "Human milk intake and growth in exclusively breastfed infants", *J Pediatr.* 1984, 104, 187-94.

[8] Saint, L. et al, "The yield and nutrient content of colostrum and milk of women giving birth to one month post-partum", *Br. J. Nutr.* 1984, 52, 87-95.

[9] Prentice, A.; Prentice, A. M., "Unilateral breast dysfunction in lactating Gambian women", *Ann. Trop. Pediatr.* 1984, 4, 19-23.

[10] Neifert, M. R. et al, "Failure of lactogenesis associated with placental retention", *Am. J. Obstet. Gynecol.* 1981, 140, 477-8.

[11] Houston, M. J., "Home support for the breastfeeding mother", in Houston (ed.) *Maternal and Infant Health Care,* (Churchill Livingstone, 1984), p. 53-4

[12] Neville, M. C.; Neifert, M. R., *Lactation: physiology, nutrition and breastfeeding,* (Plenum Press, 1983), p. 315.

[13] ibid., Chapter 13; articles by Peralta et al; Croxalto et al; Diaz et al in *Contraception* 1983, 27, 1, 1-38. Danish researchers argue that the change to progestogens and IUDs, and away from high-dose combined contraceptives, may be partly responsible for the resurgence in breastfeeding. See Hilden, J. et al, "Contraceptives and the new trend in breastfeeding: a causal connexion?", *J. Trop. Pediatr.* 1983, 29, 2, 40-4.

[14] Frantz, K., "Slow weight gain", in Riordan, J (ed.) *A Practical Guide to Breastfeeding,* (C. V. Mosbey and Co., St Louis 1983) p. 223-4

[15] Martin, R. H.; Oakey, R. E., "The role of antenatal oestrogen in post-partum human lactogenesis: evidence from oestrogen-deficient pregnancies", *Clin. Endocrinol.* 1982, 17, 4,

336-8; Anderson, A. N. et al, Suppressed prolactin but normal neurophysin levels in cigarette-smoking breastfeeding women. *Clin. Endocrinol.* 1982, 17, 4, 363-8.

[16] Many mothers of what turn out to be food-intolerant babies notice an association between breast refusal and infant distress in the pre-menstruum.

[17] Hartmann, P. E.; Prosser, C. G., "Physiological basis of longitudinal changes in human milk yield and composition", *Federation Proceedings,* 1984, 43, 9, 2452.

[12] Neville, M.C.; Neifert, M.R., *Lactation: physiology, nutrition and breastfeeding,* (Plenum Press,1983), p.315.

[18] Gezelle, H.D. et al, "Metaclopromide and breast milk", *Eur. J. Obstet. Gynecol. Reprod. Biol.* 1983, 15, 31-6; Lancet, 1981, i, 1175-7.

[19] O'Leary, R.M., "Sulpiride improves inadequate lactation", *Br. Med. J.* 1982, 285, 843-6.

[20] Neifert MR, Seacat JM, Jobe WE, "Lactation failure due to insufficient glandular development of the breast", *Pediatrics* (1985) 76: 823-8.

[21] Wood, C.B.; Walker-Smith,J.; *Mackeith's Infant Feeding and Feeding Difficulties.* (Churchill Livingstone, 1981), p.70

[22] "Truby King babies are fed four-hourly from birth, with few exceptions, and they do not have night feeds." Truby King, M. *Mothercraft.* (Whitcombe and Tombs, Melbourne 17th impression, no date but post-1938), p. 4.

[23] Miller, R.A., "Factors influencing lactation", *Arch. Dis. Child,* 1952, 27, 187-94.

[24] Frantz, K., "Ineffective suckling as a frequent cause of failure to thrive in the totally breastfed infant", in Freier, S.; Eidelman, A. E., *Human Milk: its biological and social value.* (Excerpta Medica, Amsterdam, 1981)

[25] Frantz, K., "Techniques for successfully managing nipple problems and reluctant nurser in the early post-partum period", in Freier and Eidelman, op. cit.

[26] Riordan, J. (ed.) reference 14, p. 178-9.

[27] Lawrence, R. A., *Breastfeeding: a guide for the medical profession,* (C. V. Mosby, St. Louis, 1980 edition), p. 177-86.

[28] Neuro-developmental Treatment Association, Inc., P O Box 14613, Chicago, IL. 60614, USA.

[29] Reference 14, ch 9.

[30] Dr. J.E. Aldred, Community Paediatric Practice Seminar, Werribee, Victoria, May 1982. Copy available from Victorian Health Department.

[31] Whitehead,R.G. *Maternal diet, breastfeeding capacity and lactational infertility.* (United Nations University, Tokyo, 1983); P.C. Marin Spring et al, "Fat and energy content of breast milk of malnourished and well-nourished women, Brazil 1982", *Ann. Trop. Pediatr.* 1985, 5(2) 83-7.

[32] Reference 12, pp. 221-2, 232-3

[33] Cant, A J., "Breastfeeding and eczema", *New Generation,* 1984, 3, 4, 29-30.

[34] Davis JR et al. "Nutritional vitamin B_{12} deficiency in infants", *Am. J. Dis. Child.* 1981; 135:566-7.

[35] Zimmerman, A. et al, "Acrodematitis in breastfed premature infants: evidence for a defect in mammary zinc secretion", *Pediatrics* 1982, 69, 176-83.

[36] Miranda, R. et al, "Effects of maternal nutritional status on immunological substances in human colostrum and milk", *Am. J. Clin. Nutr.*1983, 37, 632-40.

[37] Gaull, G E et al, "Significance of growth modulators in human milk", *Pediatrics,* 1985, 75, Supplement,142-6.

[38] Conversation with Dr R Jones, at the Metabolic Research Unit, Radcliffe Infirmary, Oxford, Nov. 1983.

[39] Correspondence with a mother who did not wish the gastroenterologist named.

[40] Correspondence with Chloe Fisher, September 1984. Chloe stated that at least one European gastroenterologist considered two-breast feeding to be the usual cause of fluid stools and abdominal discomfort in well breastfed babies. Does this explain the pre-occupation with 'over-feeding' so notable in manuals a few decades ago? See also Cox, S. G., "Breastfeeding one side only each feed: a solution for the crying baby", *Proceedings, ICM 20th International Congress, Sydney, September 1984.*

[41] Ferris, A M.; Jensen, R G., "Sampling and determination of lipids in human milk", *J. Pediatr. Gastroent. Nutr.* 1984, 3, 111.

[42] Reference 22, p. 65.

[43] Walker,M.; Driscoll, J.W., *The slow-gaining breastfed baby: assessment and management guidelines.* (Available from Lactation Associates, 254 Conant Rd., Weston, Mass. 02193, USA.) These need to be used not as bibles but as beginnings – a handy basis for organising our thoughts, and a stimulus to critical analysis of the situation.

FURTHER READING 1998

• Hartmann P, Sherriff J, Kent J, "Maternal nutrition and the regulation of milk synthesis", *Proc. Nutrition. Soc.* (1995) 54: 379-89.

• Purnell S, Purnell K, "Infant regulation of breastmilk intakes and the effects on milk supply and composition", *LRC Topics in Breastfeeding* (1995) set 7.

• Daly SEJ, Kent JC, Owens RA, Hartmann PE, "Frequency and degree of milk removal and the short-term control of human milk synthesis", *Exp. Physiol.* (1996) 81: 861-75.

• Daly SEJ, Hartmann PE, "Infant demand and milk supply", parts 1 & 2, *J. Hum. Lact.* (1995) 11: 21-37.

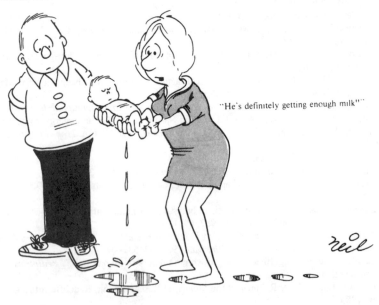

4.5. Courtesy of Neil Matterson, from *Is he biting again?* (Marion Books, 1984)

5. NIPPLE PROBLEMS

Sore nipples... are almost entirely avoidable but are still common. Not only do they drive many mothers to give up suckling but, where they are endured, they may 'unhelp' her feelings about the baby because of faulty interpretations. The attendant may say "He is a chewer" (i.e. the baby's fault not the nurse's) or worse, "He is a biter". This phrase may make the mother suspect that the baby does not love her or may even faintly suggest to her that hers is a horrible child at an early age.

- Mavis Gunther, in *Breastfeeding and the Mother*
(Ciba Foundation Symposium, 1976), p. 149

'Too little milk' is the most common reason for untimely weaning. But 'sore nipples' is the reason a significant number of women give for stopping breastfeeding. This description can cover anything from mild discomfort to perhaps the most intense pain possible outside torture chambers. How common is serious nipple pain? I'm not aware of studies investigating this scientifically, other than one UK study which was looking at the effect of restricted suckling times.[1] Their conclusion was that such practice made no difference to nipple problems – the incidence was 33 or 38 per cent during the first six weeks, or 6-12 per cent for cracked nipples. (This seems unacceptably high to me, and to other experienced counsellors.)

One would think that solutions to nipple problems would have been discovered long ago, because the pain they cause can be so unbearable. What was my experience in 1976? As a new mother, I relied on nursing staff to show me how to handle and feed my baby. This they did, at considerable length. Philip had been kept from me for 16 hours before he first suckled, and feeds were four hourly and not at night. By day two, my nipples were slightly sore. By day three, my breasts were rock hard and Philip could only suck on the nipples. That day I pointed out to the midwives how squashed my nipples looked after each feed – flattened, with a distinct stripe across it. 'Of course they do, dear, lots of women's nipples look like that, that's nothing to worry about.' By day five, I was beginning to feel a sharp pain stabbing when he first went to the breast. 'That's just tension, dear, and fair-skinned women like you often get nipples that are a bit tender.' By day seven, Philip had contracted thrush – very common in bottle-feeding nurseries, and regarded as fairly harmless. I was given medication for him, highly coloured and flavoured Nystatin drops. No mention of treating my sore nipples. I went home with very sore nipples, and battled on for three months of pain, fluctuating from agony which made me shriek to generalised soreness which made wearing even silk very uncomfortable. Naturally I was religious in following the

advice then given by the doctors I consulted, and by NMAA: keep nipples dry, lots of sunlight, use anhydrous lanolin, change positions while feeding, and so on. Perhaps that prevented the problem from becoming worse – I have seen women with bleeding cracks virtually all around the nipple – but it did not make it better.
Is that an unusual case? I think not. What was unusual was that I solved my problems, and had pain-free nipples, within *two days* of finding Mavis Gunther's book, *Infant Feeding*.[2] My local clinic sister was as astonished as I to find that there are specific, clear-cut and quite distinct types of sore nipples, for which specific cures worked like a charm (yet Gunther's ideas have been in print since the 1950s). As I have spelt out some of these details in a booklet written for NMAA,[3] I shall incorporate sections of that in this chapter. I regret having to do so twenty years after my own agony, but I still see women suffering just as I did. And there is neither need nor excuse for it.

Like many women, I would probably have had a little generalised soreness or hypersensitivity, lasting for a few days, until my breasts and nipples became fully protractile and adjusted to the new experience of a suckling child. This temporary initial soreness is partly the result of increased sensitivity and responsiveness to stimuli, which usually disappears within a week or two. It does recur at the beginning of each lactation, and similar soreness can be experienced if a woman continues to nurse a toddler after becoming pregnant, so perhaps it is at least partly of hormonal origin. Exercises to improve nipple protractility[4] have been suggested to hasten resolution of this problem, though I am not aware of any scientific studies evaluating this and there are risks of damage to sensitive tissue. One term used for this is 'nipple stretch pain'. At present I refer to this as initial hypersensitivity, as Roger Short's elegant paper showed that there is a natural increase in nipple sensitivity in the last weeks of pregnancy, peaking around day 3 postpartum, and then declining over time.

My troubles began with that 'stripe' across my flattened nipple. Had the staff been better educated, they would have diagnosed this instantly as *positional sore nipple*,[2] helped me to correct the way I was holding Philip, and that would have ended the problem – as it did three months later. In Chapter 3 I have outlined the basics of correct positioning. This cannot be overemphasised, and should be a basic part of medical and nursing education and refresher courses.

'Cracks', or nipple fissures,[2] will follow if positional soreness goes uncorrected. They may also be the result of using suction breast pumps, which are too often used ignorantly, as though dragging harder on the piston handle will increase milk outflow. A fissure is an opening or break in the skin, either on the face of the nipple or where it joins the areola. This fissure may be very fine, visible only when magnified, like a paper cut, or it may be obvious and bleeding. In either case it will cause intense pain because of the rich supply of nerve fibres in the nipple. Some mothers feel as though the baby is biting and naturally begin to resent both the 'aggressive' baby, and those who tell them what wonderful closeness breastfeeding promotes.

Fissures are commonly slow to heal if they become infected with thrush.[2] Here again, my case illustrates the then-usual treatment, which was that an infected baby was treated while the mother's nipples were ignored. At six weeks, after three courses of Nystatin drops, I tried gentian violet (0.5% in *aqueous* solution), and this cleared up Philip's mouth. But I had to treat my nipples before the problem stopped recurring. Professionals seemed to expect a nipple infection to look like the white plaques of fungus in Philip's mouth. This ignores the differences between the two environments: the baby's low excretion of antibodies in saliva, constant moisture and warmth, compared with skin with full adult defences boosted by constant flushing with human milk, with its antifungal properties. So thrush on the nipple commonly presents as slight itchiness and inflammation and tiny white traces in fissures or crevices on the nipple. It can progress to severe and obvious thrush infection, with intense inflammation, itchiness and skin flaking, and seems most likely to after a course of creams containing cortisone. What is more, it may be involved in producing mastalgia –"severe, burning, stinging pain which radiates through the breast and persists after the feeding" – as Neifert indicated.[5]

At this stage, many and varied creams are prescribed, sometimes by doctors, more often by friends who say brand x is wonderful. Nipple treatments are discussed later. What should be said here is that they, too, are a common cause of nipple pain and damage, ranging from irritation to inflammation so severe that clothes are unbearable. This is generically termed *dermatitis*,[2] or skin inflammation. It can also be also be a reaction to detergent residues in clothes, soaps, shampoos, rough or synthetic or chemically treated (e.g. 'sanitised') fabrics, Lactaid drops or oral gels given to babies, antigen in infant saliva, latex allergy, or chlorine-dipped nipple shields. To quote Gunther again, "This condition looks like a slight or definite redness of the nipple. The distinguishing features are that the mother suffering it feels pain, not only as the baby takes the breast, as with positional and fissure types of soreness, but for as long as the baby is at the breast. It differs too in that the nipple is tender if touched with the back of the hand."

So how did I solve my problems? I stopped using anhydrous lanolin – the dermatitis decreased. I used gentian violet – the thrush was gone, and the fissure free to heal. I positioned Philip correctly – the fissure healed over, and the positional stripe disappeared. This all took two days, after three months of agony.

Because of the way the fissure healed, a large crevice was left on the breast. It became the site of recurrent minor thrush attacks. If that nipple began to feel tender and irritated, I learnt to apply aqueous gentian violet. This washes off in the shower, fading to a mauve. There would then always be a tiny adherent flake, almost like dandruff, which remained a dark purple and came away after a couple of days. Try to shift this earlier, and it would cause soreness, even bleeding. I assumed that this was thrush because it was never there at other times; it always coincided with a fungal infection elsewhere in the family (tinea, vaginal thrush, etc.), and it was destroyed by gentian violet. However, I cannot prove that it was. Yet it is clear both from NMAA literature and an excellent monograph by Kay Hoover and Lisa Amir in the Lactation Consultant Series,[6] that thrush is both common and persistent, and is implicated not only in skin irritations but also in gut disturbances in mother and baby alike. In fact there are those who would see it as a major cause not only of sore bottoms, but also of food intolerance problems.[7] Obviously if this becomes accepted, it should end the casual attitude towards treatment of the whole family, and advice about prevention (low sugar diet, use of lactobacillus, care in wiping bottoms from front to back, etc.) will become routine practice. After all, the cycle may be as shown below

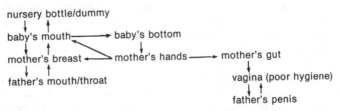

This may go on, literally for years, unless it happens that the immune systems of all family members are synchronised to destroy it simultaneously. Thrush is one of those opportunistic infections, it waxes and wanes with the individual's state of health and nutrition, but being a fungus is remarkably persistent. No one likes to talk about these things, and there are often different standards of hygiene among family members. Many women complain that they can't get their partners to take this sort of problem seriously, hence they go on suffering reinfection. In treating family members, pay attention to other objects likely to be contaminated. The discovery that 44% of dummies randomly tested were colonised with thrush[8] lends point to older perceptions of them as dirty objects!

Then there are 'white spots' on the nipple – a subject that has been raised here in Australia and in the UK,[9] usually by women who find that bouts of mastitis seemed to coincide with the appearance of white spots. Although they occur without causing mastitis, these white spots are discussed in the next chapter.

Gunther reports one final type of nipple soreness of which I have no first-hand knowledge: psychosomatic sore nipples, more recently classified as nipple vasospasm. "In this condition, the mother feels pain in the nipple when she feeds her baby and for as long as the baby is at the breast. When the nipples are examined they blanch, usually the whole face going white because of the shutting down of the blood supply. Sometimes while they are still being inspected, the blood supply is restored and the nipples can be watched becoming a mulberry colour. The mother who has this very real trouble usually has some fear or unhappy association connected with breasts or breast feeding. If someone helping her says, 'I think you must have something worrying you about breast feeding,' the mother can usually say immediately what the trouble is, such as that her mother died of cancer of the breast, that she knew someone who had suffered from an abscess of the breast or sometimes that she is unable to face feeding the new baby in front of her older children. A great fear, even without foundation, cannot be dispersed in time for the mother to feed successfully. A lesser one, if understood by the mother, can melt away and the soreness is gone."

Gunther concluded that "Most mothers with psychosomatic soreness are unable to feed their babies for long. It is best to offer them the means of stopping easily."[2]

However, reports from the National Childbirth Trust[10] and from Australian lactation consultants are more hopeful. While I for one experienced blanched nipples when feeding Philip, these were rare after I learnt how to position him correctly. For me they always indicated compression, and warmth and massage brought the blood back to them (there was no psychological component). Women who come to dread feeding or who are sensitive to cold[11] can have vasospasm triggered quite apart from feeding times; the typical triphasic colour change of the nipples is diagnostic. Psychotherapy might even prove to be useful. Some doctor lactation consultants are now prescribing nifedipine,[12] and this may well be justified in extreme and recurrent cases. However, prevention is always more important than medication. In virtually all reported cases not obviously triggered by cold or compression, severely damaged nipples preceded the development of the vasospasm. Preventing nipple damage may thus prevent some cases of vasospasm. It also seems reasonable to try topical treatments before systemic ones of unknown safety: a sample size of five mothers is not sufficient to assure us that there are no problems with powerful medication affecting the whole body. In addition, drugs do not tell us why such conditions arise. An interesting hypothesis by an Australian IBCLC who suffered this complaint, Lesley Heap, is that vasospasm is now more common because intrapartum whole blood loss is less often replaced, and so circulation is poor and peripheries colder. This could readily be tested.

However, what can we do about vasospasm here and now? If triggered by

1) cold: thermographic studies show clearly that nipples are often cold. Try the new Swedish breastwarmers[13] and any other rapid re-warming, and keep the breasts and the body in general warm (wear a hat!);

2) compression: fix the feeding technique or address the oral problem;

3) conditioned reflex responses after severe and persistent pain: explain the nature of conditioned reflexes; keep nipples warm – all after solving the underlying problems if they still exist; work on biofeedback.

In every case a full history is needed to explain to the mother the genesis of the problem she now has. Understanding can have its own curative power. In every case suspicion of thrush is warranted, as is any other cause of dermatitis: some women experience severe nipple pain with no apparent external signs other than slight inflammation, and gentian violet or mild hydrocortisone as appropriate (see below) can work wonders.

To conclude, then, nipple pain has specific, distinct causes, "quite clear cut and for the most part avoidable. Their exact diagnosis is made by looking carefully, and this is part of good practice as in other branches of medicine. Some people speak of cracks, but this slovenly word is used only by those who have not troubled to see what the injury is."[2] Amen, Dr. Gunther.

Another form of nipple soreness can be self-inflicted. Idiotic practices like the use of baby-wipes containing all sorts of chemicals and alcohol are not unknown to those who counsel mothers. Our neurosis about hygiene causes some problems (I think some people would be happier if breasts could be boiled!). As well, over-enthusiastic or just plain rough handling of breasts and nipples by partners cannot be recommended, either as sensual pleasure or as contribution to painless breastfeeding. And the abrasive effects of five o'clock shadow mimic that of sandpaper, not something recommended on delicate erogenous zones. Yet men who would not dream of sanding down a penis may get offended at being told such facts. Sometimes women declare their breasts taboo zones while feeding solely because they cannot communicate to their partners how to handle them sensitively. Men need to be aware that the sensitivity of breasts and nipples can be very much heightened during lactation; that what was once delicious may now be painful; that more gentle handling can produce equal or greater pleasure.

Knowing what caused the problem of nipple pain is half the battle. NMAA makes various suggestions which can ease discomfort and perhaps hasten healing, but these are no substitute for correct diagnosis of a specific problem. I will not repeat all those NMAA suggestions, but select a few of the more important. When your nipples hurt:

• Stimulate your milk flow – warmth, relaxation techniques, music, gentle breast massage, or using the hot jar technique (see p.154) before attaching baby. This shortens the period of summon-up suckling, which is more energetic.

• Use other measures to help with letdown – for example, breast massage, oxytocin, small alcoholic drink, and so on. Whatever works. Needless to say, in this case nipple stimulation probably won't!

• Never allow baby to find his own way on to the breast and nipple, or be distracted and pull away/look around while hanging on, or pull off the nipple himself. A finger in the mouth between the gums breaks the hold, but watch out for the baby with instant reflexes who lunges back at the breast and clamps his gums on the nipple: be sure to move out of range. Never press down on the breast or the baby's chin – he will reflexively bite down to hold on harder as he feels his grip slipping.

• Keep nipples clean and moisturised. Sunlight in small doses (avoid sunburn) may help by increasing vitamin D levels in the skin. Drying out skin is definitely not recommended in this era of the proven benefits of moist wound healing. However, there is nothing wrong with removing excessive surface wetness before applying an emollient, which is not at all the same thing as cooking nipples with hairdryers or ray lamps. Pesticide-free anhydrous lanolin such as Lansinoh is recommended to expedite healing once damage has occurred: the sceptics should try this for themselves on any painful dry skin. Research in progress suggests that there are clear reductions in healing time when Lansinoh is used on fissures due to trauma. (I confess that in one recent case I not only applied Lansinoh, but also a carefully positioned piece of hypoallergenic tape to hold the edges of the fissure together between feeds – with great results. Watch the literature for news of hydrogel use and other new techniques.)

• You may feel that you have to stop feeding from that breast for a feed or two, despite your increased risk of true infection and abscess formation if you stop baby suckling.[14] This is sometimes inevitable if the breast is just too painful. But you can help to facilitate flow from the damaged breast by holding the baby to feed on the other, with either the Kaneson pump or a wide-mouthed jar over the painful breast, and when baby stimulates milk flow on one side, the gentlest of suction will relax the nipple sphincter and allow milk to flow from the painful nipple.

These techniques should not be necessary for more than a few days at most, once the problem is properly identified, unless there is some physical or psychological problem not yet diagnosed. (An obvious one is the mother with very large nipples and a baby with a very small mouth. Tincture of time and TLC are the only cures for such physical mismatches. Fortunately babies' mouths grow very rapidly.)

Before leaving the topic of nipple pain, it might be as well to emphasise that the foregoing are the usual, minor problems of breastfeeding – minor unless mismanaged, that is. But there are other conditions which can cause nipple problems. Herpes viruses can infect the breast, and I have seen one areolar lesion that looked very much like herpes. (The mother's and father's history was positive, the father actually developed a mouth lesion a week before the breast problem developed.) Unfortunately the doctor thought the testing was too expensive and took too long, so this was not confirmed. LLLI advisers are reluctant to advise weaning a baby who has thus been exposed to herpes, as the mother is making antibodies which will be excreted in her milk, and at present that is the best medicine available. The child will almost certainly have been infected before the problem is diagnosed, or might be even afterwards, as his mother still has to care for him. Medical advice must be sought if herpes is suspected, but breastfeeding should be continued.

Another medical condition involving the nipple and areola is eczema, or atopic dermatitis. This is discussed in the older books.[15] I have known many mothers with such problems, which prove remarkably persistent unless the mothers are willing to find causes and eliminate them, whether from their diet or environment. Steroid creams are often prescribed, despite their hazards, to enable the mother to persevere with feeding. Where eczema has occurred, the babies have been older than six months, or both mother and baby were food-intolerant. The inflamed area usually corresponds to the area covered by the child's mouth: was it antigens in saliva, or relative pH, or some factor that sets up the original inflammation? Some mothers have found partial relief by bathing the area immediately after every feed in mild alkaline solutions, as mothers do when teething babies cause irritation.[16] This is another condition requiring some proper investigation and not getting it. Psoriasis too can involve the breast and nipple and make feeding difficult.

Then there are really serious problems, such as Paget's disease of the nipple, a form of cancer which may present as a small, almost insignificant lesion on the nipple that does not heal and which is often accompanied by dimpling of the breast tissue. For this reason, it is essential that even apparently minor unexplained problems should be seen by a competent doctor. Many capital cities have Breast Clinics geared towards cancer detection; these can be useful in reassuring the mother that her problem is not serious. Unfortunately, though, so little is known about the lactating breast that the advice can sometimes be unhelpful as far as breastfeeding is concerned. Weaning is suggested quite inappropriately at times; and the value of the breastfeeding relationship for both baby and family can be under-appreciated.

Nipple creams and lotions

There are all manner of creams, lotions and potions available for use on nipples. Many of these products are simply moisturisers with a few fancy additives and no scientific basis for effectiveness. Others have active ingredients which may or may not do what you want them to do (and may do things you'd rather they didn't). Nipple preparations can smell and taste repellent, clog pores, make nipples soggy and fragile, cause allergic reactions, impair the skin's natural resistance to infection, and have the baby eating all manner of ingredients never intended for human consumption. But does this mean that the only thing that should ever be applied to a breast is breastmilk or a baby?

What, if anything, should be used on nipples? Obviously, only substances that cannot harm mother or baby, or disrupt the breastfeeding relationship. There are some risks involved in the use of any chemicals, but the decision is always a matter of evaluating benefits and risks, both in general and in particular.

Nipple skin is thinner than skin on other parts of the body, and like the inside of your mouth it lacks an outer dry keratin layer. Friction from poor attachment and from repeated wet/dry exposure with breastfeeding can strip natural moisture from the skin, leaving it dehydrated and vulnerable to further breakdown and/or infection. Putting products on nipples has not been shown to prevent sore nipples or to do much for the tenderness many women experience in the first week. But when the nipple is painful, abraded, cracked, irritated or infected a suitable product may give relief, aid healing and enable continued breastfeeding.

Nipple preparations come as creams, lotions, solutions and ointments. Creams, by definition, are multi-ingredient emulsified products and most contain water. Although they may give temporary relief, moisture can't be added to dry skin from the outside without making matters worse (think about what happens if you keep licking dry lips). Lotions are generally just runnier creams, with the same problems. Solutions are active ingredients in a liquid solvent base, to be sprayed, painted or wiped on the nipple. If the base is evaporative it is probably alcohol, which will dry the skin even more. Ointments such as anhydrous lanolin or petroleum jelly have a thicker, greasier consistency. They add a protective water-resistant layer to the skin surface, helping the skin retain its own internal moisture (which normally would evaporate), and also protect the skin from surface wetness. Obviously this could be a good thing where skin was dehydrated or cracking; a bad thing where it was not needed.

What, then, are some of the risks of nipple products?

In the mother, dermatitis may develop because of sensitivity to some of the ingredients.[17] Vitamin E (alpha-tocopherol) is a common ingredient in creams and can produce both immediate allergic urticaria and delayed dermatitis.[18] Allergic reactions to tea-tree oil are becoming more prevalent, particularly in people allergic to grevillea or poison ivy.[19] Antifungal creams may produce an irritant dermatitis on skin already damaged by thrush, with irritation and dryness persisting after the thrush has cleared.[17] Other likely causes of sensitivity are fragrance mix and preservatives. Lanolin used to be a problem[20] because of allergy to the detergent residues and wool alcohols, but these have been removed to varying degrees of purity in the new modified lanolins.[21] The first of these on the market, Lansinoh, has had no reactivity reported despite intensive efforts to identify any such case.

Anything that has to be cleaned off before feeds may damage the nipple physically.[22] Alcohol, used as a solvent in some products will dry the nipple epithelial cells[2] and alter the normal osmotic balance by removing natural oils and sweat. Hot water, soaps and shampoos can also degrease the skin. Products which neutralise the natural acidity of the skin leave the cells more vulnerable to infection because bacteria thrive on alkalinised skin. Alteration of the delicate balance between skin micro-organisms may[23] also lead to an overgrowth of one or other, e.g. thrush.

An additional danger, for both mother and baby, is that some products contain quaternary ammonium compounds (such as cetrimide) which are supposedly antibacterial but are no longer used in veterinary medicine because it was realised that by changing the charge on the bacteria, they enable them to cling more avidly to the skin. (Skin normally repulses them.)[24] First aid creams containing these compounds have been found to actually delay healing. Skin is not intended to be sterilised, so products that provide antibacterial, antifungal and anti-inflammatory agents create a highly unnatural situation, and 'backlash' is not uncommon[25] once they are discontinued.

In the baby, taste or smell may cause breast refusal; I recommend you rub a product into the back of your hand and lick it off before applying it to your nipples. Anaesthetic agents may cause numbness of the lips, so that baby cannot suckle. Certain ingredients may cause problems for the baby, should the mother fail to clean off residues of the cream.[26] Elevated vitamin E levels from nipple preparations have been detected in the serum of breastfed babies.[27] There is a reported case of a baby with diarrhoea from aloe vera ointment used on the nipples.[28] Peanut oil in nipple creams and infant formula has recently been shown to cause sensitisation and anaphylaxis. Some ingredients may worsen baby's jaundice.[29] If the cream contains antibiotic agents, there is the risk of breeding resistant gut organisms in the baby.[30] These could cause major systemic disease at a later date. (Because of the different gut environment a partially breastfed baby would be more at risk of this than a fully breastfed one.)

How then do you decide whether to use, and if so, which nipple preparation? This requires you to identify first of all what your problem is and what is causing it. If a nipple preparation is indicated for treatment or relief, what is the most suitable product, what is in it, and what are the risks and benefits?

The active ingredients of nipple preparations can be roughly classified as follows:

- Moist wound healing agents – products which create a moisture barrier to prevent scab formation and facilitate healing
- General healing agents – e.g. vitamins, plant extracts.
- Antiseptic agents – chemicals to prevent the multiplication of micro-organisms.
- Antibiotic agents – drugs derived from living cells which do the same.
- Anti-inflammatory agents – agents to reduce inflammation.
- Anti-fungal agents – compounds that destroy or inhibit fungal growth.

- Analgesic/anaesthetic agents – pain-killing substances, or substances that prevent the body from registering pain.

As well, most products usually contain a cocktail of preservatives, anti-oxidants, emulsifiers, humectants, colouring, perfume and other ingredients not there for healing nipples but for reasons such as shelf-life and product stability. And all creams and ointments are constructed with a base of some sort, often lanolin or paraffin. Where lanolin is used, unless specified as highly purified, it is likely to be regular lanolin containing pesticide and detergent residues, and wool alcohols.[31] Petrolatum and paraffin/mineral oil are all petrochemical hydrocarbons. Widely used to soften the outer layer of skin, they form an occlusive, slippery film and tend to clog the pores. The idea of eating this by-product of the oil industry is fairly unappealing.

Which product to use therefore depends on what the problem is. The more specific and simple the treatment, the less likelihood there is of unexpected reactions to unsuspected ingredients. The basic idea is to interfere as little as possible with the body's own sophisticated healing mechanisms, unless these have been overwhelmed. You should, of course, be guided by your doctor if the problem is severe or persistent enough to warrant medical attention. However, there are a number of minor nipple problems that are quite commonly managed by the mothers themselves, usually with the pharmacist's help and a reliable guide such as NMAA or LLLI's literature. What follows are suggestions based on my own and other mothers' experiences, as well as on what literature I could find on the subject. I have had this material reviewed, but there are no guarantees in it. Your nipples may respond quite differently, so you need to take responsibility for care and common sense in your application of any suggestion.

In the case of 'general' soreness, I recommend your very own product: human hindmilk, expressed at the end of a feed and allowed to dry on the nipple.[32] This is 'live' human fat, with antibacterial and antiviral properties, and other immune factors which also help to protect against infection. Normal hygiene is sufficient. Excessive washing before and after feeds is unnecessary and potentially damaging, especially if soap is used on the nipples.[22]

Dry skin that needs an emollient will benefit from pesticide-free highly purified anhydrous lanolin such as Lansinoh. It is considered safe for the baby to eat residues left on the nipple.[33] NMAA and other groups have always recommend the sparing use of anhydrous lanolin (not creamed lanolin), although pesticide contamination caused it to fall from favour until a purified version became available. You can check whether you are sensitive to this, or any other product, by putting some into a warm protected crease such as groin or elbow for 24 hours. This test is not infallible, as traumatised nipple skin may react different from intact elbow skin, but if there is any redness, don't use it.

Lanolin has both advantages and drawbacks. It is probably the best of the emollients because it resembles human sebum (the fatty substance your skin exudes) and can penetrate the epidermis and help keep the skin's own moisture below the surface, supposedly making dry skin more supple. It is semi-occlusive, which means it allows skin to breathe but slows evaporation (occlusive products like oils and petrolatum can make skin soggy). Like all foreign substances, lanolin smells and tastes unlike skin; it can also go rancid under extreme conditions; and if kept in an open jar which fingers dip, it can become bacterially contaminated. Purchase small quantities at a time, as very little is needed unless you suffer from eczema or psoriasis. Preferably, nothing should be needed: if nipples are sore or dry, you need to find out why and remedy that basic cause.

Nipple preparation, once in the rule books for everyone, is now considered unnecessary. However, I have heard of a few women with very dry skin and a history of nipples that cracked open at the first sight of a baby. With the next baby, they used purified lanolin) once or twice a day in late pregnancy, and after every feed in the first week after delivery, and had no nipple problems. While unnecessary and not recommended as a routine for most pregnant women, it may help a few with a particular problem.

What about nipple fissures? For years a profitless debate went on between NMAA and hospitals. NMAA rightly said that the widespread use of compound tincture of benzoin (tinc. benz. co.) damaged nipples. Nurses swore that it helped 'cracked' nipples, and that it 'toughened' nipples for breastfeeding (along with nightmarish practices like scrubbing nipples with rough towels, nail brushes, and so on). This was all part of the "if it hurts, it must be good for you" mentality, I suspect, as removing the outer layers of skin can hardly help to prevent nipple problems. As so often in these debates, both sides were partly right. Tinc. benz. is a natural resin dissolved in alcohol. Carefully painted into the fissure only, it stings like mad (the alcohol, which sterilises) but seems to provide a temporary seal (the resin) under which healing can commence. Since discovering its virtues, I have used it frequently on other hard-to-heal skin lesions on knuckles and joints, and overlooked (and now infected) cat scratches, paper cuts, ingrowing toenails or rose thorns turning septic, with 100 per cent success. But because alcohol destroys live tissue, tinc. benz. should never be used on large areas at all or even on the healthy skin around the actual fissure – with or without oil. Many a fissure has been created by its drying effects on a slightly sore nipple. (I would add that tinc. benz. with castor oil was nowhere near as effective as the undiluted compound for the hard-to-heal cuts. Is castor oil an irritant to skin as well as to the gut?) And as Gunther said, no one should use tinc benz on anyone else: it hurts!

These days moist wound healing of nipple fissures is to be recommended. Wounds treated this way do not form a scab, are more comfortable and heal faster.[34] This is achieved by creating a moist healing environment with the use of an occlusive dressing such as a hydrogel, or a semi-occlusive topical such as Lansinoh (the purest anhydrous lanolin available). Once again, apply the product only to the fissure and make sure you are not occluding the surrounding skin. I now have enough experience of Lansinoh to recommend its use for this purpose.

Another nipple problem for which creams are often prescribed is thrush. As I have said before, gentian violet is a cheap effective remedy.[6] Get your doctor to prescribe the 0.5% aqueous solution (i.e. very little alcohol). It is messy, but equally good for breasts and babies' bottoms. (With vaginal thrush, always see your doctor, as home remedies cannot penetrate far enough to deal with the problem.) Children enjoy having faces painted around their belly button as a pay-off for being quiet while Mum paints a spotty bottom. Babies sometimes look rather startled at bright purple nipples, but others take it in their stride. It's best not to be too thickly coated with gentian violet if baby seems to object to the taste, so paint it on after a feed and then rinse off (don't rub) any excess before feeding. Baby will take off more, which is one way of applying it to his mouth! Gentian violet is also a mild anti-staphylococcal agent. Staph. germs are common on the skin, and so me are potentially very harmful. So while gentian violet will not sterilise the skin, it does reduce the bacterial population while killing off the fungus. This reduces the risk of overgrowth.

Regrettably gentian violet for human use is now available only on prescription in Australia, although veterinarians frequently have it for sale. This restriction is the result of some studies showing liver cancers (of a type not seen in humans) in mice fed large doses of gentian violet for over 18 months of their 24 month life span: a curious reason for eliminating an inexpensive and valuable agent. Even more curious was the fact that when approval for the use of gentian violet was first withdrawn, the FDA approved two exceptions: for surgeons who found it a useful skin marker; and for confectionery manufacturers who complained that no other purple worked as well! Gentian violet may well have some carcinogenic potential if used in large amounts over a long period, but what chemical doesn't? And there is no substitute for it in the treatment of thrush: reports of sensitivity to daktarin gel are numerous; and creams are ineffective compared with gentian violet. Mothers who try it are sold on it. Frequently only one application is needed to dramatically reduce pain and itch. Some mothers have need of longer treatment, usually because they have not just topical thrush but also systemic problems and only a course of systemic anti-fungals will help. Spores will survive and re-grow, but if the characteristic slight itch begins again on the nipple, another application is needed. There is no apparent likelihood of resistance developing.

Dermatitis is best prevented by not using any irritant product on your nipples. Other causes may include soaps, perfumes, detergent residues in clothing, synthetic fabrics, spray deodorants, and perhaps even the chemicals impregnated in 'sanitised' fabrics. Whatever its cause, dermatitis presents as a combination of inflammation and dry scaly skin. If it does not subside rapidly after carefully identifying and removing the cause, your doctor may prescribe an anti-inflammatory steroid such as 0.5% hydrocortisone ointment to be applied thinly after every feeding for a few days, then taper off the use and stop.[2] The hazards of cortisone are such that I would use it only as a last resort. There is a case report of an infant seriously affected by corticosteroid excess after the mother used a steroid product on her nipples for two months. I know of one case of dramatic proliferation of thrush across the whole areola and some of the breast when the woman discontinued a multi-ingredient cortisone cream. The skin had been virtually sterilised and its natural immunity depressed, so once the cream was stopped the fungus went berserk. That being said, some women with severe nipple eczema could never have breastfed but for cortisone. In situations like this when longer term use of a steroid is necessary, it may be just as effective to reduce the needed dose to once or twice a day, and apply Lansinoh after every feed and before showering. Of course, it is vastly preferable to identify and avoid the foods and chemicals to which the mother is sensitive, so healing the eczema.

What, then, of all the many other expensive special nipple preparations on the market, containing aloe or pawpaw, vitamin E or fish oil, magic ingredient a-z? Some are a regular cocktail. In eight years of breastfeeding, I needed none of them. Yet other women could consider them essential. Studies sometimes held up as proof that nothing has been shown to be significantly effective focus only on prevention and early transitional soreness. We already know that good attachment and expressed breastmilk are all that most mothers need in the early period of breastfeeding. Where are the controlled studies on damaged nipples, when continued breastfeeding is endangered, and when the benefits of using a product may outweigh the risks? The remedies I've described above can all be safely left on while feeding the baby. Any that need to be cleaned off should not be used on sore nipples, as trauma before every feed will not help healing. For this reason, too, there is no need to compulsively 'clean' breasts before feeding. In fact, where this is suggested (as it was in Nigeria) there is likely to be greater exposure to water-borne pathogens and so higher infant morbidity.

Antiseptic sprays are also not recommended – indeed concerns are now being expressed that common antiseptics may be enhancing bacterial resistance to antibiotics. An older UK spray contained one-fifth of one per cent chlorhexidine gluconate in a solution of either water and alcohol, alcohol alone, plus propellant (either fluorocarbons, which damage the earth's ozone layer and should be banned, or hydrocarbons). The percentage of alcohol is probably quite high, as a warning on the can says not to spray near any naked flame, and it dries extremely rapidly on the skin. This concoction was said to be "for the prophylaxis of mastitis and treatment of cracked nipples". How useful is it likely to be for that purpose? Obviously the alcohol will not be of benefit. That and the other inactive constituents (99.8% of the whole) can be seen as a very expensive way of packaging an antiseptic readily available in cheaper creams and lotions. But is chlorhexidine gluconate of benefit? This antiseptic is active against certain types of skin organisms, but not others, which means that it will disrupt normal skin ecology. (Perhaps the use of such antiseptics is responsible for the changed gut flora recorded at some hospitals.) Cases of skin sensitivity to chlorhexidine are on record, which means there is a risk, however slight, of dermatitis. Chlorhexidine is most active at neutral or slightly alkaline pH and is rendered less effective by blood or organic matter (breast milk presumably?). Hence, on the general grounds discussed elsewhere, as well as because of these particular problems, it seems to me that this antiseptic ingredient is highly unlikely to help with cracked nipples or to prevent mastitis. I know of no randomised clinical trials suggesting that it does. I also object to the aerosol formulation not only as extraordinarily inefficient and expensive, but also as encouraging the 'hands-off' mentality that it isn't really nice to touch those parts of one's body. If antiseptics are needed on the nipple, why spray one's whole chest so as to avoid touching the breast? I'm delighted that this product was never available in Australia – we don't need any more encouragement about 'hygiene'!

If your doctor or pharmacist recommends some commercial product as a remedy for nipple problems, be sure to ask certain questions:

• What ingredients are in it, and how do they work?
• What does it smell/taste like and is it safe if the baby eats the residues?
• How much needs to be put on?
• Should it be cleaned off nipples completely before feeding?
• How often should it be applied, and for how long?
• What should be done if a rash develops (or some other symptom)?

If your doctor hasn't time, a pharmacist can tell you this from books which he or she must (by law) have available, and you can ask to read the product literature in the package, or request further information from the manufacturer or distributor. There are some risks in the use of any medication, although these are greatly reduced if you understand what to do. And in many cases the risks are out-weighed by the benefits. Use modern medicines appropriately and sparingly, and they'll serve you well.

One final suggestion. Newton suggested that diet might influence skin health and singled out lack of vitamin A, vitamin B complex and essential amino acids as possible causes of "sub-clinical vitamin deficiency". That was in 1952. Zinc is also essential for good skin health, and women taking iron supplements can be zinc-deficient. (Eat more meat or egg yolk and skip the iron tablets.) More recent work also suggests that mothers with sensitive nipples ought to look to their diet, and it probably wouldn't hurt. Among the favourite nipple creams are ones containing fish oils (high in vitamin A), and others containing B vitamins. Those who consume vitamin supplements of course ought to be aware that fat-soluble ones such as E and A can quickly reach toxic levels in young infants, and even a few days use of vitamin E-containing oils on the nipple can significantly raise infant serum levels.[27]

It is obviously preferable to have enough essential nutrients coming through from the inside out, in diet, rather than merely applying them to external surfaces in the form of creams. All the same, if you are temporarily deficient in B vitamins, as when taking antibiotics, adding a little to damaged skin could help, provided that your skin does not react to all those *other* ingredients of the cream.

Nipple shields

In 1984 I stated that nipple shields are almost never worth the trouble they cause, especially in the newborn period. Nipple shields have improved in the last decade, becoming thinner and more flexible, less obnoxious to taste, easier to use. But the basic problems remain. It still is more difficult to position a baby at the breast correctly if she has to cope with a mouthful of rubber/silicone. Obviously, too, stimulation of the nipple and compression of the areolar area, the essential factors in feeding, are reduced, difficult or impossible with different types of shields. Further, when they prevent proper extension of the breast-nipple teat back into the baby's mouth, shields make it very likely that the nipple will be subjected to pressure by the gums and will be abraded against the rubber/silicone. The most basic problem of nipple shields is simply the problem the world would have if competing shoemakers insisted on producing average-sized shoes, according to some measure nationally assumed to be correct. Feet come in a huge range of sizes. So do nipples. But nipple shields are made in one or at most two sizes, and no one is expert at fitting them!

Then there are the usual objections to any artificial teat: the hazards of nitrosamines and metals and chemicals used to toughen the rubber/silicone; the risks of contamination; and above all, the wrong conditioning of the baby's sucking reflex and the possibility of inappropriate conditioning of the newborn suckling pattern: 'nipple confusion'. What is more, some mothers find discreet feeding is impossible – which for some mothers is devastating – and the mother may feel awkward and physically uncomfortable during feeding. All of this decreases her likelihood of perseverance (see case history 12 in Chapter 12).

Yet there are experienced counsellors who can use nipple shields successfully;[35] the *Journal of Human Lactation* devoted a whole issue to the topic in 1995. I can happily acknowledge that some people find them helpful in a crisis, while still finding their use problematic. Those who use them often talk as though their main value was either to protect sore nipples *(but in most cases correcting the cause is the key. Once attachment problems have been fixed, I haven't known a sore nipple last long enough to need a shield)* or to make an inverted flat or non-protractile nipple easier to grasp *(but I don't agree that nipples should be grasped)*. Their use in engorgement is dubious indeed, because put over the nipple on a tight distended breast, the baby may end by clamping down on the protrusion, which is the nipple shield and nipple. Ouch! They may well work best in such cases if the mother has an abundance of milk – her let-down may be sufficient (as it was in history 2) to enable the baby to receive milk without suckling. But a more satisfactory solution is to express enough to soften the breast, preferably storing the excess before putting baby to the breast. For weak suckers, nipple shields are no answer; the mother can learn to express her breast while the baby is feeding, and this has the advantage of consolidating the complex neuromuscular business of proper feeding. The Dancer technique (mentioned at the end of the previous chapter) may also help such babies.

Different types of shields exist, from these old glass/plastic ones topped with what look like a lamb's teat, to all-rubber latex or silicone ones. When in Oxford, where the thin latex shields were devised as part of an experiment to monitor milk flow and composition, I discussed my doubts about shields with midwives involved in the project.[36] I was assured that they shared my doubts; that they saw the shield as a research tool rather than as a useful aid. Even the thin latex shield they developed, clearly preferable to thicker and more cumbersome alternatives, would cause problems for most mothers and babies, reducing milk yield by 22 per cent (as against 58 per cent by thicker shields).[37] Hence they saw it as a last resort, in carefully selected cases not helped by more physiological solutions. This is the underlying attitude of competent

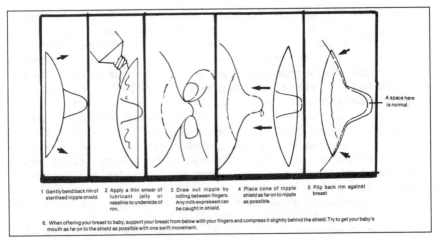

Figure 5.1 Instructions for using a nipple shield.

practitioners writing in a 1996 issue of the *Journal of Human Lactation*. Of course one of the key problems in nipple shield use is size of the shield to size of the nipple. A size seven nipple in a size 4 shield is as painful as such a misfit would be in a shoe or a glove, and the tight compression of the nipple (I've seen some white nipples in shields) would hinder milk transfer far more than a well-fitting shield. Why are nipples assumed to be standard across whole populations?

There is no longer any excuse for crazy practices such as popping ordinary bottle teats over mothers' nipples. This will not prevent them happening. In the area of breastfeeding, rationality often has very little bearing on practice. The most extraordinary devices have been used as 'aids' in the past. Dr Mavis Gunther told me in October 1983 that even after it had been demonstrated that lead nipple shields were causing brain damage in babies, and the shields had been banned completely (after almost a century of use), she discovered on ward rounds at a major teaching hospital that the nurses had merely put them into a drawer and used them when doctors were not about. People are very slow to accept that what they have 'always' done might be an appalling health risk. Yet it must be said, even the worst objects can have a use occasionally. The nipple-shield case that most impressed me was a NMAA counsellor with deeply inverted nipples on both breasts, who successfully breastfed without pain by using an old glass nipple-shield, where the breast was almost completely enclosed and no compression of breast tissue was possible (see fig. 5.5). When this broke, she tried the more modern ones and experienced agonies, as they all allowed compression of the damaged nipples. Even physiologically-defective gadgets can have an occasional use!

One thing that helps make nipple shields less harmful is a clear set of instructions for their use. There are still shields on the Australian market with inadequate instructions. I was impressed with those supplied by the Oxford midwives at the John Radcliffe Hospital (see Figure 5.1). My thanks for permission to reproduce them here.

NEW IMPROVED
BREAST NIPPLE SHIELD.

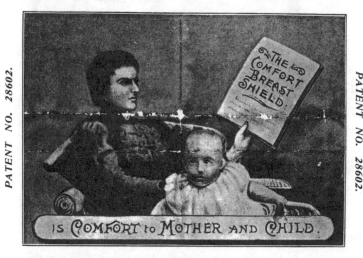

THE MEDICAL PROFESSION strongly advise that ALL MOTHERS should use a Breast Shield, especially during the first week of Nursing, as a protection against the pain arising from tender nipples.

Breast Shields are invaluable in cases where the nipples are insufficiently large for the child to suck with freedom and comfort.

——※——

The COMFORT BREAST SHIELD is THE BEST.

Combining as it does lightness and durability, is not breakable and dangerous as are the old-fashioned Glass Shields, and is more sightly than any other Shield.

The Teats are easily removed for cleansing purposes and are as simply replaced. A most essential and novel feature in the construction of the Shield are the spare Teats, two of which are supplied with every Shield so that a fresh clean Teat can be used every time of nursing.

The Shield fits close to the breast preventing suction of air by the child, also leakage, which causes such annoyance and discomfort to the mother.

Figure 5.2 Advertising for a 19th century nipple shield. Photo courtesy of Sovereign Hill Historical Park.

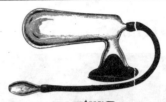

MAW'S
Nº II GLASS NIPPLE SHIELDS
FITTED WITH
Teat and India-Rubber Lining, 1/- each.

MAW'S
Nº II BREAST GLASSES
FITTED WITH
India-Rubber Lining, 1/6 each.

No. 11 Glass Nipple Shields fitted with India-Rubber Tube, 1/- each.

The advantage of the above is obvious, the India-Rubber Lining preventing undue pressure upon the nipple, and the pain consequent upon the use of ordinary Breast Relievers.

MAY BE HAD OF ALL CHEMISTS AND DRUGGISTS.

<u>Figure 5.3</u> **Nipple shield and breast glass, circa 1864.**

How did our beliefs about the utility of nipple shields arise? Was it as the result of nineteenth-century commercial claims? The advertising in this trade catalogue, Figure 5.2 (kindly supplied by the Sovereign Hill Historical Park), is very explicit. Unfortunately no picture of this particular nipple shield survives, so we cannot judge how far it was any improvement on, say, the Maws shield pictured in Figure 5.3. Perhaps it was made of wood, as some were (see Figure 5.5). But whatever it was, virtually every claim made in the advertisement would now be regarded as inaccurate and dangerous. Note that while teats were to be removed for cleaning, no mention is made of cleaning the other parts of the shield for every feed. Breastfed infants exposed to this sort of contamination, and being given other paps and cordials, were at serious risk of infection. Note, too, the invocation of the blessing of the medical profession, which has been an essential selling strategy for every dangerous new innovation in infant feeding.

The extraordinary objects shown in Figure 5.3 defy all rational explanation. As a means of promoting weaning, they must have been superb. That they were not immediately exposed as harmful must say a great deal about the number of women with bountiful milk supplies, who were able to feed their babies something despite the unphysiological appliances to which they were attached. Or perhaps it was the lack of communication between women about physical matters that enabled such a hoax to be perpetrated for so long. After all, nipple shields were still being handed out in some hospitals in 1984 (see Figure 5.4) that were merely a refinement of the Maws No. 11. Feeding bottles have improved more than breast shields.

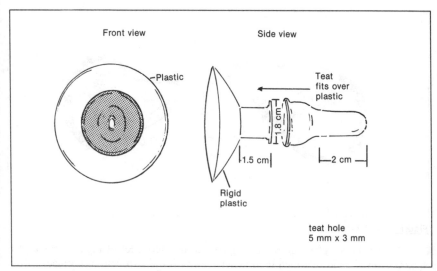

Figure 5.4 A nipple shield, circa 1984.

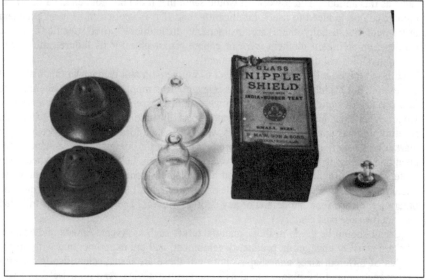

Figure 5.5 Wooden and glass nipple shields. Photo courtesy of Sovereign Hill Historical Park.

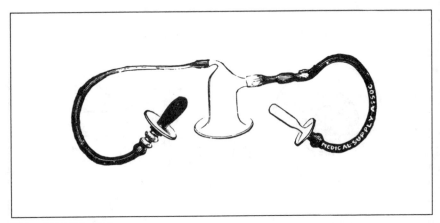

Figure 5.6 A 'tetarelle'.

Like the 'breast glass' shown in Figure 5.3. the 'tetarelle' of Figure 5.6 was "an apparatus by the aid of which the mother draws off the milk into a receptacle, from which the child can then suck it." The mother sucked on the right-hand attachment, generating flow, then plugged the other end into the baby's mouth and hoped that the flow would continue. In 1989 I purchased an Italian-made plastic model, exactly the same as this antique. Did it work? It would seem that it did not, for Jellett says, "If the mother can be induced to use it intelligently, and if it is kept clean, it is an excellent instrument but usually there are insuperable difficulties"[38] (not specified). Those careless, unintelligent mothers were of course responsible for its failure, rather than the unphysiological design of the instrument!

I have strayed a little from the subject of nipple pain and damage in this historical digression, but I think the diversion was relevant. That nipple shields have altered little in a century of rapid technological change cannot be seen as proof of their enduring value. What their largely unchanged state does illustrate is the total lack of critical scrutiny that has enabled manufacturers with half-baked ideas to create a product and market it as beneficial, without being brought to book for doing so. Would such inefficient and damaging devices have survived so long in any field of medicine where men suffered the consequences? Would men have blamed themselves for being unable to make the device work? It may be female chauvinism, but I think not. (To convince me otherwise, please send me details of any similarly useless and painful objects inflicted on men over the past century.)

Credit should be given to those manufacturers such as Avent, Ameda and Medela who are actively engaged in product development, and are experimenting with nipple shields of different sizes and shapes: but until these are tested scientifically we still cannot recommend the nipple shield as a therapeutic device. And until we can, I still believe that scepticism and use as a last resort measure is far more appropriate than gung-ho application, while at the very least we should try to develop some system of fitting shields to nipples, as shoe companies have for feet. It takes days and months to develop foot deformities from ill-fitting shoes. The consequences of ill-fitting nipple shields can be catastrophic much faster.

Not only nipple problems, but breast problems can cause extreme pain and untimely weaning. The next chapter will discuss the more common breast problems.

NOTES

CHAPTER 5: NIPPLE PROBLEMS

[1] Slaven, S.; Harvey, D., "Unlimited suckling time improves breast-feeding", *Lancet*, (1981) i, 392-3.

[2] Gunther, M., *Infant feeding* (Methuen 1970). See also Gunther, M., "Sore Nipples", in *Medical World* (1953) 79, 571.

[3] Minchin, M., *About Breast and Nipple Problems* (NMAA 1981).

[4] Hoffman, J B., "A suggested treatment for inverted nipples", *Am. J. Obstet. Gynecol.* (1953) 66, 346. This is well discussed in Riordan, J., *A Practical Guide to Breastfeeding* (C.V. Mosby & Co., 1983) pp. 11-9, together with Cotterman's device, a more intensive method of enhancing protractility of inverted nipples. The Niplette is a new and improved device that probably does work but is grossly overpriced.

[5] Neville, M.C. & Neifert, M. R., *Lactation physiology, nutrition and breastfeeding.* Plenum Press, 1983), p. 337.

[6] Amir, L., et al, *Candidiasis and breastfeeding*, LC Series #18 (Avery Publishing, NY 1995). Kay Hoover has a superb A3 colour sheet on thrush, available at low cost from her at 613 Yale Ave., Morton PA, 19070-1922. Tel/fax: 1-610-543-5995.

[7] Crook, W., *The Yeast Connexion* (Professional Books, 1983) available from P O Box 3494, Jackson, Tennessee, U.S.A. or local allergy associations.

[8] Manning, D.J. et al, "Candida in mouth or on dummy?", *Arch. Dis. Child.* (1985) 60, 381-2.

[9] *New Generation* (NCT Magazine) 1983, p. 21-2. Three cases of women who succeeded despite complete blanching of the nipple; two sounded like physical compression and the third a possible psychologically induced case. All successfully breastfed.

[10] *New Generation*, op. cit., (1984) 3.1, 21-22.

[11] In fact, sensitivity to cold has been well-documented. *Allergy in Children.*

[12] Lawlor-Smith, LS, Lawlor-Smith C, "Raynaud's phenomenon of the nipple: a preventable cause of breastfeeding failure?" *Med. J. Aust* (1996) 166: 448.

[13] Available from NMAA, or direct from Sniggles, PO Box 408, Hillarys WA 6293, tel/fax: (08) 9409 3159.

[14] Marshall, B. R. et al, "Sporadic puerperal mastitis – an infection that need not interrupt lactation", *JAMA* (1975) 233, 1377.

[15] e.g., Waller, H. *The Breasts and Breastfeeding*, (Heinemann, London 1957), p. 16-17.

[16] The standard dilution is one teaspoon of sodium chloride or sodium bicarbonate in a pint of water, cf. Horton, (letter) in *Talkabout* (NMAA counsellors' magazine) 198 v.10 no.8.

[17] Beveridge, G.W., "Skin sensitisation to topically applied drugs", *Aust. Prescriber* (1976) V.10 No. 8)

[18] Fisher, A., *Contact Dermatitis* (Lea & Febiger, Philadelphia 1986).

[19] Menz, J., speaking at ALCA National Conference August 1994, Adelaide.

[20] Breit, R. and Bandman, H.J., "A review of allergy to hydrous wool fat and wool alcohols", *Brit. J. Derm.* (1973) 88, 414.

[21] Clark, E. et al., "Lanolin of reduced sensitizing potential," *Contact Dermatitis* (1981) pp. 81-3.

[22] Newton, J., "Nipple Pain & Nipple Damage", *J. Pediatr.* (1952) V. 41, p. 411-423. Truby-King, in an earlier and influential work suggested that tinc. benz. be applied to sore nipples and cleaned off before feeds with methylated spirits! *Mothercraft*, Whitcombe & Tombs, 17th impression, post 1945, p. 87.

[23] Marples, M.J., "Life on the human skin", *Scientific American* (1969) 220: 1; 108-115. In a recent *BMJ* editorial, it was noted that the human body contains 10^{14} cells, of which only 10% are human, the rest being micro-organisms of various kinds (bacteria, viruses, fungi, etc.)! *BMJ* (1998) 316: 1255.

[24] For a breakdown of some typical creams, refer to Riordan, op. cit., p.123 or Lauwers, J. and Woessner, C. *Counselling the Nursing Mother* (Avery N.J. 1983), p. 415.

[25] This is particularly likely when creams containing steroids (cortisone etc.) are abruptly discontinued. Their use should be tapered off. Kenacomb is a common example of such creams.

[26] Gribetz, D., "Ingestion of a bismuth-containing ointment by a breastfed infant", *Mt. Sinai J. NY* (1974) v.41, No. 3, p. 498-501.

[27] Marx, C. M. et al, "Vitamin E concentrations in serum of newborn infants after topical use of vitamin E by nursing mothers", *Am. J. Obstet. Gynecol.* (1985) 152: 668-70.

[28] Mohrbacher, N., Stock, J., *The Breastfeeding Answer Book* (LLLI, Schaumburg IL, 1996 edition).

[29] Lauwers, J., Woessner, C., *Counselling the Nursing Mother* (Avery Publishing, New Jersey, 1983) p. 414.

[30] Most doctors are aware of this. Antibiotic creams are not common. The mother is usually prescribed oral antibiotics. Care is needed here too, cf. Lawrence, R., *Breastfeeding: a guide for the medical profession.* (C. V. Mosby & Co. 1980), p. 165.

[31] Martindale, *The Extra Pharmacopoeia*, 28th edition (1981).

[32] Lawrence, op. cit., p. 124, describes a N.Z. routine. This is also used in the U.K. (correspondence with Chloe Fisher)

[33] *US Pharmacopeia* 1992.

[34] Hinman, C., Maibach H., "Effect of air exposure and occlusion on experimental human skin wounds," *Nature* (1963) 200: 377-88.

[35] Helsing, E. and Savage-King, F., *Breastfeeding in Practice – a manual for health workers* (Oxford University Press, 1982), p. 144-5; Riordan, op. cit., p. 120-2; Lauwers and Woessner, op. cit., p. 418-9.

[36] Lucas, A. et al, "The nipple shield sampling system", *Early Hum. Dev.* (1980) 4/4, 365-372. Discussion with team midwives, November 1983, Oxford. A detailed set of instructions for applying the shield helped to minimise nipple abrasion and maximise normal feeding.

[37] Woolridge, M. W., et al, "Effect of a traditional and a new nipple shield on sucking patterns and milk flow", *Early Human Dev.* (1980) 4/4, 357-364.

[38] Jellett, H., *Midwifery for Nurses* (6th ed., J. & A. Churchill, London 1922), p. 349.

6.

BREAST INFECTION? OR MASTITIS?

E very book about breastfeeding has a chapter discussing blocked or clogged ducts, 'caked' breasts and breast infections. Even Riordan's generally excellent book[1] assumed that mastitis and breast infection were interchangeable terms, as did Virginia Phillips.[2] Things are looking up: in 1997 Sally Inch, a UK research midwife, was working on a review of mastitis which I hope to see published soon. It should be excellent.

But first, what do we really know about mastitis? I suspect that much of our basic understanding and underlying assumptions stem from bovine mastitis. Should it be? Cows' udders are subject to enormous stresses which human breasts are not: the stress of overdistension because of infrequent milking, trauma because of their weight and location on the animal's body and rough handling by milkers and machines, and contamination with faecal material. Not surprisingly, bovine mastitis is very often infective, and antibiotics are a staple of veterinary practice. But is human mastitis always infective, and are antibiotics always necessary? I believe not.

Let's be clear about definitions. '-itis' always means inflammation. Mastitis is the general term given to any type of breast inflammation whether caused by infectious organisms or not. Inflammation is the body's primary response to most injury, and to any foreign, or non-self, particle that invades the body.[3] During the process of inflammation, the walls of blood vessels dilate, expand, allowing cells to leak from the blood into the affected area. Some of these cells (white blood cells, leukocytes) attempt to engulf the intruder, destroying it and usually the white blood cell as well. It is the debris from this process that we call 'pus'. Other blood and tissue cells begin the immune response to the foreigner simultaneously, but it is the inflammatory response that we first notice. It usually involves pain, local swelling, redness and raised temperature, which may be localised (a throbbing finger) or general (rise in body temperature).

A breast responds no differently from a finger. But how do the foreign invaders get into the breast? And are the foreigners bacteria, or viruses, or something altogether different?

Infective mastitis

Because it is widely assumed that inflamed breasts are infected, let's begin there. Bacterial mastitis is a reality in every mammalian species, particularly so in animals that are milked only intermittently, rather than as freely as nature intended.

Live human milk is not usually a good medium[4] for bacteria to grow in, and therefore bacterial mastitis is the result of either (a) conditions that favour an immense overgrowth of disease-causing (pathogenic) bacteria; or (b) conditions that prevent the body from destroying and excreting such bacteria, and which give the bacteria access to breast tissue.

Such conditions include the prolonged use of nipple shields or clothes which abrade skin tissue; poor physical health in the mother, especially iron deficiency which causes a drop in antibody production;[5] poor nutrition[6] or possibly smoking, which alters some immune responses;[7] damaged nipples, usually caused by incorrect positioning during feeds; and the use of nipple creams or lotions which either damage the skin or alter the skin's natural defences against infection.[8] Poor personal hygiene has been suggested as a cause, though the evidence of millions of women living in poverty suggests not a common one. Overdistension of glandular tissue due to long intervals between feeds undoubtedly contributes to mother cows' vulnerability to mastitis of all kinds, hence women's oversupply problems must be taken seriously.

Bacteria can cause infection on the outer skin of the breast (superficial mastitis) or deep inside the breast itself (intramammary mastitis). Within the breast, infection may occur within the glandular tissue (parenchymatous mastitis) or the connective tissue which supports it (interstitial mastitis). These classifications are merely descriptive, not explanatory. Unless infection is quickly eliminated, the cell walls will be destroyed and a pus-filled abscess will develop. This may or may not drain through the duct system; antibiotics and surgery may be required, although feeding can often continue without incident. Intramammary mastitis can be either epidemic (infecting many women at once) or sporadic; epidemic mastitis has become rarer since the advent of antibiotics and more powerful bactericidal hospital cleansers.

Superficial mastitis, if not promptly treated, may infect underlying breast tissue. It presents as an infected wound on the outer skin of the breast, and frequent cleansing, and moist wound healing techniques are all that is needed. It is also worth taking time to understand why such a skin lesion occurred at the place and time.

Occasionally, an experienced mother will report a bout of infective mastitis which was bacterial from the very beginning: a fissured nipple or areola becoming obviously infected, red streaks radiating from that infection back into the breast, pus and blood in milk quite rapidly; severe mastitis of very sudden onset with no apparent pre-disposing factors. This is not typical of most cases of mastitis and clearly demands medical treatment immediately.

The prevention of bacterial mastitis does not consist in trying to keep nipples and breasts sterile, but in maintaining the normal balance of bacteria on the skin. Bacteria can usually be cultured in the milk expressed by healthy women, as bacteria are present in the outer nipple ducts and on the skin of the breast itself,[9] as well as on fingers, etc. Humans are not designed to feed their babies totally sterile milk – it is exposure to manageable quantities of bacteria and viruses that induces immunity in the baby. And all the many antibacterial factors in human milk enable a breastfed baby to cope with the bacteria it is exposed to. This is far more important than obsessive concern about sterilising everything the baby touches.

Similarly, many viruses have been cultivated in milk expressed by women, although in almost every case without apparently harming mother or baby: according to a 1984 review, "there are no convincing descriptions of morbidity in full-term newborns as a result of breast-milk-acquired cytomegalovirus (CMV) 'despite the fact that' 10-17% of women can excrete CMV in their milk."[10] The anti-viral activity of human milk probably helps to prevent or inhibit viral growth within the breast.[11] To my knowledge in 1984, human mastitis had not so far been attributed to viral infection by the world literature. However, it would be surprising if viruses did not cause some problems in the breast, as elsewhere in the body. I have been told of two cases of mastitis in women infected and symptomatic from mumps virus: the breasts were swollen, lumpy, and extremely painful especially at the beginning of the feed. One woman found that gentle massage with oil helped relieve the symptoms. Both women continued to breastfeed and neither child became symptomatic, although both were almost certainly well-immunised! The disease had been brought from school by an older child. After the infection receded, one woman experienced itching in the ducts; later lactations were not affected. To prescribe antibiotics for this mastitis would not only be useless but possibly harmful.

How can you know whether your fever, aches, and red painful breast are caused by bacteria or viruses? Usually you can't. If needle biopsies from the inflamed site were to be cultured and investigated, the results would come back after the problem had resolved. For this reason, almost no one ever cultures any breast tissue in cases of mastitis. However, some Danish researchers[12] have divided inflammatory symptoms into milk stasis, non-infectious mastitis, and infectious mastitis on the basis of cell counts and bacterial cultures; then in a second and larger study, they showed that milk stasis resolves with feeding, while non-infectious mastitis persists for several days, although systematic and regular emptying of the breast reduces the risk of infection developing. In infectious mastitis, specific antibiotic therapy reduced further complications and, combined with emptying, resulted in recovery in 96 per cent of patients.[13] In short, good management can be more important than drugs.

Obstructive mastitis

The Danish research cited above accords well with my long-standing belief that most cases of mastitis begin with obstruction and are usually non-infective. If some obstruction, internal or external, prevents the breast or a particular part of it from draining, milk will bank up in the ducts behind the obstruction, just as water does in a kinked garden hose. Pressure will increase in the glandular system; substances from the milk may be forced through the cell walls into the capillaries or connective tissue. Those parts of the body will react as if these substances were any other foreign invader – with inflammation. This may take the form of localised redness, and swelling and pain; and fever and flu-like symptoms if enough reaches the bloodstream.[9] There may be no infectious agent present at any stage. Needle biopsies taken from affected areas do not culture any bacteria at all,[9] although milk expressed through the (usually contaminated) nipple ducts will almost certainly grow some bacteria. (The levels of bacteria will rise dramatically if the breast is subject to ultrasound, according to a WA report.) It would be interesting to do as the veterinarians do, and check leukocyte counts: stress of any kind raises these in cows, and perhaps this could indicate the degree of the problem in humans too.[14]

Engorgement is one form of obstructive mastitis. The breast is overfull, both because of a sudden increase in milk production and because of the increased blood and lymph supply to the breast. Unless the breast can be drained effectively, the pressure reaches almost intolerable limits, with rock-hard breasts, red and painful to the touch, and fever and malaise generally. Engorgement was recognised in 1753 as causing milk fever, abscess, and even maternal death, and as being almost always iatrogenic – due to the hospital's management of mother and baby – as it was and is usual only where mothers are not allowed to feed their babies ad libitum or at night. Where hospital staff have abandoned their policies of schedule feeding and restricted suckling, engorgement is now a problem only for mothers whose supply is over-abundant for the baby's needs or who have scar tissue in the breast, which makes drainage difficult. In such cases, regrettably more common as surgeons do cosmetic surgery on younger women, some involution of those areas of the breast drained by severed ducts may occur. It is usually on the margins of the working/involuted areas that mastitis occurs. (Where surgery has included incising the areola, difficulties with feeding can be expected, although sometimes the outcome is surprisingly good. Obviously surgeons should develop techniques that minimise lactation difficulties, and women should be adequately counselled before surgery. Each case remains individual and requires skilled postpartum assessment and help.)

The old advice about perinatal engorgement was not to express too much for fear of stimulating an already overabundant supply. Nowadays many people are finding that to 'express right out' perhaps once or twice – taking all milk out of the breast, by whatever means are possible – is most effective. This probably works because removing the milk reduces the pressure in the breast, and so permits vascular and lymphatic congestion to ease rapidly. The ideal way of expressing right out is to use a safe, comfortable alternating pressure electric pump.[15] These should be standard equipment in maternity hospitals. That they are not, and that crude and dangerous hand-pumps are still in use, is another indicator of the low importance placed upon breastfeeding. A Kaneson-type hand-pump can help some women, particularly if other means of stimulating milk let-down are used. And hand expression can be very effective, though in some cases the breasts are so painful that this is impossible. Women must be warned to treat engorged breasts extremely gently; additional bruising is very easy when the breasts are in this stage, and it prolongs the problem. One simple piece of home technology is a glass jar 'pump', an idea that dates back a century or more. Use a wide-mouthed jar, three-quarters-fill it with very hot water and leave to stand for 10 minutes. Smear some vaseline on the mouth of the jar. Empty the water, then apply the jar to the breast very carefully so that you don't burn yourself. As the jar cools, it creates a gentle vacuum which, together with the warmth, will relax the nipple sphincters and draw milk from the breast. When the breast is too painful to hand express or pump, this can get the milk flowing.

So too can a warm bath or shower, or leaning over a basin of warm water and immersing the whole breast as far as possible. And crazy as it sounds, the use of cabbage leaves (simply washed, dried, and placed in the bra to cover the breast) seems to reduce oedema;[16] if left longer than a couple of hours, it may even reduce milk supply too far![17] This is clearly preferable to drugs and worth trying. (Cabbage has even reduced the swelling of bilateral hydroceles in one unfortunate gentleman, so Australian midwives are convinced it works.)

The use of drugs to resolve or reduce engorgement may very rarely be indicated. In case histories in Chapter 12, the consequences were serious; unresolved oversupply problems caused lactation failure. Clearly small doses of drugs would have been preferable to breastfeeding failure, especially as they are usually necessary only for a few days. One doctor finds that just one or two 5 mg tablets of stilboestrol will reduce engorgement without affecting breastfeeding success. Illingworth recommends this in his edition. Gunther in 1958 had recommended two tablets of 0.25 mg soon after delivery and one tablet a day later.[18] Such minute doses would be preferable if effective. Concern about the use of stilboestrol during pregnancy has made it a contentious choice, and we need to know more about possible ill-effects used postpartum. However, this is a choice of evils. Included in the decision should be the known side effects for the mother, which includes a slight risk of thrombosis, increased in women over 30, those with varicose veins or history of thrombosis, those with blood groups other than O and delivered by caesarean section.

The drug of choice in gross engorgement was thought to be bromocriptine, which had been shown to be very effective in suppressing lactation. That was until the FDA revoked its permit for sale for the suppression of puerperal lactation, after findings of stroke and psychosis in too many women for comfort. What dosage regime might be safe and best reduce engorgement without long-term harm to breastfeeding or the breastfeeding mother has not been discussed. We know now of course that careful conservative management, expressing to comfort, allows involution to occur naturally via the inhibitory feedback loop. Engorgement must damage breast tissue, perhaps making it more likely to develop cancer in later life. (It has been documented for many years that cancer tends to develop only in unsuckled breasts,[19] among women who feed from one side only. Yet few people recognise abrupt termination of feeding, or suppression of lactation, as damaging.)

Other causes of obstructive mastitis

Friends and NMAA members have had mastitis because of:
- restrictive clothing or 'trapdoor' bras;
- bruising from a toddler's elbow or a heavy-handed expressing midwife or enthusiastic partner (the breast, being very vascular, bruises easily);
- misplaced suckling at night by a vigorous baby;
- too tight a grip when supporting the breast while feeding;
- milk blister or thrush covering the nipple ducts;

- scar tissue within the breast;
- small growths such as papillomas in the duct system itself;
- a thickened 'plug' of what seemed to be milk;
- wearing bras at night (structurally bras are not designed for this and put pressure in odd places);
- delayed or too-hurried feeds;
- sleeping on one's stomach; and so on.

This list, written in 1982, corresponds neatly to some of the precipitating/predisposing factors listed by Riordan from her clinical experience. Unfortunately Riordan tried to fit these into an 'infectious' model, which is unnecessary.

Anything that disrupts the normal draining of the breast may cause an inflammation in the breast – i.e. mastitis. Some women's breast tissue is 'knottier' than others: this may pre-dispose them to mastitis. The actual location of the blockage can give useful clues as to its basic causes. It is most common in the lower segment of the breast (usually because bra straps are too loose and the weight of the breast hinders drainage) or towards the armpits (because the breast is unsupported while feeding). Pressure and blockage in the usually well-drained upper segments are frequently caused by bras that are too small or straps that are too tight. Watching the way the mother holds the baby and breast while feeding is an essential part of diagnosis. Where are her hands, fingers, the bra itself, the baby's hands? How tense are her shoulders? (Physical and emotional tension can inhibit the let-down in some – not all – women, leaving the breasts inadequately emptied.)

Here again, if a woman reports that she has mastitis, the professional needs to discover the cause. Why this, at this time? If causes are not discovered, the woman is very likely to have the problem recur. It can be only a mild nuisance, but it can also be incapacitating, even potentially fatal – unchecked obstructive mastitis could lead to fulminant infective mastitis as increased pressure opens the ducts[20] making it easier for bacteria to enter. And babies have (on very rare occasions) developed kidney infections and septicaemia as a consequence.[21] Breast abscess was until recently a notifiable disease, a relic from the pre-antibiotic days when milk-fever was a major health hazard. This problem still seems to be a major cause of concern in Europe, particularly Germany and Russia, as numerous articles published in Eastern Europe discuss how to treat acute suppurative cases of the kind now rare in Australia. Clearly management is poor, when 70 per cent of 518 women develop abscesses, 2 per cent gangrene, and 9.4 per cent sepsis! Although I can't read Russian, the English abstracts make it clear that mothers take their babies off the breast when mastitis threatens.[22] And while there is talk of aggressive chemotherapy and radiation(!) there is no mention of frequent expression/removal of milk. Small wonder that milk-fever remains an apparently major hazard in those countries, while it has been drastically reduced here in Australia, thanks to NMAA's common-sense approach.

Vasculitic mastitis?

Another distinctive type of mastitis I have christened 'vasculitic mastitis', my own term for a phenomenon that I have observed, but which has not yet been scientifically validated (volunteers, please). In obstructive mastitis generally, Gunther postulated that increased pressure within the breast forced substances from the milk into the blood. This vasculitic mastitis may be the reverse: defects in blood vessels permit substances from the blood to leak into breast tissue. Those defects may be permanent or temporary - related to complicated immune responses.

I postulated the existence of this problem from the experience of some of the 110 food-intolerant breastfeeding mothers, who were the basis of *Food for Thought*, my earlier book on food intolerance. Perhaps a dozen found that they had recurrent mastitis for which no physical obstruction could be identified, but which rarely progressed to overt infection, and which often recurred either premenstrually or before ovulation. These mothers came to realise that their recurrent mastitis was often accompanied by other symptoms of allergy or intolerance – some of them indicating that blood vessels were affected, e.g. migraine, easy bruising or purpura, hives, and/or premenstrual tension. The connection between this mastitis and breast refusal – often just before a period – was commonly noted. It would be fascinating to know more about how hormonal changes affect the response of blood vessels to chemical mediators of inflammation, perhaps in both mother and baby. Studies might be done too, to see whether such changes affected maternal uptake of antigen from the gut, or excretion via milk, or excretion of other substances.[23] In some cases breast refusal, PMT and mastitis all ended after the mother identified and was avoiding her allergens. In some cases, premenstrual avoidance of chemicals such as caffeine was all that was required to effect a total cure: and many women now associate tea/coffee drinking with recurrent mastitis. The apparent link between caffeine intake and fibrocystic breast disease tends to support this finding.[24] (Those babies who refused the breast were always colicky around that time of the month too, and the colic was food-related.) Certainly those babies could recognise some change in the milk itself, because they went to the breast eagerly, then pulled away as if being poisoned.

While I can offer no scientific studies to support this idea, there is plenty of hard medical evidence showing that this process of vasculitis does take place in other blood vessels, and that food and chemicals are common causes.[25] And having discussed it with a doctor specialising in migraine, I am now offering it for testing against the experience of those women with inexplicable recurrent mastitis. One other related possibility is that it is change in hormone levels per se which produces this effect: that changing diet altered the balance of hormones (as immune responses include endocrine responses, too). Colic/mastitis could also be due simply to increased prostaglandin levels. One scientist at the Edinburgh MRC Reproductive Biology Unit found such a correlation between colic and prostaglandin levels premenstrually. But this was never published – not being sufficiently important as a subject of scientific work (!) and anyway being only one case. Interestingly, recent research indicates that human milk stimulates prostaglandin synthesis in cultured human skin fibroblasts: perhaps the milk of some mothers has more dramatic effects on the breast as well as the baby's gut.[26]

Prevention and treatment

By outlining the likely causes of mastitis, we have covered the logical preventive steps. This is basic medicine: you do not use drugs to alleviate symptoms without looking for causes. But do antibiotics have a place in the management of mastitis? Obviously, yes. (Should they always be used? No.) Infection may develop after the first 24-48 hours of unresolved inflammation; in the rarer cases of overt infective mastitis it can progress extremely rapidly to a very nasty abscess. (How rapidly depends on many factors: the virulence of the pathogen, the immune competence of the mother, and so on.) It's therefore only common sense to see the doctor immediately – an appointment two or three days away is not soon enough – and be prescribed an antibiotic. After you have been through one bout of mastitis, and learnt how to drain the breast thoroughly, you may want to think again about antibiotics. After all, there are drawbacks in using such drugs. They disturb not only the mother's gut flora, but often, and sometimes very severely, the baby's bowels as well. Breast tissue can be a difficult place for antibiotics to penetrate in levels sufficient to be effective, and there is a danger of breeding resistant bacteria – if, indeed, bacteria are involved, and if they are not already resistant to commonly used antibiotics.

When mastitis recurred, I always got the prescription immediately but waited a day to see if the inflammation could be ended by less drastic means. I ended up with half a dozen unpresented scripts in my drawer, and in subsequent lactations never even went that far, being more aware of the early warning signs and so preventing problems of mastitis before they started. Prompt and efficient treatment of mastitis, as detailed in NMAA's pamphlet, *About Breast and Nipple Problems*, will almost always prevent infection from developing. But it is safer for the inexperienced mother to use antibiotics while learning what to do. Remember that draining the breast is the absolutely crucial key to success: where the baby is taken off the breast an abscess is statistically very likely.[27] Only two of my friends ever developed abscesses: both were consulting expensive specialists who routinely prescribed antibiotics and weaning; one of the children promptly developed cows' milk intolerance, and the other became ill with some unidentified infection (possibly because of pathogens from milk being able to multiply rapidly once the immune factors in milk were withdrawn and the gut environment drastically changed by milk encouraging bacterial overgrowth and putrefaction; see p. 52).

In this field, advances in our knowledge of sensible management have come largely from the veterinary world. In the James Herriot pre-antibiotic days we read of cows being saved by a determined vet sitting up all night to 'strip' the cow, i.e. thoroughly empty the infected teats. Then came penicillin, and it was used everywhere for cows, until it became a problem – residues in milk and cheese, sensitivity in humans, and so on. Penicillin and other antibiotics are still widely used, but veterinarians are now once again advocating constant milking and the use of oxytocin as adequate to end many cases of mastitis.[28] As Naish pointed out, most cases cleared up without abscess formation[29] even in the pre-antibiotic era. Medical advice not to feed the baby on the affected breast brought about many an abscess; this therefore is another iatrogenic problem.[30] Common sense suggests that after identifying the cause of obstruction, you remove it, and then speed up drainage from the obstructed area. Frequent feeding, ultrasound,[31] gentle massage towards the nipple when feeding, hot and cold compresses, expression of surplus milk, all may help and all are well described in standard texts. It is interesting to note that both hot and cold compresses have been found to be helpful by some mothers: cold restricts blood flow and reduces inflammation while warmth increases circulation and thus enhances immune responses. Warmth before feeds, and cold thereafter, is some women's choice of therapy, though I know of no proper trials of this. An interesting 'jacket' devised to hold ice packs in place is available from NMAA: ask about the Cool-a-bra. Pinning two knickers together can achieve the same effect: see p. 74.

To improve milk drainage from the inflamed area, choose a feeding position that allows milk to flow downhill to the baby. If the blockage is above or under the nipple, lift the breast with your other hand while feeding. If it is on the right side of either nipple, feed lying down on your left side, your right leg supported by a pillow. (Reverse for the other side.) If you have a persistent blockage below the nipple, try feeding while kneeling on all fours! The slightly older baby will look at you as though you are daft, but most get on with the business of feeding however you position yourself. This technique, however, is not recommended for the office party...

Whether to rest or not is a personal decision too. Some mothers feel so bad that they have no choice but to go to bed. Others find that rest so increases their supply that emptying the breast is difficult. They do vigorous arm exercises[32] to improve circulation in the breast, then go to bed to rest and build up their decreased supply only after the blockage is cleared. (The increased volume would of course generally help flush out the breast, but how bed rest affects supply varies among women. Because mastitis causes changes in milk composition, including increased saltiness,[33] some babies tend to refuse the breast at the very time that they're most needed. In most cases, increased supply could help reduce the salty taste.) To rest or not to rest is a decision that must be made individually. There seem to be two types of mothers: those who find that physical activity reduces their supply, and those whose supply is reduced by emotional stress. There is probably a physiological basis for this. It is useful for women to be observant and decide which factor affects them most; it helps, in such decisions, to know whether your supply will be enormous if you go to bed.

This outline of management basics may seem redundant to many of my readers. It is included because a very clever investigation by Dr Audrey Naylor, of the San Diego Lactation Clinic, revealed an incredible lack of knowledge about the appropriate management of breast engorgement. Telephone calls were made to 81 community hospitals and 23 medical centres. Callers posed as breastfeeding mothers, and asked for help: a delayed feeding and baby refusing to nurse. More than 40 per cent of the doctors and nurses gave wrong advice, nearly one in four suggesting bottle-feeding. Only

7 per cent suggested more frequent feeding; 10 per cent merely said to calm down and do nothing. Very few asked about the baby's past feeding pattern, wet nappies, stools or temperature; very few asked about chills and fever in the mother. It would be fascinating to see the results of a similar survey here. However, to conduct such a survey would probably be political suicide for whoever did it: here in Australia professionals would be likely to react very strongly against anyone who challenged the tacitly accepted assumption that of course they know how to manage breast-feeding problems. We parents are guilty of helping to maintain that fiction: I am tired of hearing mothers in various self-help groups bitterly criticise most professionals in private, then get up in public and congratulate all professionals as though their management was beyond reproach. We have a responsibility to speak the truth in justice.

Increased susceptibility to infective or obstructive mastitis may perhaps be due to stress or nutritional deficiencies. Stress reduces the bactericidal powers of blood cells and the production of antibodies. Antibody production drops dramatically, for instance, if the woman is iron deficient. (Don't take iron pills. Improve your diet, and if concerned get a doctor or blood bank to check your haemoglobin levels – very simple.) Zinc and other deficiencies also have an impact on the efficiency of the immune system, and iron fortification can cause zinc deficiency. Good nutrition, again.

For some women, identifying the basic cause of mastitis can be very important. These include women sensitive to antibiotics or women with related symptoms. Hence it's well worth taking the time to find out why *this* bout at *this* particular time. I cannot help wondering whether my son's subsequent penicillin allergy was not related to the antibiotics I took so often while he was breastfed. Once I understood the logic behind mastitis, I had no further bouts requiring antibiotics, in the next five years of breastfeeding. But what you choose to do must be your decision.

To summarise what seems to me to be important unexplored aspects of mastitis:
• The association of nipple damage and mastitis. It is commonly assumed and stated that bacteria enter through a 'cracked' (fissured) nipple and cause infection deep within the breast. If nipple tissue is always the portal of entry, why is there so often absolutely no evidence of infection *there*? Certainly, asymptomatic ascending infections are theoretically possible, though in other cases such as cystitis I suspect inflammatory responses are also primary. However, in the breastfeeding situation the pathogen must survive intact skin defences and 'swim upstream' against a flood of active bacteriostatic and bactericidal agents. The idea of primary inflammatory cause deep in breast tissue seems more likely.
• The assertion that prolonged feeding leads to nipple damage.[34] In my experience this is only so in cases of incorrect positioning. Restricted feeding may promote mastitis by leaving the breasts too full.[8]
• The assumption that cultures of milk samples expressed by the mother will reveal the pathogen. This seems quite absurd to me, on any number of counts: contamination of the specimen; the bacteriostatic and bactericidal effects of breastmilk included. The assumption that if milk samples reveal *no* pathogen the 'infection' is in connective tissue, seems equally unproven.[35]

• The assumption that fever and aching always indicate infection. This seems due for revision in the light of new immunological research on the importance of inflammation. I would add that taking anti-inflammatory medication can defeat the body's efforts at self-repair and should be reserved for inflammation that is serious and perhaps not being adequately controlled by the body. Simple comfort techniques such as tepid bathing do not interfere with the good effects of inflammation in the body; medication will. Bed, vitamin C, and chicken soup are probably preferable to anti-inflammatories.

• The assumption that a prompt decrease in symptoms when penicillin is given 'proves' the bacterial origin of the mastitis. This may also be suspect. Many women have experienced equally prompt resolution of symptoms without antibiotics, either through accelerated drainage of milk, or the use of vitamin C, or vitamin A in the form of cod liver oil.[36] These latter remedies fit the vasculitic theory: vitamin C and essential fatty acids have been shown to be important in the immune response and in keeping blood platelets normal. Of course penicillin may be effective not because of its antimicrobial action, but because it (initially) enhances the phagocytic clearance of *any* inflammation.[37] Unfortunately it seems to leave the immune system less efficient when the course of antibiotics ends – hence a recurrence of symptoms (which 'justifies' the prescription and another course?).

• Seasonal variations in incidence of mastitis in certain areas, and 'epidemics'. Could there be environmental factors (other than carriers or pathogenic bacteria) which explain these? Examples are changes in environmental allergen load, effects of agricultural chemicals, effect of temperature variations.

• Antiseptic sprays or lotions, promoted as helping to reduce the hazards of infection. Dr Whittlestone pointed out at a New Zealand conference that such compounds were no longer used for cows, but they are by human mothers. (For rational choice of nipple creams, see Chapter 5.) Even the basic underlying idea that the breast would be better to be sterile is highly questionable. It may be excessive hygiene which prevents the colonisation of the breastfed baby's gut with harmless flora derived from mother's nipples – and so leaves the baby more vulnerable to colonisation by potential pathogens.

• Whether particular types of breast structure are involved. Is poor drainage more likely in some breasts than others? How do we identify these and what helps?

• Whether particular brassiere designs contribute. Trap door bras, underwire bras, crop tops, or any bra at all: what is best for breast health? Anything that restricts lymphatic circulation would seem unwise on first principles.

The mysterious white spot

Before finishing this chapter on mastitis, I would like to take a closer look at another intriguing little problem raised in Australia and overseas. Many women report that their bouts of mastitis coincided with a 'white spot' on the nipple. Obviously if such a 'spot' obstructed a nipple duct, milk would bank up behind and eventually produce mastitis. But what are these white spots?

- Thrush is an obvious answer (see Chapter 5) and has quite clearly been related to mastitis in some women.
- A second possibility is the milk blister, which as far as I can ascertain was first described by Gunther.[9] Occasionally milk seems to accumulate beneath a layer of skin. If the breast is squeezed, the blister bulges. Rupture the skin with a sterilised needle and milk will flow, or sometimes spurt out, but may cause mastitis in the meantime by obstructing the outflow of milk.
- A third possibility is the true plugged duct: ducts with plugs of material which can be extruded as stringy material or expressed as discrete lumps. The latter are well described by one mother: "I gently tried to remove it [a minute white dot] and eventually expelled it out – it shot across the bathroom. I pressed my hand on the left side of the breast, and the milk flooded out. Relief! After this I became an expert at detecting these white granules – nearly always at exactly the same place. At times it took ages to get the granule to 'pop' – it would appear and then retreat. During one expressing session I expelled nine white granules".[38] These are almost certainly corpora amylaceae (milk bodies): concretions of casein and calcium found in the milk of dairy animals. And found more frequently in milk from traumatised or mastitic udders.

Other mothers describe strings or lengths of fatty-looking material. This may be the origin of the idea that 'blocked ducts' were caused by 'thickened milk'. While physically removing the plug may end that episode of mastitis, problems tend to recur. Lawrence found that "The condition dramatically improved by limiting the mother to polyunsaturated fats and adding lecithin to the diet as well".[39] Nevertheless, in the present state of knowledge about dietary fats and the composition of breast milk, this cannot be recommended without some major reservations. If the mother's intake of saturated fats (mostly animal) had been excessive, a reduction is certainly in order, and adding a little lecithin might be of benefit. (Too much can be toxic.) However, the fats in breast milk are related to diet. Until it is clear just what ratio of saturated: unsaturated fats is most beneficial to the baby it would seem sensible to make sure that the breastfeeding mother's diet contains both in adequate quantities and let the body balance them in milk production.

- Are nipple creams associated with white spots? Several women in British studies mentioned incidentally that they were using creams, oils, or Rotersept.[40] Because everything put on a nipple alters the skin layers in some degree, could this be a reason for the spots? If creams can clog facial pores, can they do the same to nipple ducts when injudiciously applied? While sometimes necessary, creams are certainly questionable as a routine and should not cover the tip of the nipple.

Gunther regarded white spots as rare,[8] despite very expert and detailed examination of thousands of women. Could it be changes in diet and in pharmaceuticals and their use, which makes them seem more common nowadays? Or is this the consequence of better means of communications between articulate breastfeeding mothers? Here are some questions about white spots that need answers:

- Are white spots common in your experience?
- What, if any, treatment have you tried, and with what results?

- Do these problems consistently occur at particular times, in relation to stress, hormonal changes, diet, body weight?
- Which explanation, if any, seems to fit the cases in your experience?
- Are you aware of other factors or features which are not mentioned here?
- What are the 'milk plugs'? Are you aware of anyone who has analysed them?
- Were you using any form of nipple cream or lotion, or any other medication, at the time of the 'white spot'?
- Were 'white spots' associated with mastitis, in your experience?

This whole question of mastitis really needs careful research. Let's hope some medical school will take up the challenge. Meanwhile, please report whether this explains your observations, or whether some aspect of mastitis, as you have experienced it, fails to fit this scheme. We can all learn from you!

NOTES

CHAPTER 6: BREAST INFECTION? OR MASTITIS?

[1] Riordan, J. *A Practical Guide to Breastfeeding.* (C. V. Mosby, St. Louis, 1983) pp. 149. Similarly, the very prestigious *Guidelines for Perinatal Care* of the American Academy of Pediatrics and American College of Obstetrics and Gynecology embody this unhelpful assumption and the poor management that increases the risk of infection.

[2] Phillips, V. *Successful Breastfeeding* (NMAA 3rd Edition 1983).

[3] An excellent technical account of this process is found in Berman, B. A. & Macdonnell, R. F., *Differential Diagnosis & Treatment of Paediatric Allergy* (Little Brown & Co., Boston 1981), ch. 1, and p. 60-61.

[4] Pittard, W. B. et al, "Bacteriostatic qualities of human milk", *J. Pediatrics* (1985) 107: 240-3. This showed that bacterial contamination did not significantly increase in milk left unrefrigerated for up to 6 hrs at 10-26 º C.

[5] *Parent Centres Journal* (NZ), Nov. 1974, pp. 19-20.

[6] Miranda, R. et al, "Effect of maternal nutritional status on immunological substances in human colostrum and milk", *Am. J. Clin. Nutr.* 1983, 37 632-40. There may be a particular hazard in the malnutrition of affluence (high fat, high sugar) as compared with the malnutrition of scarcity, which is what is usually defined as malnutrition.

[7] Kjellman, N. I., "Effect of parental smoking on lgE levels in children", *Lancet* (1981) 1, p. 993; Holsclaw, D. S. & Topham, A. L., "The effects of smoking on fetal, neonatal, & childhood development", *Pediatr. Ann.* (1978) v. 7 No. 3, p. 105

[8] cf. Newton, N., "Nipple Pain & Nipple Damage", *J. Pediatr.* (1952) v. 41, pp. 414-423.

[9] cf. Gunther, M., *Infant Feeding* (Methuen, 1980), p. 86-91. Dr Gunther is one of the few who have really "troubled to see what the injury is" (p. 80) in mastitis as in nipple pain. It was her observation of mastitis which is the basis of my distinction between infectious and obstructive mastitis – that and practical experience! See also Carroll, L., et al, "Bacteriologic criteria for feeding raw breastmilk to babies on neonatal units", *Lancet* (1979), ii, 732-3.

[10] Freier, S., Faber, J. "Loss of immune components during the processing of human milk", in Williams, A. F., Baum, J. D. (eds) *Human Milk Banking.* (Raven Press N. Y. 1984).

[11] May, J. T., "Anti-viral activities and viruses in milk from Australian women", paper given at International Conference on Human Milk Banking, Czechoslovakia, May 1981. (Supplied by author: Microbiology Dept., La Trobe University, Bundoora, Vic. 3083); Berger, R. et al,

"Influence of breast milk on nosocomial rotavirus infections in infants", *Infection* (1984) 12, 3, 171-4; Welsh, J. K. & May, J. T., "Anti-infective properties of human milk", *J. Pediatr,* (1979) v.94, p. 1-9.

[12] Thomsen, A. C., et al, "Leukocyte counts and microbiologic cultivation in the diagnosis of puerperal mastitis", *Am. J. Obstet. Gynecol.* (1983) 146, 8, 938-41. Thomsen, A. C., et al, "Course and treatment of milk stasis, noninfectious inflammation of the breast, and infectious mastitis in nursing women", *Am. J. Obstet. Gynecol.* (1984) 149, 5, 492-5.

[13] In the earlier study, women had been followed for the first weeks after delivery; in the second study, there was no indication as to time elapsed since birth. This may be significant, as many more varied causes of mastitis develop after the initial engorgement phase of lactation, if NMAA experience is any guide. What is more, I wonder about the wisdom of using chlorhexidine solution so vigorously (swabbing nipple and areola three times before sampling). Could it alter skin ecology and physiology to the point where infectious mastitis becomes more likely and infant gut flora abnormal? However, this group is definitely on the right track, and I hope to see the results of further investigations published soon. They do need to note the caution offered by the next footnote, however.

[14] Ballek, J., *Mastitis and milk cell counting* (Dept. of Agriculture, Government of Victoria, Jan. 1979. This stressed that "fairly high cell counts can occur in older cows, cows in very early and late lactation, and cows that have had mastitis which has cleared up" and concludes "Do not treat cows during lactation on the basis of cell counts alone." Cows with very high counts (over 1 million cells per ml. of milk) should be closely inspected; those with negligible to low counts (up to ½ million cells/ml) can be disregarded. I would fear that if this technique were applicable, it could be misused to justify automatic antibiotic consumption, however.

[15] Of those I have tried, I would recommend the Whittlestone physiological milker, and then the Medela double pumping system. All pumps should be stringently tested by independent researchers before being marketed. I have tried some which exerted great suction on the nipple, but no compression of the areola – as though human milk was extracted by suction. Some would obviously cause nipple fissures. Very few come with adequate user instructions to guard against fissures. One recent study has looked at some U.S. pumps – see Johnson, A. C., *Clin. Pediatr.* 1983, 22, 40-45. Local breastfeeding mothers' groups would probably have some ideas as to the effectiveness of national brands. Books such as Riordan, *A Practical Guide to Breastfeeding* (C. V. Mosby & Co., 1983) and Lauwers & Woessner *Counselling the Nursing Mother* (Avery Publishing 1983) also contain details of some.

[16] Roberts KL, "A comparison of chilled cabbage leaves and chilled gel packs in reducing breast engorgement", *JHL* (1995) 11: 17-20.

[17] Amir L, "Cool cabbages for hot breasts", *Aust. Fam. Phys.* (1991) 20: 1675.

[18] Gunther, M. in "Discussion on the breast in pregnancy & lactation", *Proc. Roy. Soc. Med.* (1958) 51, 308.

[19] Ing, R. et al, "Unilateral breast feeding and breast cancer", *Lancet* 1977 ii, 124-7.

[20] Neville, M. C. & Neifert, M. R., *Lactation: physiology, nutrition and breastfeeding.* (Plenum Press, N.Y. 1983), p. 54.

[21] Such cases frequently occurred when the doctors were asserting that 'suckling should, I believe, always be withheld' – Waller H., *The Breasts and Breastfeeding* (Heinemann, London, 1957), p. 54.

[22] Polonski, A. M., (Treatment experience with acute suppurative lactation mastitis.) English abstract. *Vestn. Khir.* (1982) 128(2) 50-2

[23] That women patients *do* experience changes in symptoms or sensitivity to foods that are associated with hormonal changes is documented in the "Joint Report of the Royal College of

Physicians/British Nutrition Foundation, on Food Intolerance and Food Aversion", *J. Royal Coll. Physicians* 1984, 18, (2), p. 19. And also in Minchin, *Food for thought: A parent's guide to food intolerance* (George Allen & Unwin, 1983).

[24] *Am. J. Epidermiol.* (1985) 122: 391-9.

[25] cf. Rea, W. G., "Cardiovascular disease triggered by foods", in Gerrard, J. G. (ed.) *Food Allergy* (CC Thomas, 1980). Discussion with a Melbourne physician researching food related disease (Dr Colin Little) has helped to clarify this point.

[26] Subbiah, M.T. et al, "Human breast milk stimulates prostaglandin synthesis in cultured human skin fibroblasts", *Biochem. Biophys. Res. Commun.* (1985) 129: 972-6

[27] Marshall, B. R. et al., "Sporadic puerperal mastitis - an infection that need not interrupt lactation", *JAMA* (1975) 233.

[28] Whittlestone, W. H., in *Parents Centres Bulletin* (N.Z.) 1977, vol. 70.

[29] cf. Naish, C., *Breast feeding* (Lloyd-Luke, London 1956). "...it should be remembered that the acute mastitis type could usually be cleared up in 4 days, without any abscess formation, and without taking the baby off the breast, before the modern medicinal treatments were available – always provided that the condition was treated rapidly and energetically. The essential elements are: promptness, rest, heat, and withdrawal of milk", p. 131. One interesting point Naish made was that the affected breast should be well supported and raised, to improve circulation.

[30] Newton, M. and Newton, N. R., "Breast abscess: a result of lactation failure", *Surgery, Gynecology and Obstetrics* (1950) 91, 651-5.

[31] Semmler, D., *The use of ultrasound therapy in the treatment of breast engorgement.* Paper available from NMAA. See also Shellshear, M., "Therapeutic Ultrasound in post-partum breast engorgement – clinical notes", *Australian J. Physiotherapy* 1981, 27 (1) 15-16.

[32] Brewer, G. S. and Greene, J. P., *Right from the start - meeting the challenges of mothering your unborn and born baby* (Rodale Press), p.136-7.

[33] Conner, A. E., "Elevated levels of sodium and chloride in milk from mastitis breast", *Pediatrics* 1979, 63, 910-11

[34] A controlled study at a major London hospital showed no significant difference in incidence of nipple soreness when sucking time was restricted. It did, however show significant differences in successful breastfeeding at 6 weeks – fewer mothers were successful if feeds had been restricted. *Lancet* (1981) 1, p.392-3. This simply reiterates Newton's 1952 findings (op. cit.).

[35] Niebyl, J., et al., "Sporadic (Non-epidemic) Puerperal Mastitis", in *J. Reprod. Med.* (1978) v. 20, no. 2, p. 97.

[36] *NMAA Newsletter*, July 1982, has case studies. See also Band, P. R. et al, "Treatment of benign breast disease with Vitamin A", *Preventative Medicine* (1984) 13, 549-54.

[37] Dewdney, J., "The effect of antibacterial antibiotics on immune reactions and host resistance of infection", in Lessof, M. (ed.) *Immunological and Clinical Aspects of Allergy.* (MTP Press, 1981) ch . 12.

[38] *New Generation*, (1982) 1, 4, p. 18. Later discussed in (1983) 2, 1, p. 23. The cases discussed included milk blisters, thrush, and duct plugs, though they were not always identified as such.

[39] Lawrence, R., *Breastfeeding: a guide for the medical profession*, (G. V. Mosby & Co, St. Louis, 1980), p. 129.

[40] An English antiseptic spray of chlorhexidine gluconate supposed to protect the nipples. So far I have seen no reports enthusing over its effectiveness, but several questioning it, or mentioning it in conjunction with difficulties. It is not available in Australia, which is probably just as well.

BREASTFEEDING AND THE MOTHER

7.

W hen asked to explain their choice of feeding method, mothers who bottlefeed often talk of its advantages for them, while mothers who choose to breast-feed usually cite its advantages for the baby. But are there significant benefits to the mother in breastfeeding? This is a crucial issue everywhere, and most especially in those curious western sub-cultures where babies are seen as less import-ant than their mothers, and the baby's rights and needs as in conflict with the mother's (often stated as the woman's) best interests.[1] This potential conflict has reached the point where some healthworkers and parents apparently fail to see the child as a vulnerable separate person whose fundamental *needs* are more important than their personal *feelings, inclinations* or *convenience*. This has led some Australian paediatri-cians (advocates for babies) to allege privately that midwives are sometimes too caught up in being "with woman", and too little aware of the rights and needs of the infants of those women: in short, that this peculiar western gynaecentrism is damaging children. Yet if all healthworkers appreciate what breastfeeding means for the health of the birthing woman, as well as her child, and the consequences of both for the woman's family, this dichotomy is absurd except in the most extraordinary cases.

Physically, it is clear that if a woman breastfeeds, her body will be different from the body of the non-lactating mother. Her uterus, stimulated by lactation hormones, will more quickly contract down to its pre-pregnant size. Delays in this process of uterine involution occasionally lead to embolisms, or blood clots. (The risk of embol-isms is greatly increased if a non-lactating mother is prescribed stilboestrol, as was usual before the advent of newer drugs to suppress lactation.) This rapid transition to the appropriate postpartum body state is to be seen as a major advantage of breastfeed-ing in a world where childbearing and its aftermath is a major cause of maternal death. Every year half a million women die as a result of bearing children.

Lactation will utilise the fat deposited in pregnancy to provide stores for feeding baby, provided the woman controls her diet, eating according to hunger, and does not overeat because she feels she must 'eat for two'. Breastfeeding and gradual weaning is said, too, to be more likely to result in fat being re-deposited in the breasts. (During pregnancy, glandular tissue proliferates and fat is mobilised, hence the breasts of any woman who has borne a child will no longer be firm and high but will have the typical curve of the mature breast. This happens to some degree in all women regardless of method of feeding, and probably for good reason). If fat is re-deposited, there is a greater likelihood that the breasts will resemble their pre-pregnancy size, if not shape. Lactation suppression, or abrupt weaning, sometimes results in very flat chests, which the success of plastic surgery suggests that few of us in this culture are happy with. Increasingly, questions need to be asked about possible damage done to breast tissue by sudden weaning or suppression. Does this have a permanent effect? Does it predispose to later difficulties and even cancer? There is scope for research in this area of breast size and shape after pregnancy and in relation to infant feeding. Do exercise, age, stress, use of steroidal contraception, diet, etc., influence the outcome? The enormous variability of the result, whether in breast or bottle-feeding mothers, must have some rational basis.[2]

Reduced fertility is another advantage of breastfeeding. The suppression of menstruation can be of vital importance in allowing the bodies of undernourished women to build up their iron stores, reducing the danger of anaemia (which is responsible for much maternal ill health, physical and mental). Breastfeeding, by inducing lactational amenorrhoea, or the absence of ovulation and menses, remains the world's most important contraceptive on a global scale, preventing more births than all other forms of modern contraception combined. During the 1980s, researchers reached consensus on the degree of protection against pregnancy provided by lactational amenorrhoea.[3] In the first six months after birth, provided that women exclusively breastfeed, that no other food or drink is given to the child, and that menses have not returned, the risk of pregnancy is equivalent to that of the mini-pill: less than 2%, and there is very little chance of ovulation and conception prior to the return of bleeding. In the next six months, because ovulation is more likely to precede menstruation, the risk of conception increases and alternative forms of contraception should be employed, even before menses return, and even if the child is still exclusively breastfed, when it is imperative to avoid another pregnancy. In this second half-year, frequent breastfeeding and feeding before giving other foods enhances protection, but the risk may be as high as 10%. Mothers whose babies have long night sleeps are at greater risk of ovulation, as intervals of over 6-8 hours between suckling bouts may lift ovarian suppression. However, there is still some contraceptive protection, as fertility is decreased, and even if conception occurs, an inadequate luteal phase often means that the egg is not successfully implanted, as so often in nature for a wide variety of reasons.

Overview articles on breastfeeding as a contraceptive by Professor R. V. Short[4] and Dr. Miriam Labbok[5] are fascinating. Those working in this field have seen the disastrous eighteenth century population explosion as attributable largely to the abandonment of breastfeeding under the twin pressures of fashion and industrial revolution. (No creches for working mothers then!) Certainly the huge families of the non-breast-feeding gentry helped to impoverish landed estates. The social impact of infant feeding methods has yet to be investigated thoroughly. But every drop in breastfeeding rates means an increased need for expensive technological contraception simply to maintain the national birthrate, while to increase exclusive breastfeeding would be to reduce it.

It is becoming very clear that both frequency and length of suckling, and also intervals between suckling, can affect the return of ovulation very differently in different women. (Night feeds may be necessary for some women to prevent ovulation, yet clearly are not for others. In one case I know of, just one breastfeed a day for a toddler 18 months and older suppressed ovulation, and within a month of giving up that one feed, very reluctantly on the mother's part, she was pregnant again! The other extreme is the 1-2% who conceive under six months postpartum despite exclusive breastfeeding – just as they do on the minipill.) The hunter-gatherer style of unrestricted feeding, perhaps several times an hour, is certainly responsible for the long inter-birth intervals notable in those nomadic communities, and important in their adaptation to such a demanding environment. But those who argue that the hunter-gatherer mode of feeding is somehow more 'natural', and therefore perhaps even necessary for successful breastfeeding, would do well to ask themselves whether it was not the scarcity of food and water, and the high-energy lifestyle, which made such frequent suckling necessary both to maintaining supply and to preventing early conception. Such patterns of breastfeeding are indeed what we are more used to in our nomadic evolutionary history, but humans have adapted well to a variety of environments. (Do the Inuit on a traditional diet, so high in marine fats, feed as frequently as the Bushmen of the Kalahari?) We know from research studies that supplementing maternal diet in humans does not increase infant weight gains, but does reduce suckling frequency – i.e. when baby gets enough, he goes longer before asking again. This is clearly the case in some Australian women, whose babies can be overfed (i.e., suffer symptoms of lactose overload: see p. 324 for an example) if intervals between feeds fall below four hours.

In my Australian experience, most mothers find that babies have varying intervals between feeds at different times of day: three and a half to four hours after morning feeds, reducing to one or one and a half hours in the late afternoon/evening. Only a minority have babies who suckle incessantly, and this sometimes turns out to be because of unrecognised problems such as poor positioning. Formula company spokesmen have perverted anthropological data in talking of the 'insufficient milk syndrome'[6] as though it were inevitable that in a society where constant suckling is impossible or difficult, women must fail at breastfeeding. This was well answered by members of the Cornell University Nutrition School,[7] who exposed the fallacies underlying such commercially-motivated nonsense. But the thesis has been effective in creating an acceptable, if specious, reason for breastfeeding failure that places no guilt upon medical professionals, mothers or company salesman. Hence it remained attractive enough to be summarised in the breastfeeding pages of the National Childbirth Trust's magazine, *New Generation*[8] in September 1984 without mention of the fact that the authors were company employees. The detailed critique by the Cornell people was published by the same journal as had published the original 'insufficient milk syndrome' paper (*Medical Anthropology*), but it has not been as widely circulated. (It is said that company people distributed the former to thousands of medical professionals, most of whom would never see any criticism of it or realise the key role that formula itself can play in bringing about a situation in which a mother actually has insufficient milk. The very fact of its wide circulation should have raised some doubts as to its objectivity. Formula companies are commercial enterprises, after all, and have that legal duty not to waste money on material that will not increase their sales!)

One could, however, agree with some of what the formula company doctors argued. 'Insufficient milk' is indeed a major cause of weaning, and in many cases is a real phenomenon and not just an excuse. For this reason I devoted Chapter 4 to considering real or imagined inadequate supply problems and their possible causes. The company thesis – that this is because of a lack of constant contact between mother and baby – is not relevant in most cases, however ideal such constant contact might be. The Australian women I mostly deal with include many who successfully combine long absences from their baby with exclusive breastfeeding: professionals who work and breastfeed, and so on. And even less well-educated, lower socio-economic group working mothers can also succeed with the right education and professional support[9] but without 24-hour contact with the baby or suckling 6-7 times per hour! In a western community it is the exceptional mothers who provide their babies with constant contact, and although rigidly scheduled suckling is now almost unheard of, few of those babies are feeding 6-7 times per hour on a regular basis. Australia, a highly developed urban nation where such patterns are rare, has been among world leaders in the breastfeeding revival.

Neither does the fact of virtually constant contact prevent many mothers from instantly leaping to the conclusion that they have insufficient milk whenever anything causes their baby to be unsettled. Constant maternal contact is not the rule in less-developed societies with fewer breastfeeding problems, either: many babies are minded by older children or other family members while women work hard elsewhere. I believe that constant maternal contact is not a precondition for breastfeeding success, although it may help some women maintain adequate hormonal levels, and is absolutely delightful in the early days before the weight and interests of the baby dictate some separate time to explore the world and relieve the mother's back! It seems reasonable to factor in the mother's nutritional status, rates of milk synthesis and size of breasts as storage organs, and the size of the infant's stomach, as well as his metabolic limitations and any physical constraints, in any consideration of how frequent infant suckling will need to be for maintenance of milk supply and indeed, suppression of ovulation, in any individual mother-baby pair.

I think that we need to reject the convenient company-propagated idea that insufficient milk is due to the unavoidable conditions of modern social life, such as separation of mother and baby and lack of instant infant access to the breast 6-7 times every hour. If we accept that extrapolation from interesting data gathered in another culture where food is hard-won, and allow it to be propagated, we are increasing the likelihood of breastfeeding failure in our own culture. Mothers who are anxious because they cannot provide constant contact, and therefore believe they cannot succeed, may well fail, because anxiety can be a potent inhibitor of milk production for some women, and because they will offer other foods to see if baby needs them. They will consequently have too little, or interpret all infant fussiness as indicating that they have too little, yet offer another convenient bottle to satisfy their 'hungry' baby, and by so doing set in train the decreased demand/decreased production cycle that can lead inevitably to weaning.

The companies have been very intelligent in their advertising. By identifying their product with breast milk, then stating that of course their product should be used only when breast milk is insufficient, or the mother is unable to feed for other reasons (work, social life, fatigue, illness, etc.), they have been the major beneficiaries of the breastfeeding promotion campaigns. The Vice-President of Abbott Laboratories, the largest U.S. infant formula maker, said in June 1981 at an investor seminar "the growth of breastfeeding has been good for the infant formula business and we feel it will continue to exert a positive influence... Our research shows that many breastfeeding mothers eventually use more infant formula than those mothers who start their infants on our products."[10] The more women try breastfeeding and fail, the more the sales of 'humanised' formulae grow, at the expense both of breastfeeding and of the older cheaper (once also 'perfect') products such as evaporated milks.[11] It is unbelievable how readily and widely accepted is the notion that breast milk and 'modern' formulae (less than a decade old in most cases) are interchangeable feedings. To have the same recommendations for use is absurd.

This digression into the 'insufficient milk syndrome' has taken us some distance from advantages to the mother, although it touches upon two other advantages that I would cite. Firstly, cost. As the formulae become more and more expensive, and as we realise how little extra food is required to adequately sustain lactation, it becomes clear that, financially, breastfeeding can be a significant saving at a personal as well as national level. Any true costing would of course have to assess the protective benefits of exclusive breastfeeding, or even of partial breastfeeding, in reduced medical costs, etc. Since 1984 some of this work has been done: NMAA's Lactation Resource Centre can provide further information. Julie Smith, an economist and NMAA Counsellor, provided a superb overview of this topic at the 1997 NMAA International Conference.[12]

Secondly, breastfeeding for many women strongly enhances their sense of their own bodies as fundamentally good and powerful and pleasurable. Particularly if a woman has had minor difficulties and overcome them, she is aware of how much the difficulty was corroding her sense of pride and confidence in her body as a basic biological unit. To fail at breastfeeding can be a profoundly negative and destructive experience, especially when the woman perceives the problem as having been her body being unable to do what her mind and heart wished to, i.e. to nourish this baby herself, from her own body. This is why it is important to tell women that the reason most of them failed had nothing to do with their physical capacity to lactate. (See ch. 2.) There are few women who have successfully breastfed who do not identify strongly with Ann Oakley's comment: "...the total of two and a half years I spent breastfeeding have given a satisfaction quite incomparable with any other. There is something so rewarding about sustaining and making a child happy with one's own milk. Each time each child smiled, nuzzled her or his soft head into my neck, or even thoughtfully poured the overflow down my blouse, I did feel my productivity and therefore value as a person confirmed. No other work I've done has ever made me feel quite that way."[13]

Mavis Gunther in 1976 described it as follows – "There is an accompaniment to a satisfying feed which many women experience: a deep feeling of tranquillity, a repose that restores, a confirmation of her love of the baby and her hopes that he will grow... I am unaware of it happening during bottle feeding."[14]

Too little attention is paid to the intensity of feeling generated by breastfeeding. For this reason I have decided to include several case histories which combine strong feeling with useful learning (see Chapter 12). But I would emphasise that the love and tranquillity felt by Ann Oakley are the *normal* experience of breastfeeding, to which all mothers are entitled – and which can be so intense that women are afraid to ac- knowledge it. I cannot imagine how mothers who bottle-feed can experience the same emotions so vividly in the absence of the normal hormonal stimulation of breastfeed- ing. (The rise in sales of 'self-feeding' bottles, designed to be gripped by the baby and to reduce adult involvement in feeding, suggests bottle-feeding does not provide comparable positive feedback and inducement to stay in close contact.) Breastfeeding matters more to mothers than most people will concede.

VILLANELLE, 1980

Around us grows a warm tranquillity
As the small mouth is fastened on the breast:
Feeding the child sustains a joy in me.
At home there is no need for ceremony –
Here is the baby's home, and food and rest.
Around us grows a warm tranquillity.
With the young smile reviving gradually.
Of all good I can do, this is the best:
Feeding the child sustains a joy in me.
While I have time to ponder quietly
The miracle of my congenial guest,
Around us grows a warm tranquillity.
No fellowship is like this company,
My fingers by contented fingers pressed –
Feeding the child sustains a joy in me.
This is the focus of his infancy,
Where he may lie and thrive, secure and blest.
Around us grows a warm tranquillity:
Feeding the child sustains a joy in me.

- Helen Lawrenson, Scottish mother

Some thoughts on psychology, mothers and babies

Breastfeeding is sometimes claimed to have psychological benefits. These have been said to include such things as greater psychological closeness and ease of bon- ding, and greater maternal resistance to stress. Much of the argument for such benefits is based upon extrapolation from animal studies. Because I have always believed women to be more complex psychologically than other mammals, I do not believe in citing such animal studies as proof, interesting and suggestive as they may be. Yet it is indeed highly likely that the act of breastfeeding confers significant, hormone- mediated benefits – for example, that high prolactin levels do help a mother to cope with the inevitable postnatal stresses; that oxytocin, the 'hormone of affiliation' released during coitus, birth and breastfeeding alike, assists people of all ages to bond together in ways that resist the stresses of everyday interaction (and helps explain the psychologists' insistence that a good physical relationship is important in partnerships). There are studies which show that women who breastfeed have a more positive mothering style (less controlling, less negative, more responsive and mutual) than women who feed artificially.[15] But in the absence of adequate studies, we may also be looking at a chicken and egg question here: are mothers more likely to succeed at breastfeeding if they are already more likely to be responsive and score higher on tests of mutuality and flexibility? Do more rigid personalities tend to want the control possible in bottle-feeding? Or does the experience of infant feeding influence the type of person we become as mothers, and perhaps for longer than the period of lactation? If we are brave enough to fund the studies that might address that question (and we could) then I personally think that we will find that breastfeeding, an incredibly powerful and intimate physical process that is repeated many times a day for many months and years, does make women more responsive and flexible mothers whatever our starting point.

It may well be that it is easier to be a happy responsive mother if assisted by the right mix of body hormones: these days only the ignorant or foolish would dispute that hormones influence human behaviour. But they do not govern it. Mothers can still be good mothers if they feed artificially. They probably do have to work harder to do so than if they were breastfeeding, since they are not being so positively assisted by hormones that influence mood and behaviour. More credit to them then, for their devotion. For I have no doubt whatever that women love their children whether they breast- or bottle-feed. Therefore I do not believe in actively promoting breastfeeding using such arguments, until the research has been done. They have the potential to be very counter-productive, as they can be heard (wrongly) as saying that breastfeeding mothers are better mothers. Of course both groups of mothers contain the selfless and the selfish, the controlling and the responsive, and much of how we mother has been learned from how we were mothered.

The emotional power of breastfeeding can work for good or ill. Breastfeeding certainly has the potential for enhancing mother-child relationships. What could be more rewarding than the emotional and sensual pleasure of a tiny baby snuggling against one's skin, smiling up in contentment, or dropping off the breast, satiated, into blissful sleep? But the real-life experience of breastfeeding also has the potential for seriously disturbing mother-child relationships. Mothers find it personally devastating when their child is unhappy, fails to thrive, rejects the breast, or causes intense pain. Purely from a psychological point of view, if they cannot resolve their breastfeeding problems, such mothers may have a better relationship with the baby if bottlefeeding. Yes, the baby may suffer from nutritional deficiencies and illnesses. This increased risk of infant illness (see Chapter 1) is not by itself a hazard to good mothering, though it may be to the baby's well-being. Provided that the morbidity is defined as illness (and not as 'normal' or caused by maternal tension) most mothers will be capable of intense devotion. Fortunately, mothers should rarely have to choose between the health of their baby and the relationship that they have with it. There is almost no breastfeeding problem that cannot be solved with sufficient skill and patience. Many mothers who persevered through extreme pain in the first months speak of the rewards of breastfeeding far more strongly than those who never felt a twinge.

Morbidity not defined as 'illness' may have very different results. Colic is one such case. In my own work on food intolerance, I found significantly more negative behaviour from food-intolerant or allergic infants, whether breast- or bottle-fed. That such continued negative feedback from the baby should affect maternal attachment feelings is hardly surprising. Mothers would be less than human if such were not the case, especially when they are openly or covertly blamed for their child's unhappiness. (Mothers' attitudes and ability to cope improved dramatically once they accepted that a colicky child is in physical pain.) Partly in reaction to that unfair burden of guilt upon women, a new emphasis is emerging. The baby whose behaviour from birth sets up a negative feedback cycle is indeed difficult to love and is increasingly being categorised as a 'difficult' (cf. 'easy') baby. Valid observations about infant behaviour are being translated into more dubious statements about infant temperament. This has its own dangers. Maternal bewilderment may become resentment – "Why me? What have I done to deserve such a monster?" – and gradually, blame – "You've always been a rotten kid, right from the day you were born." Our culture commonly imputes far too much intentionality to young infants; they are described as manipulative, engaged in a guerilla warfare to secure family domination, as needing mastery and subordination. This leads to inappropriate reactions to infant needs, based on false anxieties. "If I pick up my colicky newborn when he cries he'll learn how to get his own way by such behaviour. Give them an inch and they'll take a mile." This is encouraged by many influential books, including those written by hospital-based (and usually male) paediatricians, which adopt a peculiarly patronising, joking but 'empathetic' approach to the problem of the 'difficult' toddler or baby, often a problem the writer's wife coped with while the writer earned his degrees. It says much about women's position in society and their relationships with their children that they do not all find these male experts offensive, as I and so many other experienced mothers do, but lap up the disempowering absolutions handed out by these parenticians, as Anne Manne recently called them in a wonderful article in a 1996 issue of *Quadrant*, entitled "Electing the New Child".[16] Talk about 'taming' children is ultimately profoundly destructive of interpersonal relationships. The models of child behaviour that underlie such talk were well-discussed in an important supplement written by psychologist Peter Cook,[17] which was later developed into a book.[18]

It is difficult to criticise patronising books publicly, because their authors are patently nice people trying to help (and the books do provide some temporary comfort by their assertions that such monstrous behaviour is normal). But I believe that these doctors trivialise important issues. It would seem that their authors believe that there are no real solutions to such problems except in modifying parent or child behaviour, by whatever technique works and can be squared with a 20th century conscience. (Overt brutality is no longer fashionable, although emotional manipulation is.) Thus such people reinforce the idea of the normalcy of aberrant behaviour. (By aberrant I mean behaviour, such as persistent and inexplicable crying, that would cause deep concern in almost all other societies than the self-centred western ones we live in.) As well, the diagnosis of 'difficult temperament' puts an end to further detailed investigation which might discover unsuspected organic causes for infant distress, such as food intolerance. Those who dismiss colic as 'normal' have clearly never experienced such pain themselves (or have forgotten it). It never ceases to amaze me that despite medicine's history of oversights and blunders, wrong diagnoses and therapies, such medical men still feel confident enough to ascribe infant distress to maternal tension, ignoring environmental causes other than the very obvious ones, and leaving no possibility of as yet unrecognised physiological problems. Yet in cases reviewed by Lactation Clinics, serious problems such as hypothyroidism, congenital heart disease, structural abnormalities such as deviated septum and cleft palate, CNS disorders, allergy and infections have been found. Exclusively breastfed babies are not 'difficult' without reason (neither are formula-fed babies, but simply being formula-fed, with all its associated digestive difficulties and health problems, is often sufficient reason). And distressed babies make for unhappy families.

Of course heredity is an important variable in determining what a particular infant will be like. But how can we separate strictly genetic influences from prenatal environmental ones? (Babies are alive for nine months before they can vocalise and distress us: but we can affect them in that time!) It seems to me that facile talk of difficult babies and easy babies will not help mothers acquire a better understanding of an infant's needs. And by denying the mother hope of improvement through physical changes, such pigeon-holing of babies can be very harmful to maternal morale. After all, 'three-month colic' is endurable only when it has a time limit; mothers come close to despair when four or five months go by without noticeable change, because suddenly they realise that it could go on indefinitely. To talk of babies being genetically programmed to be difficult, or miserable, is to my mind irresponsible. It is unprovable and unhelpful, not to mention unscientific.

I would have written a great deal more on the subject of 'bonding' – a most unscientific concept, but very useful, in its day. However, I have discovered a first-rate discussion in *Maternal Bonding* by Sluckin, Herbert and Sluckin.[19] [The original promoters of the bonding concept have been at considerable pains to try to show that what was understood and publicised as their idea often failed to do justice to its complexities; hence I am criticising the popular notion, not the magnificent Klaus/Kennell work itself.] Anyone who mentions bonding publicly ought to read this before saying another word on the subject. The authors conclude that "early experience, far from being all-important, is no more than a link in the developmental chain, shaping behaviour less and less powerfully as age increases. Contrary to a variety of strongly held beliefs, there is no clear-cut evidence that events around and soon after the time of birth can readily or seriously distort either the development of the infant's personality or interfere with the growth of maternal love and attachment." Which, as they are at pains to say, does not mean that these events are unimportant – merely that they are not all-important, and therefore deficiencies in care in the neonatal period won't lead to insoluble problems unless mothers believe they will, in which case maternal anxiety (and the resultant behaviour) could create a self-fulfilling prophecy!

What is interesting to me is to compare the widespread acceptance by doctors of the general idea that there may be psychological benefits of breastfeeding (as yet unproven), with their widespread ignorance of the enormous proven nutritional and immunological gulf between breast- and bottle-feeding.[20] Is this perhaps because such theories accord well with this society's idealised role for women – as the primary care-giver upon whom rests all responsibility for the psychological health of her child? This is a convenient role model: if we have delinquency because maternal bonding failed, or mothers were unable to meet all their "difficult" children's needs, then we do not need to look too hard at other factors which might require significant investments of effort and money to put right. So we accept this convenient mythology. Of course if we really believed that such links could be established incontrovertibly, we would see to it that maternal education and support received top priority in social welfare policies. It is illogical, to say the least, to allow hospitals to continue with practices detrimental to breastfeeding and 'bonding', and then affirm that the early years will determine irrevocably what the person will become. And I would not be so silly as to imagine that a good beginning protects families from all the pressures of modern life!

As it happens, I believe strongly that a loving relationship with reliable and sensitive care-givers in the first few years of life establishes a personal sense of worth and self-confidence, an independence and stability, which are basic to the building of a mature adult personality. After all, I stayed home to care for my children, and never left one of them to be minded until it was clear that he/she was happy to be left; while breastfed they went everywhere with me. And I have mothered three great young adults – reasonable (most of the time), creative, independent, affectionate to us and one another, kind to little kids, and concerned about wider issues.[21] One has already gone on to birth and mother her own baby with fierce maternal protectiveness and incredibly sound instincts. However, I also believe strongly in the resilience and adaptability of human beings, and am sure that a less-than-optimal start to the mother-child relationship need never mean disaster.

This too I can document from personal experience. Our third child was born under conditions that left me physically and psychologically shattered. The only emotion I felt for weeks afterward was rage. We certainly didn't bond instantly. I felt, and recorded that I felt, complete indifference for a very long time. That didn't prevent me from meeting her basic needs for food and warmth and closeness. She, not being the slightest bit interested in my state of mind, grew and thrived. As she did, a funny little personality emerged which seduced me into a relationship with her every bit as intense as my relationship with the other two. So long as I met her needs – which were physical and basic – she had no complaints. Having had two children, I knew this would happen and didn't worry about my lack of spontaneous affection. Well-cared-for babies are lovable, gorgeous creatures; they elicit fond feelings even from bystanders. Very young babies are concerned with actions, not thoughts or feelings. Remember this when someone next starts talking about how babies can 'sense' feelings of indifference or rejection. They can, if those feelings take some physical form. *But they are not mind-readers.*

Any mother who gets off to a bad start, or misses the hypothetical bonding period, or who fails at breastfeeding, need not fear that she has done irreparable psychological damage to her child. The relationship will be the outcome of an ongoing process. If she is reasonably caring, sensitive, consistent, and available when the child needs her, the relationship will be a good one. Worrying about her deficiencies as compared with some artificial ideal can only be harmful. Each mother will do the best she can within the limits of her personality and circumstances. Those who believe mothers should do more, or differently, ought to stop preaching and get busy changing those circumstances, and providing support for maternal personal growth. Pigeon-holing babies as 'difficult', or mothers as 'inadequate', is simply another way of ignoring the real issues (give the problem a label, and forget it). And if the mother is too persistent, the doctor will give her some pills to put him out of her misery, to paraphrase Diana Wyndham's beautiful comment.[22] Less psychology, less psychotropic medication, and more common sense help, please!

In this area of psychological effects of breastfeeding we should mention other family relationships. No one suggests weaning in those rare cases where other children feel left out when the mother breastfeeds. Rather, they suggest practical ways for the mother to cope without excluding the siblings. But if a father has problems with the fact of his partner breastfeeding, or if the mother's sexual urge is diminished, weaning is all too often accepted as reasonable.[23] In some cases that the baby may be weaned for such reasons. A man and woman socialised in mid-twentieth-century philosophies may have insuperable difficulties coping with the fact that for some women breastfeeding can mean a temporary loss of interest (or a greater interest!) in genital sex. Here the problem is not breastfeeding, but the attitudes and beliefs of the couple, or one partner. Such people need help to change. Encouraging weaning in these cases may serve to cover up a problem which will indubitably show up elsewhere in family relationships. At the very least, such parents should know to what risks they are exposing their baby before they go ahead and wean. At best, they should be helped to grow into a more mature understanding and acceptance of the complexities of their sexual selves, and a greater sensitivity to one another's needs (physical and other). But they are adults who have (we hope) chosen to be parents. Having done so, they have undertaken a responsibility to another person, their child. I personally believe that no adult has the right deliberately to put his/her wishes ahead of a child's most basic needs – and breastfeeding is a basic need. Adult sexual gratification, or male jealousy and immaturity, is not a good enough reason to deprive an infant of the only suitable food for the first half-year. Sheila Kitzinger's book, *Woman's Experience of Sex*,[24] should be required reading for parents. A partner who consistently puts personal sexual desires ahead of the child's (and the mother's) needs clearly has the wrong priorities for a long-term relationship and child-rearing, and in my opinion is the sort of partner mothers do not need, and may be better off without.

It seems to be emerging from current literature that breastfeeding mothers who sleep with their babies are likely to be having coitus with their partners less often.[25] The literature clearly assumes that this is a bad thing, and that husbands are thereby feeling deprived and resentful. Where this is due to badly managed breastfeeding, colic and so on, both partners may be feeling resentful and deprived, and no wonder.

But everyone who discusses this publicly talks as though it is always males who seek genital sexual activity, and always females who restrict or deny it. Yet I have known women who have never felt more sexually interested than while breastfeeding, and the diminished frequency of coitus is because of their husband's waning interest or decreased sexual capacity – not necessarily because of the fact of breastfeeding, or feelings of jealousy of his child, but simply because of the inevitable cumulative effects of age, fatigue, and sometimes illness. So what if coital frequency declines? If both partners are getting the measure of physical contact (as distinct from genital sex) they need and want, and if coitus is enjoyable when it occurs, it may well be part of the maturing of the couple and their relationship, and an appropriate response to their circumstances. There's more to love than sex. Sleeping with your baby can be a wonderfully satisfying physical experience for either parent. If both partners are getting a lot of physical feedback from their children, their own relationship does not have to carry the whole burden of providing all the touching they need.[26] Of course physical contact and genital sexuality remain important in their own relationship, but so do other things, including their shared love of their children, their other commitments, and so on.

There are no easy answers for the woman who finds that her sexual urges exceed those of her partner. Applying pressure – whether by attempted seduction or by rational discussion – may work, but may also prove to be counterproductive. Women can fake orgasms easier than men can fake erections. What a woman decides to do about the problem may range from masturbation through sublimation to taking a lover. However, many women shrink from the latter because of the hurt it would cause, and because while they would enjoy more sex, they know that they'd end up hopelessly entangled emotionally. Most women end by accepting that they live in an imperfect world, with imperfect people; that their partner may be less interested in sex than they, but that their relationship is too good in other ways to be jeopardised by this fact alone. These women struggle at times with great frustration, and with all sorts of self doubt. ("Would he be more interested in me sexually if I were...") If any of you are reading this book, know at least that you're not alone. Regardless of psychologists' stereotypes, it is often women who would like more sex, and men who are physically incapable of providing it, but that does not necessarily mean that the marriage is doomed or that either or both are abnormal. (Or that men should risk their sight to secure an erection or two!)

If pregnancy and/or breastfeeding are the times when such discrepancies emerge, it is tempting to see a solution in the early termination of breastfeeding. Here I would reiterate my firm conviction that breastfeeding matters so much that, just as we do not currently terminate pregnancies because of sexual difficulties, so we should not terminate breastfeeding. Any marriage or relationship that can prosper only when the male dictates the terms, and which requires sacrificing one's children's best interests, is simply not worth continuing with.

Many women seem to connive at keeping alive this myth of constant male potency. Some lie to their doctors about sexual matters to protect their husband's image in the eyes of the (male) doctor. Perhaps another reason for doing this lies in the fact that a man's lack of sexual interest is almost always portrayed in popular magazines as reflecting on the woman's desirability. What does it say about our society that popular psychologists so rarely frame the converse as an explanation for why women may sometimes lack sexual desire? Sometimes women are reluctant to air these issues because they run the risk of inviting speculation about their own relationships. What women share with one another is often not reflected in the writing of those experts who assume that less coitus after childbirth has to be a health hazard or a sign of marital problems. For some people, it may be. For some of those people, that is a source of growth in the relationship. And for others, it simply is not an issue. Love is a lot more important than sex.

Possible adverse effects of breastfeeding

The usual adverse effects cited by bottle-feeding advocates include maternal fatigue, nutritional depletion, exhaustion from broken nights, restriction of mobility, and so on. These are specious arguments, hardly worth dignifying with a reply. Any experienced parent knows that artificially fed infants also have broken nights (more episodes of illness as well, and their parents miss more work because of it); that fatigue is the inevitable accompaniment of young children, however fed, in a society that provides no support systems for the nuclear family; that nutritional depletion is the result of poor maternal diet, which should not be permitted to continue as it does around the world, but which is inexcusable in affluent countries; that breastfeeding restricts mobility only because mothers are harassed by other peoples' neuroses (breastfeeding actually greatly improves mobility of the young baby).

However, no physiological process always works perfectly for everyone. The problems of breastfeeding can be considerable, even if I do think them insignificant compared to the problems of artificial feeding. We need to consider difficulties not previously discussed in relation to breastfeeding. Only by openly acknowledging any such problems, and finding solutions for them, can we prevent vested interests from publicising the problems and thus reinforcing the image of breastfeeding as hard work, requiring great sacrifice from the mother. Sometimes we breastfeeding mothers have basked in that appreciation of us as martyrs, rather than rejecting it and asserting that breastfeeding is enormously pleasurable. I thought it a joke when I first heard that wet-nursing nine babies automatically qualified one for sainthood in Greece.[27] Where was the penance in that? (Then I thought of the pain of relinquishing a baby you have suckled, and decided the Orthodox Church was quite right.)

One problem that deserves further consideration than it will receive in this book is postnatal depression and mental illness and its relation to choices of infant feeding. Studies in this area were beginning in the early 1980's and Alder provided a good contemporary overview.[28] Since then we have had studies with widely varying conclusions, and remedies rushed into (such as oestrogen patches!) to get women back to normal, as though menstruating within a few months of birth, and not lactating, had ever been normal in evolutionary history. Doctrinaire beliefs that breastfeeding women were more at risk of postnatal depression have been proven wrong. A major population-based Victorian study of over 1100 women found that factors associated with increased risk of depression included having an operative or assisted delivery, bottle feeding, and weaning before three months of age, which in Australia usually means trying and having failed at breastfeeding.[29]

However, I think all such studies need to go beyond simple variables like feeding per se to ask questions about the mothers' medical and dietary history. If, for instance, one finds a particular mother is depressed and breastfeeding, and on psychosocial grounds there is no reasonable explanation, could it be a vitamin or trace element deficiency that is responsible? Some assert, for example, that the use of the contraceptive pill causes long-term changes in vitamin B metabolism; that vitamin B deficiency is involved in depression; and that mothers on the pill may be at greater risk. So Pill usage would be a relevant factor to record in any investigation, and vitamin supplementation might be a rational course to explore in treatment. No doubt other hypotheses will emerge as the interaction of nutrients and behaviour is further explored.

The first such problem I should like to raise for discussion is the appearance or exacerbation of joint pain during lactation and its remission during weaning. Quite a number of women have recently remarked upon the fact that while pregnant, or breastfeeding, or both, they have suffered from sometimes severe joint pain – usually in one or both wrists, but sometimes elsewhere. Consciousness of such problems has doubtless grown as a result of other repetitive motion injuries in offices and factories.

One woman who wrote to me about this mentioned that her doctor diagnosed the problem as 'nursing mothers' wrist'. This implied that in his experience such problems are common in breastfeeding mothers. This was news to me, so I asked via the NMAA Newsletter for further reports of such problems. About 30 mothers replied. Many wrote in some detail about themselves, raising questions about possible relevant factors. I should like to hear from other mothers who have experienced joint pain during lactation.

Two other problems that have emerged for consideration are headaches and nausea when initiating feeding. Findings are preliminary at this stage, but some women do experience nausea and even vomit, and Swedish midwife-friends tell me that gastric hormones are the culprit and that women should eat before feeding. (In these days of weight phobia, no wonder the problem has emerged!) Headaches can be triggered by hormonal changes as well, with a fall in plasma vasopressin recorded. More in the next book, but women should be reassured that these are not psychosomatic complaints but biological responses.

In a society where breastfeeding has historically been blamed for all sorts of maternal and infant health problems, some mothers are reluctant to admit that certain problems emerged or became worse during lactation. I would urge mothers who have had such problems to write to me about them. My interest in breastfeeding is not merely to demonstrate its superiority – which I think is self-evident – but also to solve its problems, so that it can be for all women the life-enhancing experience that it was for me. My perspective ensures that your problems will not be bruited abroad to scare off other mothers, but will be taken seriously, with an emphasis on finding ways of preventing or ameliorating its effects on mother and baby. I am now involved with every major network of breastfeeding 'specialists', so I can call upon international resources of experience and knowledge to think through your problem. It may take months or years, but if there's an answer it will be found. So do write

---

NOTES

CHAPTER 7: BREASTFEEDING AND THE MOTHER

[1] In the last few years there has been a wave of such books, all stressing the need for women's needs and wishes to determine patterns of childcare. This is all very well, but most writers are utterly ignorant about infant nutrition, and as a result see little to be concerned about when the best option for the woman seems to be not to breastfeed in a society which makes that difficult. It is far more radical to insist that society change to accommodate infants' utterly non-negotiable need for breastmilk, than to suggest that infants should accommodate to society's pressures.

[2] It should be noted that not all of each breast needs to lactate, and if drainage is a persistent problem, some women will effectively have breast tissue which has lactated and breast tissue which hasn't. Enquiries about breast problems are an important part of any cancer investigation.

[3] See Saadeh R, et al (ed.) *Breastfeeding: the technical basis and recommendations for action* (WHO Geneva 1993.) pp.29-30

[4] Short, R. V., "Breastfeeding", *Scientific American* (1984) 250, 4, 35-41. "The biological basis for the contraceptive effects of breastfeeding", in Jelliffe & Jelliffe (ed.) *Advances in International Maternal and Child Health*, vol. 3 (Oxford University Press, 1983), p. 27-40.

[5] Labbok M. "The Lactational Amenorrhoea Method (LAM): another choice for mothers", *Breastfeeding Abstracts* (1993) 13: 3-4; Labbok MH, Perez A, Valdes V et al, "LAM – a postpartum introductory family planning method with policy and program implications" (review), *Adv. Contraception* (1994) 10: 93-109.

[6] Gussler, J.; Briesemeister, L., "The insufficient milk syndrome: a biocultural explanation", *Medical Anthropology* (1980) 4, 2.

[7] Greiner, T.; Van Esterik, P.; Latham, M. C., "The insufficient milk syndrome: an alternative explanation", *Medical Anthropology* (1981) 5, 2, 233-260. This concludes with a piece which purports to support Gussler & Breisemeister but which actually indicates very clearly how early supplementation (juices, cod liver oil, totally unsuitable starchy foods) damages lactation; there is also no discussion of hospital practices (other than 10% have no milk; 10% give rice cakes while in hospital) or feeding advice and habits, etc. etc. Anthropologists seem remarkably unaware of how complex variables interact when they consider any one 'biocultural explanation' sufficient to explain lactation failure. Greiner has a website accessible via links listed later.

[8] *New Generation* (1984) 3, 3, 29-30.

[9] Reported in testimony to the Congressional sub-committee on oversights and investigations of the Committee of Energy & Commerce, House of Representatives, June 17, 1981. Serial no. 97-73. (U.S. Government Printing Office, Washington, 1981), p. 25.

[10] p. 5-4, Seminar June 4, 1981

[11] ibid. "In spite of the strong position which the Committee on Nutrition of the America Academy of Pediatrics has taken against the use of cows' milk in the first year of life, a great deal of cows' milk is still being consumed... roughly 40% of all milk from all sources, during the first year of life. We view the potential opportunity here to be of such a magnitude that it can accommodate continued expansion of breastfeeding and still provide ample dollar and unit growth opportunity for infant formula." Clearly no major expansion of breastfeeding was considered likely or desirable!

[12] Proceedings of this Conference are available from NMAA.

[13] Oakley, A., *Taking it like a woman*. (Jonathan Cape, 1983), p. 87.

[14] Gunther, M. in Ciba Symposium no. 45, *Breastfeeding and the Mother*. (Excerpta Medica, 1976), p. 151.

[15] Virden, S.F., "Relationship between infant feeding behaviour and maternal role adjustment", *J. Nurs. Midwifery* 1988; 33: 31-5; De Man A., "Early infant feeding and subsequent child-rearing attitudes of French Canadian women", *Percept. Mot. Skills* 1989; 68: 879-82; Franchesini R., Venturini P.L., Cataldi A. et al, "Plasma beta-endorphin levels during suckling in lactating women", *Br. J. Obstet. Gynecol.* 1989; 96: 711-3.

[16] Manne, A., "Electing the new child", *Quadrant*, 1996; Jan-Feb pp. 8-19.

[17] Cook, P. A., "Childrearing, culture and mental health", *Med. J. Aust.* 1978, special supplement to the August 12 issue.

[18] Cook, P., *Childcare: infants and nations at risk*, (News Weekly Press 1996).

[19] Basil Blackwell, 1983.

[20] This is one of my major criticisms of some of the work published by Raphael's Human Lactation Centre. See also Sears, W., *Creative Parenting* (Dove Communications 1982), p. 96.

[21] Not three problem-free children: adolescence is the real testing ground, as my generation have discovered, and one can be very grateful for the patience and love developed in infancy by responsive mothering styles.

[22] Wyndham, D., Doctor gives me pills to put him out of my misery. *New Doctor* 1982; 23: 21-5

[23] dee Post, R.; Singer, R., "Psychological Implications of breastfeeding for the mother", in Neville M. C.; Neifert M. R., *Lactation: physiology, nutrition, and breastfeeding*. (Plenum Press, N.Y. 1983

[24] William Collins, Sydney 1984.

[25] Cable, T. A.; Rothenberger, L. A., "Breastfeeding behaviour patterns among La Leche League mothers: a descriptive survey", *Pediatrics* 1984, 73, 6, 830-5. This article provides a glimpse of what is regarded as 'normal' by US professionals. Where unrestricted breastfeeding is a normal social pattern, their assumptions are hilarious.

[26] Montagu, A., *Touching* (Harper & Row, N.Y. 1978).

[27] Paper given at the International Confederation of Midwives 20th International Congress, Sydney, September 1984, by Maria Tsitsiloni. Published in *Proceedings*, p. 648-52

[28] Alder, E., "Postpartum changes in mood and sexuality, and some implications for care", in Houston (ed.) *Maternal and Infant Health Care* (Churchill Livingstone, 1984).

[28] Astbury J, Brown S, Lumley J, Small R. Birth events, birth experiences, and social differences in postnatal depression. *Austr. J Pub Hlth* 1994; 18: 176-84.

FURTHER READING 1998

• Labbok MH, "Breastfeeding as a women's issue: conclusions and consensus, complementary concerns, and next actions", *Int. J. Gynecol. Obstet.* (1994) 47 (Suppl): S55-S61, and any other publications, all well-researched and woman-centred.

• Cook, K. The implications of breastfeeding for a sexual health practice. *Venereology* 1995; 8: 92-102.

• Coombes F. Postnatal depression and the breastfeeding woman. *LRC Topics in Breastfeeding* 1996; set 8.

• Stuart-Macadam P, Dettwyler K. Breastfeeding: biocultural perspectives. Aldine de Gruyter NY, 1995

• All and any research by Kerstin Uvnas-Moberg , of the Karolinska Institut in Sweden, who has investigated the role of oxytocin and other hormones in breastfeeding women.

8.
BREASTMILK AND THE HOSPITALISED CHILD

The many advantages of breastmilk are particularly important for a hospitalised infant. It seems strange, then, that there should ever be any difficulty about a breastfeeding mother staying with her child (i.e., in the same room, not in a separate house over the road). Despite enormous advances in this area, the sterling work of the Association for the Welfare of Children in Hospital (AWCH), and the development of the Baby-Friendly Paediatric Unit Guidelines by the Australian BFHI National Steering Group, it remains unfortunately true that mothers are often needlessly separated from their children. I don't want to discuss the whole question of hospitalisation – this has been well done by other writers – but I want to make a few points that are rarely, if ever, emphasised, and which have emerged from the experience of food-intolerant and breastfeeding families.

Firstly, in some hospitals, sick breastfed babies are still being arbitrarily weaned on the orders of ignorant doctors, who seem to think all milks the same. This is most common in cases of gastrointestinal disturbance, particularly if a Clinitest reading shows 0.5% reducing sugars. Lactose intolerance is *assumed* to be the primary or major problem. And Mead Johnson's heavy promotion of lactose-free formulas seems to have increased the number of doctors who think that lactose intolerance is diagnosed by treatment: taking the baby off lactose-containing foods such as breastmilk. Yet good evidence shows that even in acute diarrhoea, babies do much better when breastfeeding is continued.[1] But it happens, too, in other cases of infection or disability. Sometimes for practical reasons – it's too difficult to handle the baby normally, and why go to any bother. Sometimes for psychological reasons – 'we staff feel uncomfortable with a mother breastfeeding a baby over 3, 6, 9, 12, 15 months old, there's no nutritional benefit, and the mother must be obsessive'. Sometimes it grows out of the wider staff-parent relationship – we're in charge here, we can't control and measure breastfeeding, it means the mother is always hanging about and we feel uncomfortable dealing with the children when there's an observer around. Sometimes, as we were told after Philip's surgery at just under the age of four, "we can't develop a close relationship with the child when a parent is always there." How typical these experiences were or are, I have no way of telling. That they happened at all is inexcusable.

Secondly, babies are being weaned because of some hospital routines, and lack of facilities for expressing and storing milk. Prolonged periods when nursing is impossible, combined with the stress of the situation, and obviously hostile or disgusted nurses, can cause total lactation failure in some women. This is often not the aim of the staff, but when they insist that a mother should breastfeed or express only at certain times, in certain places, with the nursery curtains drawn and special screens around her, they communicate quite clearly a negative attitude to the whole process. Experienced nursing mothers will of course disregard all such silly restrictions, very nicely, telling the staff how awkward they are, and if need be discussing the issue with nursing and medical supervisors. If breastfeeding in public is not a problem for the mother, others have no right to foist their peculiar hang-ups upon her and jeopardise the health of her child.

Thirdly, breastfed babies scheduled for operations are being put at risk by being fasted for four to 12 hours before the operation; and their mothers are often put under the intolerable strain of holding and comforting a baby screaming with hunger, who cannot understand why the milk he can smell is unavailable. Human milk is not the same as any other food. Some doctors believe that a child could quite safely be breastfed two to four hours before anaesthetics:

• Because that is the normal stomach-emptying time. Lawrence, in fact, quotes one and a half hours as the normal gastric emptying time for breastfed babies.[2] Cavell confirms that the half-emptying time for breast milk is 48 minutes; for some formula, 78 minutes.[3]

• Because even if the baby were to vomit and aspirate – an unlikely event – mother's milk would not cause the same problems as alien proteins unless of course the baby was highly allergic and the mother had not identified and avoided problem foods. Animals that die of anaphylactic shock when alien milk is put on to their larynx do not react at all to species-specific milk. Indeed, as we have said, it may be necessary to the induction of tolerance for babies to inhale breast milk. Mother's milk is less irritant to human lung tissue than glucose solutions. (A 1997 study actually assessed whether human milk or formula was more irritant to *rabbit* lungs and concluded that breastfeeding should not be permitted in *human infants* too close to surgery because it damaged rabbit lungs….: the appropriate comparison would have been of rabbit milk and bovine milk in rabbit lungs, of course!) One could even argue that *all* babies scheduled for anaesthesia could be given a feed of human milk. By reducing their distress due to fasting, this would leave them physically better able to cope with the stress of surgery. In Scandinavian countries mothers' milk *is* used in this way for sick babies. Some children become so distressed by the usual long fast that they end up ketotic, dehydrated and unable to be operated on that day. In 1984, hospitals restricting breastfeeding also urged the use of lemonade, cordials, and other sweet drinks four hours before operation. Did this cause any reactive hypoglycaemia? What were the effects of the chemicals on an empty stomach? Did the high osmolarity promote dehydration?

Similarly, it's hard to justify long delays after operations before re-feeding with human milk. It's quite clear from physicians working with LLLI, who handle many breastfed babies, that restricting breastfeeding before and after operating is quite unnecessary. Some allow mothers to feed ad lib right up until the baby is sedated; others observe a two-hour rule,[4] which is at least humane in its regard for the physiological hunger pangs a child will be experiencing.

Efforts to get paediatric authorities to establish a set of guidelines based on physiology and detailed knowledge of human milk have proved unavailing to date. So what happens to babies will continue to be as variable as the knowledge of the doctors in charge of each case. Parents should inform themselves, and make their concerns known to both the doctor and the anaesthetist. I for one would not permit any child of mine of any age to be forbidden breast milk when sick.

Fourthly, sick older children could benefit from the use of human milk. This is logical on academic grounds: its unique nutritional bioavailability, decreased metabolic load, increased immunological value, and so on. It is true on clinical evidence, as I for one can attest. When our son was almost four, he had an appendectomy. (The problem actually was mesenteric adenitis due to food and chemical intolerances.) He had recurrent bowel obstructions on a convalescent diet of chocolate-flavoured cow's milk and orange juice. Over 10 days and much surgery, he lost more than 30% of his body weight, finally developing stools so fluid and acid that his whole back blistered when a nurse could not be found to bring a bedpan and the liquid stools seeped along the plastic bed linen. Because I was concerned by his condition, I asked for nutritional support for him. This was not possible, as the surgeon felt cows' milk and juices to be the correct diet. Hence in desperation, and after discussion with the dietitian, I threw out the chocolate-flavoured cows' milk and substituted expressed breast milk. Diarrhoea and obstructions never recurred, and he came home. Coincidence perhaps? (From my later reading on lactose intolerance, cows' milk sensitive enteropathy, and so on, I very much doubt it.) Six months later we discovered that Philip's stomach and joint pains at night – 'normal' since nine months – ceased when we took him off cows' milk. Probably his colic, 'normal' too, was the precursor – more severe because the gut was less mature; by nine months of age he could tell us verbally that he was in pain.

But the evidence for therapeutic benefits of human milk is stronger than that family anecdote. It is not yet extensive, because extensive trials have not yet been done, despite the strong probability that this could be of benefit to many categories of the patient, but already there are reports of benefit to older children with chronic intractable diarrhoea,[5] and children with resistant enteric pathogens (giardia,[6] rotavirus,[7] clostridum botulinim[8]), as well as very young or premature or immunodeficient infants.[9] In Sweden, where prematures have always been fed human milk, necrotising enterocolitis is non-existent according to the Chief of Milk Banks in Malmo, Sweden. Another Swedish unit, using non-pasteurised human milk even for trans-pyloric tube feeding, has a mortality rate of 0.95% on an average of 3000 babies each year.[10] Closer to home, the Queen Victoria Memorial Hospital in Melbourne had remarkably successful breastfeeding rates for even the smallest babies, and the incidence of necrotising enterocolitis is very low for babies fed human milk. These rates are slipping as the companies intensify their marketing efforts for premature formulas, supplying it in handy little ready-to-feed sizes at subsidised prices. The Colombian experience described in the 1984 UNICEF Report illustrates how dramatic the effect of exclusive breastmilk feeding can be in less-affluent communities.

With such evidence of benefit, why is human milk not used more widely? Some are concerned about theoretical hazards of cross-infection or adverse immune reactions, and so they urge caution. Such concerns are valid, although when balanced against the actual hazards of alternative feedings, and the experience of Scandinavian countries, they seem a trifle illogical. If doctors wanted to solve those potential problems, they would have done so by now. Parents are not unreasonable and, if given a properly informed choice, must accept the consequences of a choice (which should be theirs to make) between alternative therapies. (I'd opt for human milk any time if the criteria for donors excluded those taking social or other drugs.) But it is useful to be able to raise the spectre of transmissible diseases if basically one does not wish to alter the status quo or have to become involved in mobilising community resources to supply donated milk. It's so much easier just to accept a can from a company which asserts that its product is as perfect as it can be. Even if each can costs $35-40, and at least 10 per cent of children will be unable to tolerate it (as is true of the most sophisticated feedings), it seems easier to use artificial milks than begin the potentially risky and labour-intensive task of organising a milk bank. Besides, the company would have to bear the liability for any mishap with its formula. As the government pays for the most specialised infant formula, there is no incentive from parents or hospitals to change the status quo; and as speciality milks increase their share of the formula market,[11] so do company profits increase. How expensive must those formulas become before we realise that human milk may be both cheaper and better? Not all cultures have had our reluctance to use human milk for anyone except babies; it was commonly believed to be ideal for the sick and frail elderly[12] as well, and was used for that purpose. And here in Australia, I know of a gang of shearers who congratulated one country wife on her scones, not knowing that she (24 km from town) had used frozen human milk because the cartons ran out. Curious, yes. Disgusting, no. She was a good deal cleaner than any cow! (And sportsmen are swallowing bovine colostrum!!)

The fifth point that emerged from parents' experience of hospitalisation was that significant numbers of staff seem to be incapable of understanding either children or parents; much less the value of constant parental presence to the child, the need to take seriously parents' requests or observations, and the ways in which parents can relieve the nurse's workload. What was even worse, there were staff who seemed to perceive the whole issue as being one of their authority and power being challenged by usurpers. While we ourselves found most of the nurses to be good-hearted and well-meaning, we found only one who seemed capable of understanding Philip's perspective on the situation. Naturally she supported us in staying with him, showed us what needed to be done, and then got on with the job of looking after all those other children who needed her. At the other extreme was Nurse Bossyboots, a childless authoritarian female who did her level best to confine our presence to daylight hours, tried to exclude us from all 'medical' procedures (though we knew best how to calm Philip and explain what was happening, and he was angelic through many unpleasant procedures while we held him), and so on. As time wore on, it became clear that no one could complain that we made life more difficult for either Philip or the staff; so then we heard that our presence was "preventing them from developing a close relationship…" etc. I nearly retorted, "Stiff cheese! My child doesn't exist to provide emotional gratification for nurses. If that's what you want, go work on a relationship with the kids who keep crying all day!" But unlike those unhappy children without their parents, Philip was attractive, i.e. bright and cheerful when not in intense pain (which they repeatedly suggested he was 'putting on' because we were there. Knowing our child, we insisted on getting the doctor and saved Philip from bowel resection due to delayed recognition of yet another obstruction). Staff doted on our extrovert two-year-old daughter when she came to visit, taking time to play with her, and she happily responded. They commented that 'she would be no trouble', implying that Philip was, simply because most of the time he ignored them as irrelevant. More than any other comment, that revealed the depth of their ignorance of children. We, knowing Catie, knew that she would be a hopeless patient at that age because she could not understand what was going on. In fact, for years afterwards she was incredibly frightened of medical procedures; not until five or six was she able to control herself and permit unpleasant minor medical procedures. The impact on her of Philip's hospitalisation was devastating; despite her smiles and charm, and our best efforts, we could not protect her from the reality of Philip's pain; and not understanding, she became afraid of the places and practices associated with it. Philip, by contrast, has a mature understanding and acceptance of what happened, though he has not forgiven the staff who promised solemnly that if I were needed one night they would fetch me, and then refused to do so. Next morning he told me how he had then climbed out of the cot (i.v. drip and all) and began pushing it along the corridor to where I was sleeping, but they stopped him. The nurses' evasiveness confirmed that this was no nightmare, as did a newly bandaged arm. We would never again accept the offer of a bed, but stay on a wooden chair or the floor. Trust once broken can never be mended, alas.

Was ours an isolated experience? Hardly. I've since heard of children having severe allergic reactions as the nurse disregards the mother's warnings about forbidden foods; of parents being forced to leave despite their child's distress (which may have been what killed young Matthew Davey, a child who was hospitalised for tonsillitis), of drugs being prescribed which contained substances the child was known to be intolerant of. Most professionals will privately admit that of course such things happen, that with constant overwork and staff changes they are almost inevitable. That is why each child needs its parents, or someone special there to act as informed advocate, as well as emotional crutch. Parents too, were often disturbed by the variety of tests and procedures to which their children were subjected. When these had been clearly explained, they were usually well accepted, although parents sometimes complained that later on they were never asked about the consequences for the child in anything but the immediate post-test period. For example, with food-intolerant children, 'challenges' were seen by some parents to result in difficulties for a considerable time later. Some said it took months to get the child back to where he had been prior to the challenge. When a UK senior immunologist[13] has stated that he believes Australia's policy of frequently challenging children explains why fewer (than in the UK) truly outgrow food intolerance one wonders why the challenges continue. They are thus wasting money both immediately and long-term, as children with chronic problems will cost the taxpayer far more than those given dietary supplements for longer without challenges. Of course, at present challenges are necessary to academic research and publication; but parents should be aware that there is a tension between what is necessary strictly for their child's sake, and what is necessary for the researcher to be able to write a paper which may (or may not) help others at a later stage. To co-operate in a research project is fine, so long as the parents understand clearly what they are doing. To subject one's child to risk simply because of bureaucratic demands for verification at given intervals is less acceptable.

And finally, a number of parents (and their children) were put under great stress by health hazards in the hospital environment. One of these has happily improved in the last decade: hospital 'no smoking' policies are no longer so frequently flouted by visitors and staff alike, as they once were. This was inexcusable, given the incontrovertible evidence of harm due to passive smoking. Perhaps hospitals should consider supplying nicotine chewing gum to nurses still so addicted that they are unable to survive their shift without smoking and coming back reeking to care for a child who is sensitive to the vile smell: assuming that nicotine gums are effective substitutes for addicts. But the strengthening attitude to passive smoking that is evident in some countries and institutions is by no means universal.

This depressing litany of some hospital failings is not the only thing that could be said about hospitals and their staff. Many have dramatically improved care for the breastfeeding family over the last decade. Parents are willing to accept that they too can make life difficult for staff, who are almost always grossly overworked in the cost-cutting, profit-making 1990's. Parents accept, too, that it is probably unrealistic to expect the childless to be able to empathise fully with either parent or child, though surely such skills should be part of professional training? And curiously, the very young trainees and nurses often seemed to have more instinctive kindness than some more experienced nurses and doctors. (Perhaps there is an emotional fatigue that sets in?) Parents are deeply grateful to those staff who have been kind and treated them as equal human beings, explaining what they need to know clearly and patiently. Be that as it may, there is such a substantial element of dissatisfaction within certain sections of the community that it seemed necessary to raise these issues publicly, in the hope that they may stimulate improvements. Once again, I do not expect to be particularly popular for saying publicly what so many parents say privately to one another. Perhaps enough caring professionals will hear what I am trying to communicate, and work even harder to improve these matters. And so perhaps we shall soon see full implementation of Kangaroo Care[14] practices in all children's hospitals, and moves towards full implementation of the BFHI and its Baby-Friendly Paediatric Unit, the basic criteria for which are set out in the following pages. If we are concerned about quality of life issues for children, these standards are evidence-based minimal requirements that should soon be normative, except where impossible for strict medical reasons. And even there they can be modified in most cases.

11 Steps to Optimal Breastfeeding in the Paediatric Unit

Step 1. Have a written breastfeeding policy, and train health care staff caring for breastfeeding infants in skills necessary to implement the policy.

Step 2. When the sick infant is admitted, ascertain the mother's wishes about infant feeding, and assist mothers to establish and/or manage lactation as necessary.

Step 3. Provide parents with written and verbal information about the benefits of breastfeeding and breastmilk.

Step 4. Facilitate unrestricted breastfeeding and/or frequent breastmilk expression by mothers who wish to provide milk for their children, regardless of age.

Step 5. Give breastfed children other food or drink only when age-appropriate or medically indicated.

Step 6. When medically indicated, use only those alternative feeding methods most conducive to successful breastfeeding, and restrict the use of any oral device associated with breastfeeding problems.

Step 7. Provide facilities that allow parents and infants to remain together, 24 hours a day, that encourage skin-to-skin contact as appropriate, and that avoid modelling the use of artificial feeding.

Step 8. Administer medications, and schedule all procedures, so as to cause the least possible disturbance of the breastfeeding relationship.

Step 9. Maintain a breastmilk bank that meets appropriate standards.

Step 10. Provide information about community breastfeeding support groups to parents at the time of the infant's discharge from the hospital or clinic.

Step 11. Maintain appropriate monitoring and data collection procedures to permit quality assurance and ongoing research.

Using the Self-Appraisal Questionnaire to assess policies and practices

A Self-Appraisal Questionnaire was developed originally for use by maternity facilities, to evaluate how their current practices measure up to the Ten Steps to Successful Breastfeeding elaborated in the 1989 WHO/UNICEF Joint Statement, *Protecting, Promoting and Supporting Breastfeeding: The Special Role of Maternity Services*.

An Australian working party of paediatric specialists has developed this equivalent Eleven Steps to a Baby-Friendly Paediatric Unit, and devised this questionnaire, to protect, promote and support breastfeeding in paediatric units, whether free-standing paediatric hospitals or units within maternity or general hospitals. This is in keeping with WHO and UNICEF's encouragement of family-friendly national initiatives incorporating local experience. The Nutrition Unit of WHO Geneva has acted as a resource in the development of these criteria.

Any paediatric unit that is interested in becoming Baby Friendly should appraise its current practices vis-à-vis these Eleven Steps. The checklist below permits a quick initial appraisal or review of a unit's practices in support of breastfeeding. Eventually it is hoped that a process of external assessment will be available.

PAEDIATRIC UNIT DATA SHEET

Date: _____

Unit Name: _____

Address: _____

_____ **Telephone:** _____

Chief Hospital Administrator: _____

Senior Medical Officers (or other personnel in charge):

For the Hospital: _____ Telephone: _____

For the Paediatric Unit : _____ Telephone: _____

For Community Liaison: _____ Telephone: _____

Type of Unit(s) being assessed. Tick all that apply	☐ Government	☐ Public/Private (Mixed)	☐ Private
	☐ General Hospital	☐ Paediatric Hospital	☐ Maternity Hospital
	☐ Teaching	☐ Other	
	☐ Level 1 nursery	☐ Level 2 nursery	☐ Level 3 nursery
	☐ Paediatric ICU	☐ Paediatric unit	

Hospital census data:

Annual number of deliveries: _____

Total bed capacity: _____

_____ in the Level 1 nursery

_____ in the Level 2 nursery

_____ in the Level 3 nursery

_____ in the paediatric wards

Other (please specify) _____

If no such area exists in the paediatric facility, write "none" in space provided.

Total admissions in the year 199__:
Total admissions of children 0-2 years old in the year 199__:

_____were in paediatric wards

_____were significantly preterm (< 35 weeks)

_____were in Special care nurseries

Infant feeding data from admission records:
Numbers of:

_____ artificially-fed infants 0-6 months admitted in the past month

_____ mother/infant pairs bottle-feeding at discharge in the past month _____%

_____ breastfed infants 0-6 months admitted in the past month

_____ mother/infant pairs discharged breastfeeding in the past month _____%

_____ breastfed children older than 6 months admitted in the past month

_____ children breastfeeding (or breastmilk-fed) from admission to discharge in the past

month _____%

Audit results:
Children of all ages breastfeeding at admission who were no longer breastfeeding when discharged in the past month _____ %

Relative risk by feeding group for admission to hospital (compare percentages of breastfed and artificially-fed children in hospital with data from local community figures for breastfeeding and artificial feeding) _____

How was the infant feeding data obtained?

From records _____

Percentages are an estimate, provided by: _____

Paediatric Unit Self-Assessment Tool

(Please circle the appropriate response)
STEP 1.   **Have a written breastfeeding policy and train all health care staff in skills necessary to implement it.**

1.1   Does the paediatric unit have a written policy that addresses all 11 Steps to Successful Breastfeeding in a Paediatric Unit?
Yes   No

1.2   Does the policy protect breastfeeding by prohibiting all public promotion of breastmilk substitutes, feeding bottles and teats?
Yes   No

1.2   Does the policy promote safer bottle feeding by mandating individualised parent instruction in the use of breastmilk substitutes, feeding bottles and teats?
Yes   No

1.3   Is the breastfeeding policy available to all staff who take care of mothers and infants, and can staff refer to it?
Yes   No

1.4   Is the breastfeeding policy posted or displayed in all areas of the health facility which serve mothers, infants, and/or children?
Yes   No

1.5   Is there a mechanism for evaluating the effectiveness of the policy?
Yes   No

1.6 Are all staff aware of the advantages of breastfeeding and acquainted with the facility's policy and services to protect, promote and support breastfeeding?

Yes   No

1.7 Are all staff caring for women and infants oriented to the breastfeeding policy of the hospital on their arrival?

Yes   No

1.8 Is training on breastfeeding and lactation management given within six months of their arrival to staff caring for breastfeeding infants?

Yes   No

1.9 Does the training cover the Eleven Steps to Successful Breastfeeding in a Paediatric Unit?

Yes   No

1.10 Is the training on the hospital's breastfeeding policy at least 8 hours in total   for registered healthworkers caring for breastfeeding infants ?

Yes   No

1.11 Has the healthcare facility arranged for specialized training of specific staff members in lactation management or appointed a relevant specialist?

Yes   No

STEP 2. When the sick infant is admitted, ascertain the mother's wishes about infant feeding, and assist mothers to establish and/or maintain lactation as necessary.

2.1 At admission, is the child's past and current feeding history ascertained and recorded, and the breastfeeding mother assured that continued breastfeeding is valuable and will be supported by staff?

Yes   No

2.2 Are staff members or counsellors with specialized training in breastfeeding and lactation management available to advise mothers during their stay in the unit and in preparation for discharge?

Yes   No

2.3 Does a woman with breastfeeding problems receive immediate attention, consistent advice and support from the staff?

Yes   No

2.4 Do staff offer mothers assistance with breastfeeding within six hours of admission?

Yes   No

2.5 Are most breastfeeding mothers able to demonstrate how to correctly position and attach their infants for breastfeeeding?

Yes   No

2.6 When necessary, are mothers of infants unable to breastfeed shown how to express their milk or given information on expression?

Yes   No

STEP 3. Provide all parents with written and verbal information about the benefits of breastfeeding and breastmilk.

3.1 Do staff inform parents about the benefits of breastfeeding?

Yes   No

3.2 Do records indicate whether breastfeeding has been discussed with parents?

Yes   No

3.3   Are staff informed about the particular benefits of breastfeeding for sick or hospitalised children and their mothers?
Yes   No

3.4   Is visual and written promotion of breastfeeding obvious within the unit and the whole facility?
Yes   No

3.5   Is visual, oral or written promotion of artificial feeding prohibited within the unit and the whole facility?
Yes   No

3.6   Is instruction about artificial feeding given only on an individual basis to all family members and caregivers for whom it would be appropriate?
Yes   No

3.7   Are mothers of infants who are artificially fed encouraged to take responsibility for feeding their children wherever possible, and supported appropriately?
Yes   No

STEP 4.   Encourage unrestricted breastfeeding and frequent breastmilk expression by mothers who wish to provide milk for their children, regardless of age.

4.1   Do staff show parents that they are aware of the importance of unrestricted breastfeeding?
Yes   No

4.2   Provided that there are no medical reasons to restrict intake, are mothers advised to breastfeed their children whenever their children want to breastfeed, whether for food or for comfort?
Yes   No

4.3   Are mothers of sick children unable to breastfeed helped to initiate and/or instructed to maintain lactation by frequent expression of milk?
Yes   No

4.4   Are mothers of sick children of any age permitted to give their breastmilk to their infants if the mother wishes to do so?
Yes   No

4.5   Are suitable facilities available for a mother to breastfeed her older child without physical or psychological discomfort?
Yes   No

4.6   Do staff actively support the mother breastfeeding an older child?
Yes   No

STEP 5.   Give breastfed children other food or drink only when age-appropriate or medically indicated.

5.1   Are staff aware of the few acceptable reasons for supplementing or complementing newborn breastfed infants? (See Acceptable medical conditions, Annex 1: The Global Criteria).
Yes   No

5.2   Do breastfed infants under six months of age receive food or drink other than breastmilk **only when** this is appropriate?
Yes   No

5.3 Are infants older than six months given appropriate complementary weaning foods and their mothers encouraged to continue breastfeeding?

Yes   No

5.4 Are older children given suitable food but also permitted to continue breastfeeding if they wish to do so?

Yes   No

5.5 Are any breastmilk substitutes (including specialised formulas) used in the facility purchased in the same way as other foods or medicines?

Yes   No

5.6 Do health facility and all health care workers refuse free or low cost* supplies of breastmilk substitutes, but pay close to market price?

Yes   No

5.7 Has the facility set up a system to monitor the use of breastmilk substitutes to prevent misuse or wastage?

Yes   No

* *Paying for supplies of infant formula and setting up simple accounting systems can both reduce the unnecessary use of breastmilk substitutes. The Australian BFHI National Steering Group has defined low-cost as being less than 80% of the wholesale price. Breastmilk substitutes intended for experimental use or professional evaluation should also be purchased at 80% or more of wholesale price.*

STEP 6. When medically indicated, use only those alternative feeding methods most conducive to successful breastfeeding, and restrict use of any oral device associated with breastfeeding problems.

6.1 Do staff avoid feeding breastfed infants using bottles with artificial teats whenever this might interfere with the establishment or maintenance of lactation?

Yes   No

6.2 Are staff familiar with and skilled at feeding infants via teaspoon, cup, tube, and breastfeeding supplementer?

Yes   No

6.3 Do staff minimise the use of dummies to preterm breastfed infants able to be given "Kangaroo care"* or to breastfeed?

Yes   No

6.4 Are breastfeeding mothers informed by staff that they should not give any teats or dummies to infants having problems with breastfeeding?

Yes   No

6.5 Does the hospital refuse free or low-cost teats, bottles, and dummies, and gift packs containing these, thus avoiding inadvertent promotion of these to mothers?

Yes   No

* *Kangaroo care is described in the UNICEF Video of the same name. It consists of keeping the baby constantly warm and upright against the mother's skin, close to her breasts where the infant can breastfeed ad libitum.*

STEP 7. Provide facilities that allow parents and children to remain together, 24 hours a day, that encourage skin-to-skin contact as appropriate, and that avoid modelling artificial feeding.

7.1 Do facilities enable parents to remain together with their children 24 hours a day if they wish to?
Yes   No

7.2 Is skin-to-skin contact encouraged for all clinically stable infants ?
Yes   No

7.3 Is Kangaroo Care facilitated for all clinically stable small or sick infants?
Yes   No

7.4 Does the unit provide simple washable slings to facilitate parental contact with their infants as appropriate?
Yes   No

7.5 Is all promotion for infant foods or drinks other than breastmilk absent from the facility, including waiting rooms, pharmacy and wards ?
Yes   No

STEP 8. Select medications, and schedule all procedures, so as to cause the least possible disturbance of the breastfeeding relationship.

8.1 Are relevant staff aware of the effects of drugs on the initiation and/or maintenance of breastfeeding, and do they consider this when prescribing and administering?
Yes   No

8.2 Do staff inform parents of the effects of drugs on the initiation and/or maintenance of breastfeeding, and encourage mothers to continue during any temporary difficulties?
Yes   No

8.3 Is the role of breastfeeding in pain control explained to staff and parents?
Yes   No

8.4 Are breastfed infants fasted for no more than 3 hours before elective surgical procedures?
Yes   No

8.5 Are infants able to be put to the breast as soon as they are willing to after medical and surgical procedures?
Yes   No

STEP 9. Maintain a human milk bank that meets appropriate standards.

9.1 Does the unit encourage mothers unable to remain with their breastfed children to express their milk and send it to the hospital?
Yes   No

9.2 Does the unit provide collection and storage facilities for breastmilk?
Yes   No

9.3 Are facilities for milk expression attractive, comfortable, equipped with appropriate technology, and close to all wards housing infants or children under 5?
Yes   No

9.4 Is it possible for a mother to express milk close to the infant's bedside?
Yes   No

9.5 Do collection and storage facilities meet appropriate microbiological standards?
Yes   No

9.6 Does the hospital permit the use of donor breastmilk for small or sick infants where parents insist on this?

Yes   No

STEP 10. **Provide information about community breastfeeding support groups to parents at the time of the infant's discharge from the hospital or clinic.**

10.1 Does the hospital offer education to key family members so that they can support the breastfeeding mother at home?

Yes   No

10.2 Is involvement with breastfeeding support groups advocated to breastfeeding parents?

Yes   No

10.3 Does the hospital routinely refer mothers to the existing maternal and child health services in their area?

Yes   No

10.4 Does the facility encourage and facilitate the formation of special interest mother-to-mother or healthworker-to-mother support groups?

Yes   No

10.5 Where the mothers request it, does the facility allow breastfeeding counselling by lactation consultants or trained mother-support-group counsellors able to work as part of the care team ?

Yes   No

STEP 11. **Maintain appropriate monitoring and data collection procedures to permit quality assurance and research.**

11.1 Does the facility maintain detailed records of the child's feeding history at admission, during hospitalisation, and at discharge?

Yes   No

11.2 Are these records routinely evaluated and appropriate action taken as part of an ongoing quality assurance programme ?

Yes   No

11.3 Do staff have access to this and other available research and are they encouraged to initiate and participate in research as appropriate?

Yes   No

11.4 Where appropriate, does the facility periodically attempt to evaluate breastfeeding duration after discharge?

Yes   No

GLOSSARY OF TERMS

• **Breastfeeding supplementer:** any device designed to permit the flow of additional nutritional fluid from an external container into a child's mouth when the child is breastfeeding.

• **Breastmilk substitute:** any food marketed or otherwise represented as a partial or total replacement for breastmilk, whether or not suitable for that purpose (International Code Article 3)

• **Child:** a person young enough to be admitted to a paediatric unit for care and generally older than 12 months of age. (In some cases in this text "child" and "children" naturally refer also to infants, indicating their relationship to their parents, as well as to older children: e.g., Step 4 and 5.)

- **Infant:** a person aged less than twelve months
- **Infant formula:** a proprietary product meant to provide adequate nutrition for infants, which meets all the requirements of Australian Food Standard R7 or any other relevant Food Standard.
- **Kangaroo care:** described in the UNICEF Video of the same name, this consists of keeping the baby constantly upright and warm against the mother's skin, close to her breasts where the infant can breastfeed ad libitum.
- **Free or low-cost supplies:** any supplies of infant formula provided to the hospital at less than 80% of the normal wholesale cost of the product. (Australian BFHI National Steering Group definition)
- **Relative risk by feeding group for admission to hospital:** this figure is derived by comparing the percentages of breastfed and artificially-fed patients, with data on breastfeeding and artificial feeding rates in matched control groups from the community served by the hospital. While exact relative risk figures may be hard to ascertain, a hospital has a responsibility to make the community aware that artificial feeding puts children at increased risk of serious illness needing hospitalisation. Conversely it can be demonstrated that children at risk of serious illness because of other factors such as parental smoking are actually protected to a degree by breastfeeding. Breastfed children of smokers are less likely than bottle-fed children of smokers to be admitted to hospital with severe bronchiolitis, for example: once the relative risk figure is established and the additional community cost of bottle-feeding calculated, motivation to protect, promote and support breastfeeding increases. Not all paediatric units may be in a position to establish this risk ratio, but every effort should be made to do so.

Addendum: A simple baby sling

Baby slings can provide comfort for distressed young children and should be commonplace in hospitals. Most slings are rather expensive, the cheapest being NMAA's Meh Tai. But here is a pattern for a simple baby sling, which you can make out of any sturdy soft fabric you have on hand.

The basics
Two large rectangles, 38 x 33 cm (15 x 13 inches)
Two long straps, 178 x 13 cm (70 x 5 inches)
Two short straps, 18 x 13 cm (7 x 5 inches)
Two rings, about 5 cm in diameter

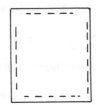

1. Pin the two large rectangles together (wrong side out). Sew, leaving space at all four corners for straps; turn inside out.

2. Fold straps in half, sew along their length, turn inside out.

3. Insert long straps into top corners, sew and reinforce with several lines of stitching. (Use different colours if you like.)

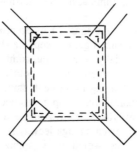

4. Insert short straps into bottom corners, sew and reinforce.

5. Fold bottom straps over ring, sew and reinforce.

6. Take in a tuck if necessary.

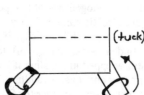

To use

1. Put the sling against your body, long straps over your shoulders; take right top strap over to left ring, left top strap to right ring, thread through, and tie straps together loosely at your waist.
2. Slide the baby up under the sling, and hold there with one hand until you can pull straps very tight with the other hand. Adjust baby's position so that the edge is tight across the nappy-padded bottom, without cutting into the baby's legs.

If baby is very little, take a tuck in the sling: fold a pleat along the whole width of the sling, as in the diagram, then pin or sew the tuck. (Big safety pins will do, and can be more easily removed, if you have no sewing machine.) Let out this pleat as baby grows.

You can also take in a tuck lengthways, if you want to have the sling going through baby's legs – which is safer, but sometimes less comfortable. (And this depends on how you use the sling: if you have one hand free all the time, to catch baby if he slips, and are not doing anything strenuous, the under-bottom hold is quite adequate so long as the sling is comfortably tight.)

The very long straps and rings on this model combine to give it a number of advantages:

- It will fit any figure and does not need to be 'adjusted' between husband and wife, as the Meh Tai does.
- The long straps allow you to use it in hospital beds – tied very loosely. Baby can sleep beside you without fear of falling. But don't use it for this if you're taking sedatives or drugs with sedative effects, such as antihistamines.
- The straps can be tied at back or brought to the front, eliminating the knot-in-the-back discomfort of many slings when you sit down.

Some people say that their babies don't like being put into a sling. Many do protest vigorously at first, but I have yet to meet a baby whom I cannot get to sleep in a sling. The trick is in tight straps and rhythmic movement, especially side to side, combined with rapid gentle back-patting. It sounds strenuous, and sometimes is – both of us remember jogging with colicky Philip. We found that changing movement, smoothly rather than jerkily, was best, though sometimes rapid running on the spot was needed to stop the first squawks. Philip also would respond to swaying sideways; his head had to be partly supported to stop neck strain or damage, but given enough leeway so that he could feel it getting heavier and heavier. His eyes would track something backwards and forwards until he found it easier to shut them altogether – at that point victory was in sight! Another five minutes, with his head gently turned sideways so that his ear was against my chest, and he would be fast asleep. While colicky, if put down he would wake in ten minutes, so I would find a book and go off to a comfortable chair. Other children could be put down still wrapped in the sling if I was careful about taking it off. So don't give up on the first few attempts. Swaddling like this can only be good for babies, even if they protest at first. Many a mother (or father) has found that the baby they thought would never tolerate a sling can be very comfortable in one. Ask another mother to demonstrate. And take no notice of the critics who say you're spoiling the baby: the Balinese believe that a baby should be in someone's arms for the first 6 months of its life.

No sling is safe for use in a car, even with the seat belt between mother and baby, and baby in a sling 'outside' the seat belt. (Seat belt over baby in sling would cause baby to be crushed in even a minor accident.) However, all risks are relative. While a sling might simply rip apart in an accident, a baby in a sling would not be thrown out in a minor braking or impact at very low speeds. Unrestrained children have been killed in stops at 20 km/h. Ideally, everyone has and uses a car seat or capsule for babies. But as a parent who had to fit three children into a small station wagon – we had to buy a new car – I know that there are situations when capsules cannot be used, or afforded. While I'm definitely not encouraging you to use a sling when travelling by car, if you do use one make sure that: (1) the seat belt is between you and baby; (2) you sit in the back seat; (3) you never use it when driving yourself; (4) you put enough pillows in your lap to take baby's weight and reduce back strain.

Remember, a sudden stop increases baby's weight by 20 times: a 5 kg baby suddenly weighs 100 kg. Never let anyone sit and hold a child, however short the trip. Even if the person's reflexes were quick enough to try, his or her muscles wouldn't be strong enough to hold any child, however small. Many fathers, in particular, seem to believe they could. A sturdy sling is vastly preferable to no restraint at all.

Slings, like any heavy weight carried for a long period, can damage your back. The higher and closer the baby, the less the strain on your spine. Some models allow babies to lean back and away from the parent's body – the leverage exerted will strain back muscles. Keep babies tucked in tight and high, at chest (not stomach) level.

NOTES

CHAPTER 8: BREASTMILK AND THE HOSPITALISED CHILD

[1] Khin-Maung-U, et al "Effect on clinical outcome of breastfeeding during acute diarrhoea", *Br. Med. J.* (1985) 290, 587-9. Lactose intolerance is discussed at some length in the 1985 edition of *Food for Thought* (Allen & Unwin, Sydney).

[2] Lawrence, R. A., *Breastfeeding: a guide for the medical profession* (C. V. Mosby & Co. 1980, p. 200.)

[3] Cavell, B. "Gastric emptying time in infants fed human milk or infant formula", *Acta Paediatr. Scand.* (1981) 70, 5, 639-41.

[4] Countryman, B. A., quoted in Brewster, D. P., *You can breastfeed your baby – even in special situations* (Rodak Press, 1979), p. 314. This book has an excellent chapter on hospitalisation and breastfeeding.

[5] MacFarlane, P.I., Miller, V., "Human milk in the management of protracted diarrhoea of infancy", *Arch. Dis. Child* (1984) 59, 260-5.

[6] Gillin, F. D. et al, "Killing of giardia lamblia trophozoites by normal human milk", *J. Cell. Biochem.* (1983) 23, 1-4, 47-56

[7] Berger, R. et al, "Influence of breast milk on nosocomial rotavirus infections in infants", *Infection* (1984) 12, 3, 171-4.

[8] Arnon, S. "Breastfeeding and toxigenic intestinal infections: missing links in crib death?" *Rev. Infect. Dis.* (1984) 6, suppl. 1, 193-201.

[9] Narayanan, I. et al, "The value of human milk in the prevention of infection in the high-risk LBW infant", *J. Pediatr.* (1981) 99, 3, 496-8.

[10] *J. Pediatr.* (1981) 99, 3, 496-8

[11] This has been "the fastest-growing segment of the formula market", according to the Vice-President of Ross Abbott. (20% of formula sales in 1979 compared with 2% a decade earlier. That added up to $120 million dollars of the 1980 total of $700 million.

[12] Fildes, V., "Putting Mum in the picture", *Nurs. Mirror* (1979) 149, 3, 22

[13] Dr J. Walker-Smith, at a meeting of the British Society of Immunology, St Mary's Hospital, London, November 1983.

[14] Ludington-Hoe, DS, Galant SK *Kangaroo Care: the best you can do to help your preterm infant* (Bantam Books, 1993) See also Lang S *Breastfeeding Special Care Babies* (Bailliere Tindall 1997); most other standard texts, and the UNICEF video on Kangaroo Care. Lang's book is simply wonderful, and should be required reading.

9. BREASTFEEDING AND DENTAL HEALTH

Experiments in vivo and in vitro support the hypothesis that under normal circumstances **milk** is not cariogenic and may have anti-cariogenic potential. This should not be surprising for **milk** is man's first and probably most important food, and if it were highly cariogenic, then man could probably not have evolved with teeth.

E. C. Reynolds and E. Storey, "A review of the effects of milk on dental caries",
Aust. J. Dairy Technology, Dec. 1979, 179.

What a sensible summary! The only problem is that the milk referred to as man's most important and first food seems to be cows' milk, which says something about the authors' mindset. At present women are being told that breastfeeding at night can cause rampant dental decay. Unfortunately those who tell them this seem extraordinarily ignorant about breastmilk. Just what are the risks?

The rampant tooth decay of bottle-mouth syndrome is certainly a serious problem. By now all parents should know that the practice of giving babies sugary drinks, including milk and formula (certain formulae being notorious, at one time, for their high sugar content), may cause terrible destruction of the child's front teeth: black rotted stumps in extreme cases. Those who don't know a great deal about breastfeeding have been quick to assume that because breastmilk contains lactose, a fermentable sugar, mothers should not nurse their babies to sleep or allow them to suckle freely at night. Once again, human milk is seen simply as another food, and breastfeeding as equivalent to drinking from a bottle. Neither is true.

Even worse, some dental authorities (whose studies are often funded by relevant commercial dairy and processed food interests) suggest that cow's milk may be less likely to produce caries than human milk, because of the undoubtedly higher protein, calcium and phosphate[1] levels of cows' milk (these serve to buffer teeth against acid formed by bacteria). They also state that human milk sours in 30 minutes to one hour, whereas it take three to five hours for cows' milk to sour.[2]

Those figures I find quite surprising. Country milk cartons used to warn us not to leave cows' milk unrefrigerated as, being days old already, it could sour in less than an hour in warm conditions. Pasteurisation reduces bacterial contamination, but does not eliminate it, and the heat used destroys many of cows' milk's bacteriostatic and bactericidal properties, so that given warmth the remaining bacteria multiply very rapidly in cows' milk. Human milk (unlike cows' milk consumed by humans) is a live milk, which is, as we have seen, far more than the sum of its nutritional components. It is designed to support a totally different gut and oral[3] bacterial flora than is a ruminant milk. (Bacteria that cause disease in humans may be necessary to digesting cellulose in cows.) Its bacteriostatic and bactericidal qualities are unimpaired, unlike those of cows' milk. In fact, it contains antibodies to "all normal streptococcal inhabitants of the human oral cavity, including those which colonise the neonatal oral cavity in significant numbers".[3] Milk banks allow for this in the instructions they give donating mothers: none suggests that milk is sour within hours of expression! A recent paper[4] on sick babies being tube-fed breast milk stated that there was no increase in bacterial contamination during 24 hours of refrigeration or four hours of room-temperature infusion. I personally have fed breast milk to a very sick post-operative three-year-old in small sips from an unsterile glass over some hours in a warm room. The taste of the milk did not alter (I checked) and the child neither complained about taste nor became symptomatic from infection. While I would have preferred to have access to refrigeration, I would do the same thing again: after that he began to improve and had no further relapses.

And how have the researchers established that human milk can cause problems similar to artificial formulae? By citing examples of diseased teeth in children who had once been breastfed or who are being partly breastfed at the time: the old medical assumption that 'breastfed' equals 'receiving any human milk' or 'ever having received breastmilk' which has so confused comparative morbidity statistics. The case reports of such ever-breastfed children are rare, but none of the children were being exclusively breastfed. This is hardly surprising, given that nursing bottle caries emerges between one and three years of age! The researchers failed to investigate other carbohydrate intake (including fruit juices or cordials), family history, use of fluoride and other prophylactic measures. Nor did they investigate the nutritional and immune status of mother and baby alike, e.g., to check for possible low antibody levels in human milk because of maternal anaemia, or decreased secretory antibody in the child's saliva because of stress. They saw a very few children who had been or were being breastfed in what they seem to have regarded as an excessive fashion; they saw caries, and they linked the two. How can researchers be so careless?

The historical and cultural fact is that most of the world's children have been breastfed ad libitum and at night, for periods ranging from one to five years, and did not suffer from bottle-mouth syndromes. My three children are a proof of that – and no, I do not have perfect teeth, but a mouth full of fillings! Nor do I know a nursing mother (and I know hundreds) whose children have suffered rampant caries, whereas in lower socioeconomic groups in Brisbane, "up to one-fifth of children under six show 'bottle caries'". As one Dr Brown put it, "Caries in breastfed children is in all likelihood a very small problem indeed compared with children who are bottlefed".[5] This is true because not only are the milks different, so is their method of delivery. This is well described in an article by Wendy Sih, from which Dr Brown's statement is excerpted.

Milk does not pool in the mouth (against the teeth) when a child suckles the breast. Milk is ejected at the back of the mouth and throat, spilling over the epiglottis (which covers the larynx) and stimulating a swallow reflex immediately. When milk flow stops, because baby has fallen asleep, the nipple is removed from the mouth by changes in maternal and infant position. Simply because the baby stops suckling, the breast and nipple retracts from being an elongated 'teat' to its normal shape. Before he can again milk the breast, the baby must reshape it by drawing it into his mouth. If we ever do find a truly breastfed child with caries, it would possibly be useful to look closely at the suckling patterns and positions of any breastfed child developing rampant caries. And at his mother's milk supply: has she an overabundant supply, resilient nipples that the baby hangs on to, 'leaking' high-lactose milk during night-time comfort suckling?

Of course some formerly or partially breastfed babies may develop dental caries. But this is no justification for blanket statements like "it would appear wise to warn mothers that, while nursing caries is relatively rare, care should still be taken to avoid prolonged suckling once the child has teeth".[6] Prolonged suckling may be very important to some mothers and some babies, whether as a source of low-allergy high-quality food, a medicine, a contraceptive[7] or a gob-stopper/sleep inducer/only way to get some peace. (Curiously, the German word for breastfeeding is *stillen*, which also means 'to silence'.) It is irresponsible for dentists to discourage physiological, individually responsive breastfeeding because of an admittedly rare risk. This, in effect, was the conclusion reached by the dental authors of a review article, "Can Breastfeeding Cause Dental Caries?"[8] Their paper reviewed the "six reports of twelve specific cases" relating prolonged breastfeeding to rampant caries. (Of such enormous statistics are media scares born.) Because the children's ages ranged from 14 months to more than two years and because they were not reported to be malnourished, one can agree with the authors that "it is reasonable to assume that all these children were consuming some foods other than human milk", and that "more comprehensive reports [of dietary intake] would have been useful".[8] Such wonderful understatement!

Among the details of that "comprehensive report" I should like to see an investigation of the possibility of malabsorption, of food allergy and intolerance, and of gastric reflux. Some milk-fed children, for example, may be receiving an adequate mineral intake but not utilising it effectively.[9] Several parents have raised the query as to whether allergy may contribute to poor dental health, as in their families (of three to five children, usually) the most food-allergic child stands out as being the one with dental problems. In the families I know of, dental problems are not the result of parental dietary restrictions: the idea of allergy is a recent one, and diagnosis and dietary changes came after the established fact of dental disease. Of course, early inadequate dietary intakes of essential minerals could contribute to create the problem, which is one of the reasons why parents concerned about allergy should seek professional help with dietary changes. This might particularly be the case when allergy causes reflux: repeated exposure to acidity damages teeth.

The paper referred to above also reviewed some of the epidemiological evidence relating infant feeding to dental caries. As could be expected, every single study showed that breastfeeding was associated with *decreased* caries prevalence. Some of these studies date back to the 1960s, before everyone became concerned about sugar; one was published in 1940, when it was middle- and upper-class women who were bottle-feeding. Yet so reluctant are scientists to be seen as advocates for breastfeeding that the authors partly explained away these consistent findings by stating that "breast-feeding is more prevalent in higher social classes", therefore "it could be the lower prevalence of sugar-eating habits that is the main explanation" of the uniform advantage of breastfeeding in these studies. The authors do not attempt to ascertain whether it was indeed the "higher social classes" who breastfed on the Isle of Lewis in the 1930s nor whether those classes had any different pattern of sugar intake, nor do they investigate historical and cultural correlates of rampant caries.

In assessing any such reports and their recommendations, parents need to keep in mind the undoubted influence of commercial interests. Of course, the researchers are honourable men. But like the rest of us, they live in a society subject to heavy propaganda from vested interests, they accept the pervasive myths that no one must be made to feel guilty, and that accurate information will necessarily induce guilt; they depend (sometimes) on funding from very diverse sources; and 'extremists' are rarely funded. There are no vested interests to defend breastfeeding; there is no money available from a breastmilk industry; it is thought to be 'extreme' to advocate traditional and physiological patterns of infant feeding, with weaning by mutual consent at whatever age.

With that in mind, certain other aspects of the paper by Hackett et al. can be reviewed. The "cariogenic potential" of breastmilk – its ability to dissolve enamel and lower pH – was assessed. The in vitro test for enamel dissolution involved incubating enamel, milk and saliva for 24 hours. This showed that some enamel dissolved with both human and cow's milk, but "bovine milk was considerably more protective to enamel dissolution than human milk".[8] This was probably because of its high calcium and phosphorus content – which means that those infant formulae which for safety's sake (to protect infant kidneys and brains) have had their excessive mineral loads reduced probably are not as good as human milk in protecting against caries. It does seem a trifle odd that the dentists go on comparing cows' milk and breast milk when no baby under six or twelve months of age is supposed to drink cows' milk. Perhaps dentists are not aware that babies should not be fed cows' milk? Perhaps they do not realise that infant formulae are all very different in their choice of carbohydrate, too. Obviously, they should do some studies on real infant formulae, not whole cows' milk. I'm sure that those formulae which, over a month, supply the baby with 1 to 1.5 kg of sugar[10] would not fare as well. Whether corn syrup and other formula carbohydrates are as bad has not, to my knowledge, been tested.

Human milk was more protective than other sugar solutions under these artificial conditions, but did cause some loss of enamel. So what? Even if a baby were to be suckling continuously for 24 hours, it would not replicate the conditions of this experiment. The child would have in its mouth freshly-made human milk, which does not sour, is full of antibacterial factors, and so on. Human milk has been shown to destroy the streptococcal bacteria responsible for dental decay. So what does this in vitro test prove? That if you were to extract your child's teeth and leave them to soak in stale breastmilk they would lose a little enamel. (Do the same with certain soft drinks, and they might have dissolved.) Not really very relevant information, is it? So why was it published?

An earlier report has emphasised the rapid clearance of breast milk from the child's mouth and argued against giving advice to curtail physiological breastfeeding.[11] Hackett et al. agree that breastfeeding beyond four to six months "does not inevitably cause rampant caries" but fail to mention one single good reason why continued breastfeeding might in fact be beneficial, as it clearly is. This negativity may be the result of ignorance, but it is depressing to see dentists intent on protecting dental enamel and unconcerned about other aspects of child health. The authors of the review are actually quite positive about breastfeeding: "in virtually all cases" feeding past four to six months does not cause rampant caries. And their conclusions are relatively moderate: "there is only cause for concern for the dental health of those infants who undergo prolonged 'at will' breastfeeding, particularly during the night; who possibly take other undesirable foods, and may also have poor oral hygiene and low fluoride intakes". But what an unbalanced presentation this is, with its emphasis on the "extreme behaviour" of prolonged breastfeeding,[12] and its neglect even of other feeding-related dental considerations such as malocclusion.

Malocclusion is, in simple terms, when the top and bottom teeth don't meet properly. It requires expensive orthondontic correction, and is nowhere more common than in America, where mass bottle-feeding is of longest standing. As far back as 1950, in the results of a study of over 300 cases of all ages, it was concluded that "nursing in the first 6 months may control a person's facial contours for the rest of his life".[13] This has now been confirmed in a major study involving 10,000 American children: orthodontic defects were much more common in those bottle-fed that those breastfed for more than six months.[14] There is good reason to suspect that bottle-feeding is the cause – both directly because of the unnatural oral mechanics of artificial feeding, and indirectly, because the bottle-fed child requires far more non-nutritive suckling from inanimate objects and is more likely to suck a pacifier, thumb, knuckle or whatever else he becomes attached to. Breastfed babies, too, have non-nutritive suckling needs, but these can be built into the breastfeeding experience itself. The human nipple conforms to the shape of the baby's mouth, rather than causing the baby's mouth to become conformed to its shape. No one believes in the importance of this more strongly than the makers of orthodontic teats, which they falsely claim mimic exactly the shape of the breast during feeding (see Chapter 3 for discussion of such claims).

In a brochure published by the makers of some orthodontic teats, the claim is made that use of other teats (or even the incorrect use of their teats) can lead to everything from adenoids to mental disorders. How can we allow such harmful products to continue to be sold, if this advertising is accurate in its representation of the hazards of improper sucking and oral habits? Or if this advertising is not accurate, how can we allow such exaggerated and frightening nonsense to be freely circulated as a means of boosting commercial profits? If advertising standards worthy of the name exist, why has there been no scrutiny of these and many other claims, such as those of formula companies about the ease of bottle-feeding, or their products (all different) all being 'closest' to human milk? The *International Code of Marketing of Breastmilk Substitutes* allows for scientific and factual information to be advertised: but this nonsense

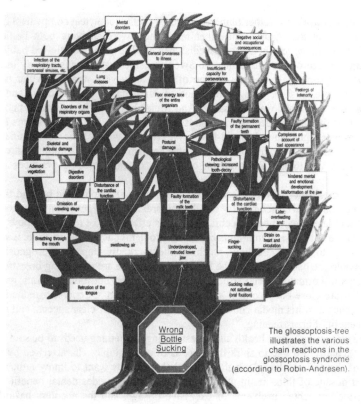

The glossoptosis-tree illustrates the various chain reactions in the glossoptosis syndrome (according to Robin-Andresen).

<u>Figure 9.1</u> **The "glossopathy tree" as published by a major manufacturer of orthodontic teats. Courtesy Mapa GmbH.**

hardly qualifies under that heading. Only in Australia has NUK been asked to justify this nonsense – or end it.

I should certainly like to see independent laboratory testing and clinical trials of all existing teats and pacifiers, including the 'orthodontic' ones. Ardran[15] in the 1950s criticised many as badly designed, too rigid, and more likely to result in an exhausted starved baby than in an overfed one. The size of the hole in the teat was often such as to cause the baby to push most of the milk back into the bottle, rather than out into the mouth. Many mothers thought their babies were feeding well because of the vigorous mouth movements they made, but in fact the babies were getting little or no milk. Ardran thought that most babies should only take a few minutes to empty a bottle, as breastfed babies receive the bulk of their feed within the first five minutes, and other baby animals are even faster. The clear implication is that bottle-fed babies have to work a lot harder for their food than do breastfed babies: it may be this excessive and unphysiological exercise that results in malocclusion. To support the idea that breastfed babies work less rather than (as alleged by orthodontic teat companies) more, I would point out that Ardran and other researchers were studying both bottle-fed English babies and largely-breastfed Swedish babies. The wholly bottle-fed babies all made frequent vigorous jaw motions; the Swedish babies varied considerably in their behaviour, and some gave the impression of using only very weak muscular movements. These, presumably, were babies whose mothers had a good let-down and who did not realise that work was necessary. And Meier has now demonstrated that premature babies find bottle feeding more stressful.[16] Whatever the facts, it seems to me that Jelliffe was right when he said back in 1978: "In view of the commonness of malocclusion and the cost, discomfort and time for its correction, additional attention needs to be given to the investigation of details of early feeding practices in its etiology."[17]

The oral mechanics of breastfeeding may also have an importance beyond that of ensuring normal facial structures. By developing oral and facial muscles, breastfeeding contributes to later clear speech in children.[18] This effect is most marked in boys, who are less mature at birth, and in infants born with problems such as cleft palate. It would be interesting to investigate how much of the markedly improved prognosis for Downs' syndrome babies is due to the fact that many more are now being breastfed[19] – which helps to normalise facial structure, provide optimal nutrition for brain growth, and also ensure close body contact and sensory stimulation. Of course a reduction in infections such as otitis media could also be important in later clear speech, and this is another benefit of breastfeeding.[20]

While discussing dental health and breastfeeding, something needs to be said about fluoride. Actually, I'd like to shirk this one, as of all the topics characterised by irrationality of discussion, fluoride is the worst. What parents want to know is basically this: what dosage of fluoride, in what form, and when, provides dental benefit while avoiding the undoubted problems of excessive dosage, and the needless hazards of artificial colours, flavours, etc. What parents get is an absolute mandatory statement to use a certain amount at a certain age, regardless of body weight, diet, environment, and much else. Or, from another camp, an equally absolute statement that fluoride is poisonous (which it is) and should never be given.

On the evidence presented to me in 1984, I thought oral fluoride supplementation of babies under 6 months of age was a dubious practice. I had hoped to be able to support moderate supplementation, to spare myself the wrath of important vested interests who are heavily committed to the idea, but could find no evidence to support it. It seems that by 1998 paediatric authorities agree: no one is recommending fluoride supplementation any more: why was that so obvious to me but not to them at the time?

What was the reasoning behind the advice to use supplementary tablets or drops of fluoride for breastfed babies? Certain dental authorities believe that an adequate intake of fluoride has two different types of effect: systemic, and topical.[21] Systemic effects include improving the "pit and fissure morphology of the developing primary molars" and strengthening parts of those baby teeth which are not calcified at birth. These are effects from the inside out, so to speak, improving the actual shape and structures of the teeth from within, so that they are less susceptible to decay. Even in 1984 I found this part of the claim somewhat amazing, and there were well-informed dentists who considered any effect on tooth structure and shape totally unproven; or if possible, also possibly dangerous to bone formation. By contrast, topical effects work from the outside in: the local application of fluoride via toothpaste is seen as hardening and strengthening the outer surfaces of the tooth enamel – once teeth have erupted. This is more readily demonstrated, but obviously there is no point taking fluoride before teeth have erupted for topical effects.

But what is an adequate intake? Too much fluoride can cause fluorosis, which in very mild cases consists of some mottling and discolouration of tooth enamel. Until now, parents asking questions about this in their children have probably been told merely that the benefits outweigh what is a minor cosmetic defect. However, many dentists argue that far from being a minor cosmetic problem, this is "a sign of chronic fluoride poisoning affecting the whole body, especially the bones".[22] Even the pro-fluoridation lobby accepts that this is too common to be ignored, and one article calls for further carefully controlled investigation of infant fluoride intake and metabolism, on a geographical basis. "Because of the variability of the fluoride content in infant formulas and other foods, the [bottle-fed] patient's age and the level of fluoride in the drinking water remain the most important factors to consider in prescribing supplemental fluoride."[21] In babies whose teeth have not yet erupted, "the important topical effect of fluoride is not achieved." In addition these bottle-fed babies will be receiving some dietary fluoride, perhaps 80-150 times that of the breastfed baby, and actively accumulating it, whereas the breastfed baby is actively mobilising it from his bones and excreting more than he ingests.

There were American babies, and American formulae, discussed in a fairly moderate article in *Caries Research* in 1978. What we need is an Australian discussion of a similar kind. The authors, Adair and Wei, assessed the fluoride content of some human milk, cows' milk products, and commercially available infant formulae, prepared with and without fluoridated water; concluded that infants being fed commercially prepared formulas may be receiving fluoride well in excess of recommended daily dosages; and stated that "downward revision of earlier recommendations for the younger infants is in order". (This later happened in the United States.) They also stated that "although the infant appears to possess a tolerance to high levels of fluoride, no supplemental fluoride appears to be necessary for infants up to six months of age". Fully breastfed infants, even in fluoridated areas, receive only very small quantities, so the authors recommended only a very low dosage, based on bodyweight. The possible influence of maternal diet on levels of fluoride in breastmilk was not discussed. In a nation of tea drinkers (tea contains fluoride) this could be relevant, as could other dietary and environmental factors. Czechoslovakian studies showed that children living near smelters take in more than 2 mg. daily from air, water, plants and animals, even though their water supply was not fluoridated.[23]

Since this 1978 study, however, other studies[24] have shown that the breastfeeding baby seems to be actively protected from fluoride: despite deliberately increasing the amounts in maternal diet, only a tiny amount was present in breast milk. Because this is not a new chemical compound, and because other chemicals of similar structure are excreted in milk in amounts related to diet, this might suggest that in evolutionary terms babies are not intended to get fluoride supplements until they're on a mixed diet. (Or it may be one of mother nature's quirks that have no beneficial effect.) But the fact that the breastfed baby excretes more than he or she ingests – as the baby does with radioactive strontium – makes me incline to the former view rather than the latter.

Other things have changed since 1978. Fluoride was once considered an essential element for humans. In 1976 this had been modified to "essential or probably essential"; then in 1979 the US FDA deleted even that definition. So the belief that fluoride is essential has been altered, yet that belief underlies many assumptions about the safety of dosing children with a known toxin. As for infant tolerance levels, how do we know what they are? If we are looking only for gross effects we may overlook more subtle problems. Fluoride is known to interfere with enzyme functioning, and I do wonder whether this may be one contributory factor in the increased incidence of food intolerance problems in children. Dental fluorosis may itself by a major problem, of course: it was apparently normal for pre-war teenagers in Nhill, Victoria, to have their 'mouldy looking fluoride teeth removed before entering the marriage market'. The bore water of Nhill contained four-fifths of the recommended 1.0 ppm that is to be imposed on many other areas, and other sources of environmental fluoride were less. I am told that the white mottled areas on teeth may later become unsightly brown stains, which can cause serious social and psychological problems. This is unnerving for me, for like most conscientious mothers in the mid-1970s I dosed some of my children. The results are not yet clear enough to be any guideline for others. Philip, the intensely food-intolerant oldest child, was given from birth the standard (now excessive) dosage then recommended, in the neat coloured and flavoured pill. His teeth are just like mine as far as pits and fissures go, but maybe the enamel is tougher – after extremely frequent day and night-time feedings, he had by 18 months developed one tiny spot on one upper front tooth. The tooth fell out when he was seven with that spot of decay barely changed. His teeth are mottled, and the front incisors that emerged at seven are fairly discoloured; still, he was caries-free after that very early one until adolescence.

Mottling of his teeth was apparent by the time our other children were born, and because no dentist I knew would provide references to explain the subject – they simply argued very emotionally – Katie received almost no fluoride supplementation. Elizabeth got none. We lived in unfluoridated areas until the children were 10, 8 and 6. The girls' teeth are not mottled, and each had had just one very small filling by the ages of nine and eleven respectively: despite frequent day and night feedings to 15 months of age, and in Elizabeth's case, no early fluoride at all. Nor has the children's dental record been due to obsessive oral hygiene. They hurt their gums when they used dental floss (and so did we), so didn't use it much; and although they clean their teeth before bed, they do not do so after every meal. However, for nutritional reasons their early childhood diet included very little refined sugar, almost no soft drinks because of preservative sensitivity, and plenty of fresh fruit and vegetables: they drink a lot of (charcoal-filtered) water. Their diet is, if anything, low in calcium by Australian standards, so really they should be prime candidates for 'nursing caries', having begun life with such 'extreme' behaviour as ad libitum breastfeeding. I said in 1984 that until all three had their second teeth I wouldn't be sure which of them, if any, has been injured by too much or too little fluoride. In 1998, when they are 22, 20, and 18, I can say that dentists have advised me that fluoride made no difference to the genetic structure of their teeth; that Catie has the best natural tooth structure; that Lizzie and Philip should have had their secondary teeth polished and sealed to overcome the fine surface fissures natural to them. So my worries were for nothing and it seems I might just as well have ignored all the directions about fluoride.

On the credit side, ad libitum breastfeeding has done them no harm in the other areas of dental health mentioned. None has needed major orthodontic work, which is just as well because we couldn't afford it. All three speak clearly and distinctly, and have done so from an early age – partly because of the excellent development, by breastfeeding, of muscles involved in speech, partly because they have never had the ear infections and hearing loss so common in bottle-fed infants. (In the first 21 child years, we had had perhaps three bouts of earache.)

If I had my time over again, would I take or give fluoride in tablets or drops? On the present evidence, no. Living near an aluminium works which discharged fluoride into air and water, I became more concerned about excess than deficiency. This was the conclusion of the Quebec Government enquiry into fluoridation. We do still use a fluoride toothpaste, but the amount on the brush is miniscule, as this is a significant source of fluoride intake (especially if children copy the advertisements by using inch-long strips, or even "a small pea"). Although some fluoride will be absorbed from the mouth, it seems to me more logical to apply fluoride topically than to swallow it, as its deposition in the bones may cause some problems. Talking to farmers about the increased fracture rate and other animal problems after a smelter began operations nearby is not reassuring, although scientific studies have reported mixed results in relation to fracture rates in the elderly. (I hope tea drinking was controlled for!) We have installed a reverse osmosis drinking water filter and all drink more water.

However, if recent supplementation might have been effective for the elderly, has it been excessive for those less likely to be suffering from osteoporosis? What is the effect, not just on elderly bones, but on adolescent kidneys? I would emphasise that I'm not recommending any particular course of action to someone. We all have to consider the information we can find and then make decisions for ourselves. But the more we talk and question, the more likely it is that definitive information will emerge. I promised in 1984 that if such information came to hand, I would see it publicised, and invited critical responses. Not one dentist to date has argued with what was written in this book. And the trend is away from excess...

Mass fluoridation of water supplies is a separate issue which I do not wish to discuss in depth, as it has little to do with breastfeeding. But I would like to put on record that there are many intelligent and thoughtful parents who, while supporting fluoride prophylaxis in general, and using fluoride toothpastes, are strongly opposed to or have major reservations about the wisdom of that water fluoridation. The article by Geoffrey Smith, a Melbourne dentist, in *New Scientist*, should be prescribed reading for politicians intent on fluoridation. It concludes "...at last scientists appear to be taking a long hard look at fluoridation and the uncontrolled, indiscriminate use of fluoride-containing dental products." It may be that in another 50 years, fluoridation will be seen as yet another mistake make by enthusiasts interfering with natural processes on the basis of inadequate information.[25]

Parents' concerns are genuine, and have not been adequately addressed in a debate polarised between two extreme camps. One can even believe that fluoride might be helpful in preventing caries without wishing to increase the fluoride intake of elderly people, particularly women, who may be consuming large amounts in their beloved cups of tea. And to ignore the ambient fluoride pollution from aluminium smelters and from superphosphate (said to be 2% fluoride) when deciding whether to fluoridate local water supplies seems rather extraordinary. Are we once again accepting that if something is good, more of it is better? This is untrue of fluoride, a potent poison, as it is of anything else. How do we monitor the inevitable build-up of fluoride in soil, in vegetables, and so on? Why has there been a retreat from fluoridation in almost all west European countries? And so on. Public statements showing a fall in caries incidence without controlling the sample population for other factors such as dietary changes, greatly increased environmental fluoride, and oral hygiene habits, do not answer these questions. Dismissing questioners as lunatics does not inspire confidence either.

One particular area of concern is whether fluoridated town water should be used for the artificially-fed infant whose formula must be made up with water. No health authority has addressed this. It seems as though it has been agreed that no one should publicly address this issue, on the grounds that to do so might undermine general confidence in water fluoridation. I have to disagree. Surely parents can see that what is safe for older bigger children may not be safe for infants whose sole diet is made up with fluoridated water? Surely we could make unfluoridated water available for making up infant formula for the first four months of an infant's life, when there are no other foods in the diet? Country folk could be advised to use rainwater; and water in supermarkets could be labelled with its fluoride content as well as other mineral load, so that parents could know whether the water was suitable or not for infant feeding. At present some parents are using highly unsuitable mineral waters, and there is no relevant labelling to guide them. In Israel, infants have died as a result.

Why is nothing being said about the risks of fluoridated water for bottle-fed infants? Does it relate to the realities of artificial feeding: is the unspoken truth that many poor families could not afford to buy water as well as formula, and we do not want to create even further pressures towards government subsidies of artificial feeding? Yet if we go on doing nothing structurally to encourage breastfeeding in disadvantaged communities, we owe it to them to reduce the hazards of artificial feeding. Water quality is one such area of risk. And in many rural and urban communities water quality is dangerous to artificially fed infants in very many ways.

It now seems quite clear that the earlier recommendations about fluoride for infants were excessive; they have been revised downward; and they are still subject to intense, well-informed criticism by many professionals, who have established that bottle-fed babies receive doses perhaps 80-150 times that of breastfed infants.[26] We now know too, that the kidneys of adolescents and children have difficulty in handling fluoride.[27] Will someone publicly admit that the earlier recommendations were wrong?

Professionals rarely admit to making major errors, especially when they can merely revise until they have reversed the once-accepted dogmas of the past. What is referred to as evidence-based medicine is changing this pattern, but only slowly.

To return to breastfeeding and summarise this complex relationship between breastfeeding and dental health: my conviction remains that physiological mechanisms and behaviours developed over millennia of evolution must be intrinsically safer and more compatible with good health (dental and otherwise), than arbitrary substitutes and routines dictated by inadequate research. There may well be problem areas, and individuals at risk. But blanket restrictions and panic-mongering are inexcusable. For mothers to be told by dentists or women's magazines not to breastfeed frequently, or at night, is outrageous. I wish there was some way of conveying to such people the enormity of their advice, and their responsibility for its consequences. Breastfeeding is too important ever to be discontinued for frivolous reasons.

NOTES
CHAPTER 9: BREASTFEEDING AND DENTAL HEALTH

[1] This high phosphate content, which in the laboratory glass protects teeth from decay, is precisely the ingredient which in the baby can lead to neonatal fits as a result of the decreased absorption of calcium. Infant formulae have had the phosphate content lowered for this reason. Depleted calcium intake is unlikely to promote strong teeth, either: perhaps the caries epidemics of the 1960s and 1970s among bottlefed children were due to high phosphate/low calcium formulae? (As well as sugar syrups, sweetened pacifiers, and so on.)

[2] Reynolds, E. G. & Storey, E., "A review of the effect of milk on dental caries", *Australian Journal of Dairy Technology* (1979) December, 175-9

[3] Eggert, F. M. Gurner, B. W. "Reaction of human colostral and early milk antibodies with oral streptococci", *Infect. Immun.* (1984), 44, (3), 660-4

[4] Wright, L. et al, "Effects of temperature, tubing and time on bacterial contamination of breast milk infusions", (Abstract) *Ped. Res.* (1984).

[5] Sih, W., "Breastfeeding and dental health", *Breastfeeding Review* March 1983, no. 2, p. 44.

[6] Letter from chairman of Dental Health Education Committee of Victoria, to a concerned mother who raised the issue, late 1983.

[7] cf. Short, R. V., "Breastfeeding", *Scientific American* (1984) 250, 4, 35-41.

[8] Hackett et al. "Can Breastfeeding Cause Dental Caries?", *Human Nutrition: Applied Nutrition* (1984) 38A, 23-28. (Excellent list of references.)

[9] Hypocalcaemia, which occurs only in bottlefed infants – because of the poor bioavailability of calcium in some formulae – can cause defects in dental enamel. cf. Stimmler, L. et al, "Dental defects associated with neonatal symptomatic hypocalcaemia", *Arch. Dis. Child.* (1973) 48, 217.

[10] Data supplied by Mead Johnson advertising literature, criticising competitors' products. Collected at ICEA Convention, June 1984.

[11] Abbey, M. A., "Is breastfeeding a likely cause of dental caries in young children?" *J. Am. Dent. Ass.* (1979) 98, 21-4.

[12] One could more readily describe as extreme the behaviour of those who think it normal to leave babies to cry in darkness and isolation, rather than to feed them as is normal in less 'advanced' communities.

[13] Pottenger, F., Krohn, B. "Influence of breastfeeding on facial development", *Arch. Pediatr.* 1950, 67.

[14] Labbok, MH; Hendershot GE, "Does breastfeeding protect against malocclusion? An analysis of the 1981 Child Health Supplement to the National Health Interview Survey", *Am. J. Prev. Med.* 1987; 25: 116A.

[15] Ardran, G. M., et al, "A cineradiographic study of bottlefeeding", *Br. J. Radiol.* (1958) 31, 361, 11-22.

[16] Meier P, Anderson G, "Responses of small preterm infants to bottle- and breastfeeding", *MCN* (1987) 12: 97-105.

[17] Jelliffe, D. & Jelliffe, E. F. P., *Human Milk in the Modern World* (O.U.P. 1978) p. 268. See also Simpson, W. J. and Cheung, D. K. "Developing infant occlusion: related feeding methods and oral habits", *J. Canad. Diet. Assoc.* 1976. 42, 124; and Finnochi, L. L., "Breast Feeding, Bottle Feeding and their impact on oral habits: a review of the literature", *Dental Hygiene* (1982) 56, 11, 21-5.

[18] Broad, F. E., Duganzich, D. M., "The effects of infant feeding, birth order, occupation and socio-economic status on speech in six-year-old children", *N.Z. Med. J.* (1983) 96 (734) 483-6.

[19] Aumonier, M. E., Cunningham, C. C., "Breastfeeding infants with Downs' Syndrome", *Child: care, health and development* (1983) 9, 247-255. Danner, S., *Breastfeeding the Downs' Syndrome Baby* (cf. p. 125).

[20] Saarinen, U., "Prolonged breastfeeding as prophylaxis for recurrent otitis media", *Acta. Paed. Scand.* (1982) 71, 567-71. Schaefer, O., "Otitis Media and bottlefeeding: an epidemiological study of infant feeding habits and incidences of recurrent and chronic middle ear disease in Canadian Eskimos", *Can. J. Public Health* (1971) 62, 411.

[21] Adair, R. & Wei, Y., "Supplementary fluoride recommendations for infants based on dietary fluoride intake", *Caries Research* (1978) 12, 76-82.

[22] Correspondence with Dr P. R. N. Sutton.

[23] cf. Smith, G., "Fluoridation - are the dangers resolved?", *New Scientist* (1983) 98, 1356, 286-7. Sardines contain a certain amount; bone powder used by the milk-intolerant as a source of calcium, is also fluoride rich.

[24] Ekstrand, J. et al, "No evidence of transfer of fluoride from plasma to breast milk", *Br. Med. J.* (1981) 283, 761-2. Spak, C. J. et al, "Fluoride in human milk", *Acta Paed. Scand.* (1983) 72, 5, 699-701. Esala, S., et al, "Effect of maternal fluoride intake on breast milk fluoride content", *Br. J. Nutr.* (1982) 48, 201-4.

[25] *New Scientist*, (1983) 98, 1356, 286-7, see also *Med. J. Austr.* (1985) 143: 283-8.

[26] Sutton, P. R. N. "Bottlefed infants are overdosed with fluorides", *Breastfeeding Review* (1985) 5, 38-40 cf. also. *Br. Med. J.* (1982) 283, 761-2

[27] Spak, C. et al, "Renal clearance of fluoride in children and adolescents", *Pediatrics*, 1985, 75: 75-9.

FURTHER READING 1998

• Murad P, "Breastfeeding and dental caries", *New Beginnings* (1994) 11: 56-9.

• LLLI, *Breastfeeding and dental caries* (1996). Bibliography also available.

• Johnston T, Hale KJ, Cox R, "Dental caries in the infant and toddler", *NMAA Newsletter* (1997) 33: 4-8.

• Labbok M, Hendershot G, "Does Breastfeeding protect against malocclusion?" *Am. J. Prev. Med.* (1987) 3: 227-232.

• Wyne AH, Spencer AJ, Szusler FS, "Infant and child feeding practices: a preliminary investigation", *Aust. Dent. J.* (1997) 42: 54-8.

10.   THE HISTORY AND POLITICS OF INFANT FEEDING

The composition of breastmilk and the method of supplying it to the infant have been evolved by Nature over an extremely long period, and on general principles we should hesitate to abandon a well-tried method. There are many ways in which we interfere with nature, but the evidence in favour of giving antibiotics, operating on pyloric stenosis, growing better cows or wheat, and for using umbrellas in the rain is much more solid than the evidence for a widespread change to bottlefeeding. The history of bottlefeeding is marred by mistakes...[examples given]...Near perfection may now have been claimed, but the history of infant feeding suggests that this remains unlikely, and that babies would be safer if they were breastfed. 'Humanisation' of preparations for bottlefeeding has led to some uncritical comparisons between breastmilk and modern cow's milk based preparations.

- C. B. S. Wood and J. A. Walker-Smith, *Mackeith's Infant Feeding and Feeding Difficulties* (Churchill Livingstone, 6th edn, 1981), pp. 96-7.

Infant feeding has been recently discovered as a fertile field of inquiry by some very able historical researchers, and some old ideas are changing. Anyone interested in this area must also read *Dream Babies* by Christine Hardyment,[1] which I cannot recommend too highly as the ideal new parent present. Valerie Fildes' books and articles[2] also make fascinating reading and are highly recommended. So too is Palmer's *The Politics of Breastfeeding,*[3] and Rima Apple's writings, referred to throughout this chapter. Here I can present only a rough outline. Because it is such a long and complex topic I have divided it into two parts: the first looking at the issue on a global scale until the early 1980s; and the second concentrating on world developments as they affect Australia and on how Australia has dealt with world issues since that time.

1 – "Think Global": Infant feeding until the International Code

The popular idea of infant feeding is that in other societies, and in past times, babies were either breastfed or died. This is substantially true, but it conceals enormous diversity in feeding habits. In Western Europe over the centuries, most babies were breastfed because their mothers had little or no alternative, and simply assumed that babies should be breastfed. Some commentators remarked upon the health and vigour of such babies of poorer families by comparison with the children of the wealthy.[4] Poor Irish in England breastfed their babies and the children were so

213

healthy as to cause comment by sanitarians, who deplored their living conditions yet recognised that "a comparative fewness of Irish in a town could improve the infant death rate". Jewish districts also had lower infant mortality rates despite overcrowding and poverty, and this was attributed to breastfeeding.[5] Of course infant mortality rates from all causes, especially weanling diarrhoea, probably resembled those of today's developing societies. But even if babies were breastfed, they were rarely exclusively breastfed. Every society had a long list of foods, fluids, and herbs which were deemed especially suitable for newborns and their mothers; every society had its prescribed routines and rituals to purge or stimulate or protect. In India it was butter and honey, in Bali premasticated rice and banana, in Peru a syrup of wild endive and chicory.[6] Given what we know now about the effects of such decoctions on the bacteria of the gut, and the long-term impact this can have, it is reasonable to assume that much of the mortality among breastfed infants was related to such food fads interfering with the protective mechanisms of breastfeeding.[7]

Many babies were breastfed but not by their own mothers. Wetnursing has been an age-old tradition and remains[8] a very successful way of rearing an infant whose mother cannot or will not feed it. Given that not all women can breastfeed without painful problems, this is to be expected – perhaps even encouraged in some situations, despite the HIV paranoia. The popular idea of wet-nurses (irresponsible poor women whose own babies were neglected as they sought comfortable employment) is being shown to be largely false for England in the period before the industrial revolution of the eighteenth and nineteenth centuries. Rather, there were three different types of wet-nurses: "the parish nurse who took in infants and was usually receiving poor relief herself; the nurses of the London Foundling Hospital who worked under the supervision of inspectors; and the privately employed nurse for whom wet-nursing was a significant and continuing occupation for which she received a good wage".[9] Wet-nursing was a cottage industry carried on by respectable married women in their own homes. Their care for their charges was often first rate, and many of those who wet-nursed orphaned children for the London charitable foundations kept in touch once the children went back after weaning, and tried to secure the children as apprentices, or even adopted them, within the family. (Evidence for the bonding effects of breastfeeding, perhaps?) When other opportunities for gainful employment came to rural areas, wet-nursing declined as an occupation. As the supply of such respectable wet-nurses dried up, so to speak, the desperate poverty and exploitation of the less-fortunate increased. In the eighteenth century, more women were forced to resort to wet-nursing as one of the few ways of staying alive. That their own children were sometimes farmed out and neglected, doped with laudanum or gin, was due to the harsh conditions of employment imposed by genteel families who used wet-nurses. More humane families permitted the wet-nurse to keep her own child and breastfeed both. This was perfectly possible for many women, especially if they lived as some wet-nurses did, well-fed and with few chores or responsibilities and little physical exertion. The experience of one eighteenth-century wet-nurse would certainly suggest that there was no need to insist on mother feeding only one child:

One of the most remarkable wet-nurses of all time was surely Judith Waterford. In 1831 she was written up in both medical and lay newspapers. She celebrated her eighty-first birthday by demonstrating that she could still squeeze from her left breast milk which was "nice sweet, and not different from that of young and healthy mothers". Judith was married to babies. She fed six children of her own, eight nurslings, and many children of her friends and neighbours. In her prime she produced two quarts [over 3 litres] of breastmilk unfailing every day, but admitted sorrowfully that after the age of seventy-five she could not have managed to breastfeed effectively more than one infant at a time.[10]

Similarly, Budin in 1907 showed that milk output by one wet-nurse rose from 700ml when suckling two infants to 1750 ml when suckling five, over a period of only four days. Wood and Walker-Smith record that in one nineteenth-century royal household a wet-nurse "was still giving milk lavishly thirty years after the birth of her last child".[11]

Probably such cases represent the capacity of a small minority of women, but there are modern parallels – the diminutive Cambodian refugee mother who fed five babies in a camp without other supplies, despite her own malnourished state, for instance. Many other examples are on record. NMAA mothers have successfully fed twins and even triplets while doing far more than a wet-nurse was ever expected to, in a household without maids, cooks and other servants. Some Western Australian mothers, for instance, have produced 1-2 litres daily.[12] Women with only one functional breast exclusively breastfed to seven months. And as I emphasise elsewhere in the book, oversupply is a common cause of difficulty here in Australia, as it obviously has been elsewhere, given all the early 20th century concern about "overfed" breastfed babies (i.e., those suffering from benign lactose intolerance and possetting.)

Another reason why wet-nurses were employed in the seventeenth and eighteenth centuries was because doctors who served the wealthier classes forbade coitus during lactation. Men who put themselves before their children therefore insisted breastfeeding had to end. Mary Wollstonecraft asserted that "There are many husbands so devoid of sense and parental affection that... they refuse to let their wives suckle their children".[13] While medical advice has changed, there are still partners who regard the infant as usurping 'their' territory, and put pressure on for early weaning.

Wet-nursing began to decline in the eighteenth century under the twin pressures of alternative employment and medical disapproval. Cadogan's *Essay upon Nursing and the Management of Children* in 1748 argued strongly for maternal breastfeeding. The example of the Duchess of Devonshire and other noble ladies caused routine wet-nursing to fall out of fashion in England long before it declined in France and Germany.[14] Methodism, too, like all other dissenting religions, argued strongly for maternal breastfeeding (Methodism became a major social force in the late eighteenth century). The philosophy of the Enlightenment, and Rousseau's back-to-nature theories, were all agreed on the necessity of maternal breastfeeding – somewhat curious on the part of Rousseau, whose five illegitimate children were all "left to the tender mercies of the foundling hospital".[15] This was not to be the last occasion when men of no firsthand experience confidently told women what to do with their children. Indeed,

Cadogan's Essay, written for the use of nurses in the London Foundling Hospital, begins: "It is with great pleasure that I see at last the Preservation of Children become the Care of Men of Sense. In my opinion this Business has been too long fatally left to the management of women, who cannot be supposed to have a proper knowledge to fit them for the Task".[16] Some of his rules for wet-nurses (scheduled feeds, for example) did untold damage when translated into maternal breastfeeding situations by Men of Sense. All the same, between 1756 and 1761 of the 15,000 babies cared for at the Foundling Hospital, one-third survived infancy. This was very good for the period. Even babies breastfed by their mothers had first to survive the effects of purges, wine (or whisky and oatmeal in Scotland),[17] oils or gruels, in the first few days of life; and later "tea, coffee, spirits, anything", even opium in order to make them sleep. Opium and alcohol were used as routinely as sedatives and anti-histamines now are, and were as freely – but more cheaply – available, and over-used. No doubt this helped to produce some 'cot deaths' too! Infectious diseases were rampant in filthy overcrowded cities. Foundlings not wet-nursed had almost no chance of survival – only 45 children survived of over 10 000 babies admitted to the Dublin Foundling Hospital between 1775 and 1799.[18] Changes in the Poor Law systems, a greater readiness to experiment with other foods for infants, and many other factors affected the mortality rate of infants; and many other factors also affected the rate of decline of wet-nursing in particular areas.

Thus it was that by the early nineteenth century respectable wet-nursing had seriously declined. Yet wet-nursing certainly continued in London throughout the nineteenth century, as Smith documents.[19] The wealthy used lying-in hospitals and workhouses as employment agencies, selecting vulnerable women who had perforce to abandon their own babies – "sacrifices to lucre and fashion", as one concerned London doctor said. How many of these women were hapless servant girls and how many semi-professionals who became pregnant in order to enjoy the relative comfort of the wet-nurse's life, is unlikely ever to be known. Certainly the job was reasonably well paid, beyond the reach of poorer families. Artificial feedings of various kinds were being used more often by those mothers unable to breastfeed or to find or afford a suitable wet-nurse. (The enormous families of this period were also related to breast-feeding patterns and failure, and the loss of its contraceptive protection.)[20] The nine-teenth century, too, saw an increase in leisure for some, leaving middle-class mothers more time to invest in child feeding and care. There was an explosion of literature[21] dealing with how to do it right, from every conceivable viewpoint, sentimental, utilit-arian, Evangelical, and medical. In spite of that (or perhaps because of it) in 1840 roughly a third of all children under five died, an improvement over earlier times probably related in part to the increase in maternal breastfeeding (80-90 per cent of bottle-fed children still died).[22]

But commercial and industrial influences became more pressing towards the end of the century. New, patented baby foods and bottles, all recommended by male authority figures, all 'perfect', were appearing. Women, too, perhaps in reaction against the con-striction imposed by large families, revolted against the idea of breastfeeding now that they were assured by 'authorities' as potent as Isabella Beeton that artificial foods were "as good as, if not better than, breast milk". The concept of infant feeding 'choice' emerged at this time, and it was spread by means of the printed word, which leisure and literacy made all-powerful. The anti-breastfeeders of this period were often women who knew "of no greater misery than feeding a child",[23] considered by some to lead to female alcoholism![24] Doctors rapidly adapted to the new situation, finding painless rationalisations designed to keep their patients happy (later, guilt-free). The arguments used are still in vogue today, so it's worth quoting a few.

Mrs Panton, a popular female guru of child care, agreed that breastfeeding may have been natural once, "but we don't live in that time now, and we must adapt our doings to the age in which we were born... Let no mother condemn herself to be a common or ordinary cow unless she has a real desire to nurse... Women have not the stamina they once possessed". This fits in well with the 1970s 'insufficient milk syndrome' theory of breastfeeding failure.

Another guru of the day, perhaps the most eminent 'expert' on infant feeding, was one Dr Pritchard. Said he: "Lactation is far more likely to go wrong in a woman than in the teetotal, vegetarian, nerveless cow".[25] (Guess who'd never been a farmer!) Women were to become as cow-like as possible, restricting social life, eating a boring diet and resting. Other doctors warned that 'sexual emotion' spoiled the quality of the milk, a development of the insidious doubts raised by Lydia Child's advice that mother's milk might appear plentiful, but have no nutritional value.[26] Both these latter ideas still enjoy currency today, despite their obvious error.

Other difficulties were created by the increasing habit of scheduled feeds, breast and nipple anomalies resulting from wearing tight stays, and the complicated supplementary formulae the doctors urged. "From the first moment the infant is applied to the breast, it must be nursed on a certain plan. The baby must take a little thin gruel, or a mixture of one-third water and two-thirds cows' milk, sweetened with loaf sugar, until the breast milk is fully established"[27] (which of course it might never be, thanks to such supplementation).

Wet-nursing had not died out altogether. As late as 1890 there was a directory for wet-nurses at the College of Physicians in Philadelphia,[28] and a book on midwifery[29] published in 1922 spelt out the essentials for a wet-nurse, one of which now was that she wean her own child. Expense was becoming a major problem: as industrial wages increased, and the supply of wet-nurses decreased, the costs rose at the same time as cheap infant foods were becoming available and were being recommended as safe. I would emphasise that it was not until the nineteenth century that the idea of using babyfoods by choice, in place of breastfeeding, began to take hold. Previously the recognition that 'breast is best' was universal. (As an interesting sidelight, it is possible that cot deaths emerged, in one physician's experience, between 1839 and the 1860s. Initially Dr Chavasse urged mothers to continue the eighteenth-century practice of sleeping with their babies for nine months. He later reduced that to "a few months" and warned of the dangers of suffocations.[30] Presumably he was seeing infants dying unexpectedly in bed at about four months of age. If infant feeding is a contributory factor, this could be expected, given the ever-increasing use of artificial substitutes.)

How could such a dramatic change come about when centuries of experience indicated clearly that artificial feeding was intrinsically more hazardous, and when medical men had for decades inveighed against anything but maternal breastfeeding? There are a number of interlocking variables, and all have present-day parallels.

Constant urging to breastfeed, without the help to make it possible, inevitably sets up a backlash (now, as then). The anti-breastfeeders had the means and the leisure to express their views; other women had the means and leisure to consider these views and respond. (Improved transport and communications were part of this process.) Failure to breastfeed and emotional distance from children went hand-in-hand in late-nineteenth-century England; whether one caused the other is debatable. This was the first era of the nanny,[31] not the wet-nurse; it was the era of 'scientific' mixtures and the beginnings of control by 'experts'. (A hundred years later in Australia, this cycle is coming full-circle as the affluent employ nannies and other household servants once again.) Some of the general developments of the nineteenth century – sanitation and safer water supplies, improved food handling, refrigeration and railways – made it possible to conduct such experiments on babies without catastrophic increases in infant mortality. (Infant mortality did rise in this period, but people expected many children to die in infancy. And in any case, detailed statistics documenting changing mortality were not widely kept or publicised. The parallel for us is our refusal to document and publicise the steeply-increased morbidity among babies put into childcare.) Female factory employment was another contributing factor. Attempts to prevent mothers working for some time after childbirth were fruitless: those who worked needed to do so, in most cases; and the 1891 Factory Act made little difference. Of course there were no childcare facilities. Many infants were heavily sedated with opium while the mother worked, and many died from its effects. But as Smith points out, to keep that in perspective we might remember that "200,000 children under 11 were being doped with doctor-prescribed tranquillisers in Britain in 1974".[32] And chloral hydrate and much more potent drugs are readily given to Australian infants. According to Dr Schlebaum,[33] half of Australia's children under five were on regular medication in 1981, and much of that was such things as valium syrup and sedating antihistamines (freely available over the counter in chemists).

As commercial milk technology improved, America pioneered the mass use of bottle-feeding, one of the most devastating aspects of America's impact on the rest of the world. Condensed milk was first developed in 1853; evaporated milk in 1885. Both were widely used; evaporated milk until the present day. Condensed milk is now causing the same problems in developing countries as it did in American, British and Australian working-class families in the nineteenth and twentieth centuries: malnutrition, rickets, diarrhoea, intellectual deficits, death.[34] The first patented substitute for breast milk was probably von Liebeg's 'perfect infant food', a mixture of wheat flour, cows' milk, malt flour, and potassium bicarbonate. This was such a commercial success that various other products rapidly appeared – some made of dried cows' milk, cereal and sugar (Nestlé Food and Horlick's Malted Milk); some form of malted carbohydrate (Mellin's Food); some simply pure cereals to be used mixed with fresh cows' milk (Eskay's Food, Robinson's Potent Barley). Most of these were nutritional disasters, some lacking or excessively high in protein, vitamins, minerals, even fats. But then as now, that did not stop any of them claiming to be entirely suitable for infants, "the most perfect substitute for mother's milk". The existence of these patent foods was one of the reasons that doctors felt they should take firmer control of the whole business of infant feeding.

By the 1890s enough was known of the crude composition of cow's milk and human milk for doctors to begin modifying cow's milk. Dr Rotch, of Harvard University, developed a technique of diluting cow's milk, then adding sugar and cream. He and his followers tried to tailor this to the needs of each individual child, varying the proportions as the child grew. The percentage feeding method was unbelievably complex. Mothers around the world grappled enthusiastically with such 'scientific' methods: as Hardyment says "What was odd was that they were not driven back to their breasts in despair!" Obviously specialised knowledge and skills were required, so mothers were pushed further out of the process of infant feeding. The process of developing 'scientific' formulae was well under way. Rotch established a special laboratory to prepare modified cow's milk formulae according to the doctor's orders, and then deliver the formulae to customers. Milk Laboratories were established in various cities throughout the United States and Canada, and even in London.[35] But individualised formulas were time-consuming and expensive and could not hope to compete with widely advertised instant foods. Nor were they reliable: prescriptions were not always filled accurately and were given to the wrong infant. Even doctors were intimidated by the responsibility and complexity of Rotch's system, and many recommended patent foods. The idea of improving breastfeeding knowledge and skills was simply not entertained.

The medical profession tried to assert its authority. In 1893 Dr Rotch stated: "it would seem hardly necessary to suggest that the proper authority for establishing rules for substitute feedings should emanate from the medical profession, and not from non-medical capitalists. Yet when we study the history of substitute feeding as it is represented all over the world, the part which the family physician plays in comparison with numberless patent and proprietary foods administered by the nurse is humiliating and one which should no longer be tolerated".[36] Mothers could buy the patent products without ever seeing a doctor. This was seen as undesirable medically – the child needed medical supervision – and financially, for artificial infant feeding could be "the portal of entrance to a large practice"[37] (unlike successful breastfeeding, one might add).

The progress in food technology and science, outlined here, was undoubtedly an improvement on earlier, even less satisfactory ways of feeding infants whose mothers could not breastfeed. Unfortunately, as Hambraeus has said, such progress also included intensive commercial promotion, which led to a rapid decline in breastfeeding.[38] By the early twentieth century this was causing alarm among doctors, and the formula companies recognised both the validity of the doctors' fears – who could trust mothers? – and the power they could choose to exert. The companies began to court the medical profession's approval. Directions were taken off the labels, so mothers could buy the product but had to ask a doctor how to use it. (Too bad about those who couldn't afford a doctor but bought the product, still widely available, anyway.) The doctor usually told the mother to come back in six weeks to have the formula changed. The company gave the doctor feeding calculators, formula blanks and other freebies, and stressed that "the physician himself *controls* the feeding problem".[39] Similarly in 1915 the new product, SMA (Simulated Milk Adaption), was unveiled at a meeting of the American Pediatric Society and thereafter promoted exclusively to doctors.[40] Other products rapidly followed. Lactogen was produced by Nestlé in 1924 to be "sold only on the prescription or recommendation of a physician". Feeding directions were supplied only to doctors. By 1932 an AMA Committee had denounced the *unsupervised* use of artificial formulae and "the promulgation of feeding formulas in advertising to the laity" (not the widespread advertising of the product: only the communication of how to use it). This left companies free to maximise sales, and doctors free to control their use, a mutually satisfactory compromise. Very few influential people queried whether this shift from natural to artificial feeding could have deleterious consequences for society, or whether advertising *of any kind* was ethical. An honourable exception was the Philadelphia Pediatric Society which in 1923 urged the American Medical Association to stop advertising formula in its lay journal, *Hygeia*, because this implied AMA recommendation and undid the work of doctors trying to persuade the public "that infants cannot be fed in this indiscriminate manner".[41] Parents followed trustingly where scientific and medical advisers seemed to lead. Many doctors, finding that control of artificial feeding meant regular infant visits, even began to feel that breastfeeding might be less desirable because the baby did not return regularly for check-ups. Earlier weaning soon began to be encouraged, 'now that our present formulas are almost as good'. A familiar line?

It is not doctor-bashing to say plainly that the speciality of pediatrics owes much to the infant formula companies. It is the simple truth, and imposes on doctors a major responsibility to undo the legacy of harm created by naive co-operation in the past. It is also true that the infant formula companies could never have penetrated the American market so thoroughly without the legitimacy given to them by the AMA's Seal of Acceptance for their products and their close co-operation with doctors. Withdrawal of the Seal of Acceptance was a significant factor in the demise of the one infant food manufacturer whose crime was *to refuse* to remove feeding tables from his advertising. Brand names adopted at this time have persisted through many composition changes; this is obviously designed to provide assurance that the products were and are 'as close as possible' to human milk. To change brand names with every change in formulation could undermine public confidence in the persistent perfection of the product.

The economic depression of the 1930s, and fierce internecine competition, gradually reduced the number of American companies promoting infant formula. The major firms emerged as Abbott (Ross Laboratories), Bristol Myers (Mead Johnson) and American Home Products (Wyeth).[42] When smaller firms attempted to enter the lucrative US market in the 1960s and 1970s, they were squeezed out. The method chosen by Ross and Mead Johnson was to begin supplying formula to hospitals completely free, rather than at a lower cost, and to increase their services to professionals.[43] There were conditions attached to such 'free' gifts (often worth thousands or even millions);

for example a free pack of company products was to be given to each mother in a hospital receiving free formula and supplies from the company. Eventually Ross and Mead Johnson were charged with breaching U.S. anti-trust legislation by a third company; the lawsuit was settled privately, and terms were never disclosed. While small quantities doubtless had always been given, this was the origin of the practice of providing free and low-cost supplies as a marketing technique. It has not yet been eliminated in the USA, and was instrumental in defeating the Carnation challenge of the late 1980s.

What of sunny Australia? In the nineteenth and early twentieth century diarrhoeal diseases were so prevalent that it was standard medical advice not to wean in summer, when foods were most contaminated. The NSW Department of Public Health produced a pamphlet of infant care in summer, which stated "The first duty of a mother is to her baby... You should never let your breast milk disappear in summer. It may be the means of saving baby's life if diarrhoea should occur."[44] (Continued breastfeeding through diarrhoea is once again urged by international health authorities, but somehow during this century many doctors picked up the idea that a child with diarrhoea should be taken off the breast.)[45] It was this incredible mortality from diarrhoeal disease, and the realisation that correct nutrition and hygiene could prevent it, which was the basis of a newly emergent infant welfare system. And the companies were to build their market through that system too, by providing helpful leaflets, booklets, and advice about the use of their product for breastfeeding mothers when breastmilk was 'insufficient'.

In England and in Australia breastfeeding was seen as advantageous mainly because human milk was uncontaminated (untrue then, as now: breastmilk *beneficially* exposes a baby to manageable doses of a wide variety of environmental pathogens). So while breastfeeding was recommended, attempts to provide hygienic milk supplies were seen as being just as important. In England milk depots were opened in a number of towns. "Attendance at a milk depot meant that the children were closely scrutinised: they were weighed once a week, their homes were visited by health visitors who reported their progress to the Medical Officer of Health, and the mothers were provided with cards on which to record the weight of their child."[46] Clinics were a natural outgrowth of these depots, and in England they became the chief source of cheap, relatively clean, artificial powdered milks such as Glaxo. In the U.K., a National Dried Milk powder was available at very little cost for decades. This has been since discontinued as it was one of the high-solute mixtures implicated in the annual epidemic of hypernatraemic dehydration in artificially fed babies. Formula manufacturers also supplied mothers with literature. Glaxo's *The Baby Book*, immensely popular, sold 800,000 copies between 1908 and 1919.[47] It is very clear from the pages of testimonial that Glaxo had a policy of supplying doctors, nurses and groups such as the Ladies' Health Association[48] with generous quantities of free samples, rightly guessing that such promotion would pay dividends. The 1919 edition recorded that 1400 of Britain's 1750 municipal baby health centres regularly used Glaxo; that the Ministry of Food had purchased 4000 tons in 1917-18. In theory, of course, both milk depot and clinics praised breastmilk. In practice, "they encouraged attendance to obtain [low-cost] cows' milk so that the child could come under observation".[49] The British medical profession also seems to have been sure that a child is healthier if artificially fed but medically supervised, than if breastfed but rarely seen. Deaths were regarded as being a consequence of poor personal hygiene,[50] rather than social deficiencies such as poor sanitation, poverty and substandard housing. This continued the theme of the incompetent mother, whose ignorance was responsible for her child's ill health, a theme that remains very much alive in medical writing, despite the warning of 1917 that this was "a comfortable doctrine for the well-to-do person to adopt... It goes far to relieve his conscience in the contemplation of excessive suffering and mortality among the poor."[51] (We may smile, but how many studies of more recent date consider an association with maternal ignorance, age, or marital status, sufficient explanation for infant disease, and talk of 'standards of mothering' rather than 'the actual milk' explaining the consistently lower morbidity and mortality in breastfed infants?) 'Mothercraft' was the solution; and while in Australia breastfeeding was seen as important, the fact that it was supplemented soon after birth with all sorts of inappropriate foods meant that its potential benefit was undermined. (Sago, arrowroot or cornflour were almost universally used, 'due to the belief that the milk by itself was an inadequate food'. Cornstarch is still used, despite the evidence that it is of no benefit and poses some risks, for reflux babies.) And now we have regular infant formulas with added starches!

This naturally made the transition to processed milks and patent foods easier and earlier. Among the varieties available here in Australia were condensed, evaporated and dried milks, similar to those still in use today for infant feeding by those who cannot afford infant formula. Roller- and spray-dried milk was even being exported from the 1900s on; Glaxo, a New Zealand product, was basically full-cream milk powder "standardised in the proportions the highest medical authorities recommend". The dairy industry in both Australia and New Zealand was quick to see important new markets opening up. Patent foods, too, similar to those described earlier, were readily available and widely advertised. In the 1890s the medical profession discussed the issue and gave limited approval[52] to several such foods, including Nestlé, Mellin's and Benger's, but only for children over six months old – a crucial distinction, but one that few parents took seriously, then as now. These were, however, an improvement over the almost-pure starchy mixtures such as boiled grated flour or cheap condensed skim milk.

The main thrust of the infant welfare clinics was seen as the promotion of breastfeeding. Artificial substitutes were "only advised when it is... necessary to complement the breast milk", although then as now such advice was often given far more frequently than that. It has been generally accepted that this early-twentieth-century breastfeeding crusade did help to increase the proportion of wholly breastfed babies in certain areas.[53] It is undoubtedly true that a sympathetic knowledgeable nurse can help mothers to continue to breastfeed even under adverse social conditions. It is also true that many nurses were far from sympathetic or knowledgeable about breastfeeding. The hierarchical nature of medicine meant that nurses were subject to the doctor's authority – as doctor and as male. This contemporary style of exercising power was mimicked by nurses, in their relations with those beneath them in the medical hierarchy. The ignorant, incompetent mother has always been the lowest point in the scale, and attitudes towards her have ranged (and still do) from censorious to patronising in a kindly manner. Many women found it utterly intimidating to subject themselves to the scrutiny of the clinic sister when things were not going well with the baby. If baby was cheerful and thriving, sister's authority gave the mother an official stamp of approval, bolstering her confidence. If baby was not thriving, or was colicky, the nurse's questions usually implied that the fault was the mother's. (Because many of the original clinic sisters had no children, their assumptions that maternal defects caused infant problems had never been challenged by personal experience.) Given the lack of accurate information about management of breastfeeding problems and the doctrinaire ideas then in vogue, many mothers must have had difficulties resulting in the clinic sister handing them a sample tin of some 'medically approved' substitute. For in Australia too, the clinics were distribution points for all sorts of free samples.

One of the areas that needs close investigation is how far the work of such clinics promoted artificial feeding. At this stage, I don't think anyone could give a balanced picture. But I am quite certain that we need to question the assumption that all clinics were and are unequivocally promoting breastfeeding. On the contrary, even today, some actively urge inappropriately early weaning and serve to legitimise the infant formula industry. Many community midwives and MCH nurses have spoken to me of their concern about the way commercial forces influence what other clinic sisters do, and how they label as 'extreme' those who try to promote exclusive breastfeeding.

The same links between medicine and commerce, apparent in the United States, were gradually forged here. To their credit, Australian doctors were generally slower to accept that artificial substitutes could be 'almost as good' as mothers' milk. (Unfortunately, some of those who were slow to be converted to the idea that modern formulae are almost as good, are similarly slow to accept the newer information about breastfeeding, so in some instances this may indicate innate conservatism rather than native perspicacity.) Before the Second World War, Australia was a less-developed country, too, with a much smaller, more conservative population. So conversion to the use of expensive perishable infant foods was naturally slower. Promotion was much less aggressive in the pre-war era, but nevertheless the formula companies consolidated their position as reputable ethical bodies concerned – as were doctors – with the relief of infant suffering; willing to contribute handsomely to professional journals through advertising; or willing to finance research, professional conferences, and the like. There seems to have been little uneasiness within the medical profession over any possible conflict of interests, such as Jelliffe discussed.[54] But then no one could foresee the enormous post-war expansion of the formula industry world-wide, and the development of its marketing and advertising networks.

Little has been documented in any detail about the patterns of infant feeding after the Second World War. By 1960, 80 per cent of bottle-fed infants in America were being given home-made evaporated-milk formulae.[55] It may be pure coincidence that by the late 1950s and early 1960s Americans were concerned about the decline in national IQ levels; indeed, they may have been inaccurate results/tests... But as these milks have been condemned as unsuitable for infants and were certainly deficient in some elements necessary for brain growth, some curiosity would seem in order. (My next book will review this connexion between infant feeding and cognitive development.) Only since the 1960s have factory-made products taken over. Indeed, considering the major changes to formulae in the 1970s and since, one could say that many formulae currently in use are less than a decade old. And yet everyone believes they have a product to use that has proved itself over generations...

Breastfeeding steadily declined in Western nations after the war. In America it halved between 1946 and 1956, dropping to 25 per cent at hospital discharge in 1967.[56] And the West exported our style of infant feeding to the urbanised elites of less-developed countries. During the 1950s and 1960s various missionary and health workers began to be alarmed by the apparent effects of the decline in breastfeeding. In some countries, such as Chile, it was quite spectacular. Largely through the well-intentioned but misguided efforts of baby health clinics distributing free milk powder, by 1969 fewer than 20 per cent of Chilean babies were being breastfed for as long as two months.[57] This rapid decline in developing countries was often due to the simplistic aid programmes of the late 1940s and 1950s, which distributed surplus skim milk powder to developing countries. As Jelliffe has said, this "could only have appeared as endorsement of bottle feeding, with a resulting displacement effect of breastfeeding."[58] Between 1951 and 1960, low-income families in Singapore were exposed to rapid modernisation influences, and the breastfeeding of infants to three months decreased from 71 to 42 per cent; by 1971 it was perhaps 4 per cent.[59] In any society, rich or poor, such a change will have a marked impact on infant morbidity and mortality. Studies in the 1930s in England and America illustrate this clearly, and the topic has been reviewed well by Cunningham.[60]

Infant formula advocates now advance some curiously contradictory arguments. We should trust current formulas to be good because they have the same name as products used over generations. But current products cannot fairly be compared with the older milks once sold as perfect foods under those names, and now considered unsafe: current formulas have not been demonstrated to do any harm. And even though we condemn the older formulas as unsuitable, neither they nor current formulas are guilty of having caused any harm to babies. I have not seen any such extreme statements by senior executives of or men employed *directly* by formula companies, perhaps because they are aware that 'in real life' their products have proved to be both "nutritionally inadequate and dangerous". There are two points that should stressed here.

Firstly, we cannot yet assess what harm the very latest formulas do. Why not? Because in the complete and continuing absence of randomised controlled trials of the safety and efficacy of individual products, we have not been using them, much less using each brand exclusively, for long enough to know. Because in addition we do not know the inter-generational impact of the infancy bottle-feeding of those women who are now breastfeeding. And because rarely have studies considered exclusively bottle-fed and exclusively breastfed children (the influence of the bottle being so pervasive by the mid 1970s that almost all babies have been given at least the odd bottle).[61] Dugdale, for instance, so frequently quoted by the formula manufacturers, failed to consider these and other variables.[62] Yet many of the changes to formula are potentially very significant. For example, once it was cheaply available as a by-product of cheese manufacture, companies increased their use of bovine whey, which contains many of the most potent milk allergens. I know of no study assessing outcomes in terms of allergy on a population basis, where casein-dominant formulas are compared to whey-dominant ones. Perhaps both are as bad as one another: but perhaps not. They do result in different plasma amino acid levels in infants, after all. That could affect not only immunological but also cognitive outcomes. Similarly, companies are now using egg phospholipids in infant formula (to improve neurological outcomes, we hope) without monitoring rates of egg allergy in children exposed so early to egg. Where are the independent voices of paediatricians and allergists protesting such changes without appropriate RCTs proving safety and efficacy? We were reassured for years that peanut oil was safe in formula: now it has been shown to cause anaphylactic shock and deaths, it is to be banned – in Australia, anyway, if no major objections are raised (on the grounds that this might restrict trade, for example). Common sense critics[63] who raised such concerns years ago were pooh-poohed. And allergy continues to increase in Australia...

Secondly, the splendid new super-duper formulas, which we are again told are closest to mothers' milk, are too expensive to be used properly – even if mother had the clean water, fuel and other necessities of hygienic bottle-feeding – by any but the very rich, in every country where government subsidies are unavailable. In the mid-70s, the cost of fresh cows' milk for a fully-fed Indian infant would have been equal to 76% of his mother's monthly income.[64] Surveys have shown that poor mothers can afford to spend at most 10% on infant food; so formula being even more expensive than cows' milk, that 10% buys even less and it is diluted to last longer. Things have not improved. In 1982, the cost of artificially feeding a baby on the *cheapest* substitute available in the Philippines was 25% of the official minimum wage. (Many workers get less.) In Nairobi, it was 46-75% of the official minimum wage. Clearly, even if these products were as safe and adequate as their manufacturers claim them to be, *they cannot be used safely* by the vast proportion of the world's population who have living standards less than that of the affluent middle class. Even in American cities affected by economic recession, overdilution of formula leading to infant sickness and death has been documented. There would undoubtedly be even more such malnutrition if the federally funded Department of Agriculture WIC (Women, Infants and Children) programmes were not supplying infant formula, at a cost subsidised by taxpayers, to many of America's poor. The WIC programme is the largest buyer in the world, spending over a billion dollars on formula each year. This has been a triumph for the major formula companies. Similarly in Australia, many poor families rely on free formula or else feed cheaper mixtures. A week's supply of formula costs around 10% of the 1997 unemployment benefit – which is about to be cut significantly for many people as under-25s are put onto a new, lower 'Youth Allowance'.

Of course there are wider ecological and social implications for the world and especially for poorer nations: the diversion of resources to feed energy-wasteful cows; the foreign debt generated by formula imports; and so on. In the Philippines in the early 1980s, almost $90 million annually went to pay for such imports. This also helps to impoverish families and depress wages in such countries, as governments raise taxes to meet their debts.

Breastfeeding is in fact a central social and political activity, a symbol of all that we have done and are doing to the Earth our mother. Yet what environmental statements look at the costs of artificial feeding – the unnecessary grass-consuming, methane-producing, maternally-deprived cows and their luckless calves; the energy and metals used in manufacture and packaging; the paper consumed in labelling and advertising and industry-sponsored books designed to persuade healthworkers; the plastics and chemicals used in the process of bottle feeding; the resources consumed by sick children and mothers as a consequence of artificial feeding; the resources lost to the world from their untimely deaths...[65]

Combine the cost/income factor with the widespread belief that most milks are equally suitable for raising healthy children, a belief held not only by credulous mothers but apparently also by a nutritionist from John Hopkins University, who stated publicly in the late 1970s that sweetened condensed milk was "probably the safest and least expensive nutritionally adequate substitute for breast milk".[66] Department stores in many countries have walls of milk products – almost all with pictures of babies advertising everything from dried skim milk to the most sophisticated formula. Many poor mothers buy the cheapest, and overdilute what was unsafe to begin with. The formula companies and the medical profession are now trying to dissociate formula from animal milks, but a century of propaganda is not easily undone... and if mothers cannot afford formula, what is the point of telling them how harmful dried milk products are? What will they use instead?

The results were becoming obvious to field workers by the 1950s and 1960s. In 1970, amid concern about increasing commerciogenic malnutrition, WHO and UNICEF convened a meeting in Colombia. Industry representatives were there, and the question of unethical marketing created a stir. In 1972 the UN's Protein Calorie Advisory Group drafted a statement suggesting action to resolve the obvious problems.[67] By 1974 consciousness had increased after New Internationalist and War on Want (WOW) had made widely publicised statements. A Swiss group translated WOW's *The Baby Killer* as "Nestlé Kills Babies" and were sued for libel. The World Health Assembly unanimously adopted a resolution calling for governments to review and regulate marketing practices, and in 1975 the International Pediatric Association passed a similar resolution. Church-based groups, aware of the problem through their overseas members, began research and concerted action such as resolutions from stockholders at company annual general meetings, and withdrawal of church funds from industries believed to use unethical marketing practices.

In November 1975 the Nestlé case began. In many ways this was exactly the forum that was needed. Sworn testimony from medical experts around the world was made public, and popular concern mounted. Although the Swiss consumer group was found technically guilty, they were fined a derisory sum, which made clear the judge's moral verdict. Shortly before the trial, the major formula manufacturers had formed the International Council of Infant Food Industries (ICIFI) and issued a voluntary Code of Ethics which was denounced as too weak even by Abbott/Ross – who withdrew from

ICIFI and adopted their own code. (They could afford to give up direct consumer advertising, increasingly seen as too expensive and less effective than promotion to naïve healthworkers and through the medical system. They were at that time the American market leader, and direct-to-parent advertising was not necessary to maintain their market share. In fact, it was probably their entrenched power in the US institutional market which in the late 1980s led to the emergence of widespread consumer advertising as the only commercially viable route of entry for new brands by companies such as Gerber (supplied by Bristol Myers) and Carnation, seeking to carve off a chunk of the highly profitable US market for themselves.)

Another US company reacted differently. In a company report, Bristol Myers denied promoting formula in hazardous conditions. The Sisters of The Precious Blood filed a lawsuit charging the company with false reporting, and with the deaths of babies. The case was settled out of court on a technicality, but it too had served to publicise the issue, and both Abbott and Borden promptly announced changes in their marketing practices. US consumers continued to file stockholders' resolutions. The Rockefeller and Ford Foundations supported such resolutions, greatly increasing the power of minor ethical stockholders such as the ecumenical Interfaith Centre for Corporate Responsibility (ICCR). This avenue of protest and change was not possible with privately owned companies such as Nestlé which at that time controlled the lion's share of the 'Third World' market. Hence a boycott was begun by a group formed in Minneapolis in July 1977, the Infant Formula Action Coalition (INFAC). They stated that Nestlé was targeted because of its position in developing countries, and because the United States was their biggest market for other products. This first boycott was to last until January 1984, when Nestlé signed an agreement to comply substantially with the WHO Code.[68] It was one of the most successful consumer actions in history, not simply because of its effects on Nestlé but also its wider consequences internationally. A variety of interpretations and perspectives on the Boycott are now available in print, for readers wishing to know more.

In 1976, the US Congress had called for an investigation. Hearings were held in May 1978 – the Kennedy hearings. It became clear that US industry was obdurate, believing that their responsibility was to produce the product, not to monitor how it was used. This attitude has long characterised vested interest. In 1899 a medical deputation to the President of the UK Board of Agriculture asked to have skimmed, concentrated and condensed milks compulsorily labelled "not fit food for children or invalids".[69] The reply epitomises unbridled-enterprise philosophy: "If the public liked to buy a thing they must be allowed to buy it." Note how a proposal to educate the consumer to choose wisely is interpreted as a restriction on sales...

Senator Edward Kennedy requested that the World Health Organisation do more. This led to the historic October 1979 Geneva meeting, at which government, industry and consumer groups were all represented. This meeting agreed, inter alia, that a code of marketing practice should be formulated. In the meantime, everyone agreed that promotion of bottle-feeding to the public should be prohibited, a fact that explained the sudden and total absence of advertisements in Australian women's magazines for formula, bottles, teats, and so on for a short period. (Infant formula was not to reappear until Mead Johnson's 1991 campaign for a follow-on product, but advertisements for teats and bottles have since proliferated.)

The non-governmental organisation representatives at the Geneva meeting formed an umbrella group, the International Baby Food Action Network (IBFAN), to represent their views to the WHO, as the WHO officials struggled to find a compromise solution acceptable to everyone. IBFAN rapidly developed a wide network being serviced by paid and volunteer staff in a few key centres: then Minneapolis, Geneva, Penang and Cambridge. Money to support these centres came from a wide variety of sources, including governments, development agencies and public donations elicited by the Boycott campaign, as well as the sale of products. By March 1981 a draft code which seemed acceptable had been developed, though no one was very happy with it. In May 1981 the World Health Assembly met. There was extraordinary pressure from industry. It has been publicly stated[70] that delegates were wined and dined, offered free trips; fraudulent letters from fictitious organisations wasted time; a company lawyer posed as a Guatemalan delegate; ICIFI hired public relations firms and even, at an undisclosed figure, a retiring senior WHO official to lobby for them. Despite this, the WHO adopted the Code as a recommendation. The vote was 118:1 with three abstentions (Korea, Japan and Argentina). The one anti-vote was, ironically, the United States. An election had brought Reagan to power, and sweeping changes in top administration were to follow. But the US 'No' vote made world headlines, and probably did a great deal to raise public consciousness of the issue, as well as persuade many governments to adopt the code.

Public reaction in the US was outrage. Congressmen reported getting 100 letters a day for a week. In June 1981 Congress condemned the Administration and announced its intention to pass legislation enacting the Code. Reagan's attempt to appoint Ernest Lefever as Assistant Secretary of State for Human Rights failed when it was revealed that his Ethics and Public Policy Center had received a $25,000 grant from Nestlé and $10,000 from Bristol Myers, both formula manufacturers. Some of this money had resulted in the publication of an article in *Fortune*,[71] which smeared formula activists as 'corporation-haters' (many were investors) and 'Marxists' (many were Catholic religious sisters). While this sort of tactic was readily exposed, I believe that it was effective at the time in certain middle-class circles – effective in creating a perception of ALL formula activists as rabid political extremists, rather than as a broad-ranging coalition of people concerned about child health and industry accountability, with only a minority of those more concerned about multi-national industry than about infant health. The initial reluctance of some breastfeeding groups in the early 1980s to become involved in this aspect of the breastfeeding issue is more readily understood when this tactic is taken into account. Green politics have always been somewhat left of centre; only a decade later are we seeing environmental causes as acceptable to the mainstream. Certainly this was part of the reason for the refusal of one breastfeeding group to own and publish a book of mine, written for them, which contained IBFAN information about Code monitoring: by working as and promoting IBFAN I was seen as 'radical'. As indeed I hope I genuinely am, in the sense that, like every good historian, I try to get to the root of things!

Infant feeding became a highly volatile and emotive issue in the United States by 1980, partly because a number of further disasters with US infant formula had helped to sensitise Americans to some of the hazards of bottle-feeding in their own country. In 1978 some batches of Enfamil with iron powder were bacterially contaminated.[72] In 1979 Wyeth had to recall 300,000 cans of SMA because of a homogenisation problem that had made infants sick.[73] This was what the industry described later as an "elegance problem": problems such as fat separation or protein agglomeration which might make babies vomit but which left the formula 'safe', i.e. bacteriologically uncontaminated and able to provide 'adequate nutrition'. As a mere mother, aware of the speed with which babies can become dehydrated and die, I am a little puzzled by the industry recommendation that formulas with 'elegance problems' should not be recalled.[74] How can a formula provide 'adequate nutrition' if it has been vomited? Would adults want to eat foods with 'elegance problems'? Industry urged the FDA that recalls of formula with problems of such a minor nature tended to reduce the efficacy of recalls of formula with major, potentially fatal defects; they did not refer to the possible effect on consumer perception of the product as 'perfect' and thoroughly reliable.

Parents were to learn that lesson the hard way. The Neo-Mull-Soy/Cho-free disaster became public knowledge by late 1979. There were many disturbing features about this incident.[75] The publicity it received was almost entirely due to the fact that among the damaged children were two whose parents had all the requisite skills to find out what was happening and then to prevent the matter being quietly forgotten. Carol Laskin was a health care management consultant whose clients included the Department of Health and Human Service. Lynn Pilot was an attorney with experience in Congress as administrative and legislative assistant. Alan Laskin was a management consultant with wide knowledge and contacts in the media. Larry Pilot was an attorney then employed by the FDA, specialising in food and drug law. With that sort of expertise it was natural that they turned to the FDA for confirmation that the formula was responsible for their children's hospitalisation. They were staggered to find that in July 1979 the only requirements for infant formula manufacture were: "(1) the product must be manufactured under sanitary conditions, and (2) the label must reflect what is in the can. There were no up-to-date requirements concerning the nutrient composition of the formula, nor were there requirements for quality control procedures to ensure that the formula contained the ingredients it was intended to contain." Two weeks after their enquiries, months after the first reports and FDA enquiries, the company recalled its formulae from the market-place. Both the FDA and Syntex (the manufacturers) treated this as a routine matter, "with little attempt to ensure the effectiveness of the recall."[76] (FDA had asked Syntex for information in May. At the November hearings Syntex were criticised for withholding much of the vital information requested by the FDA, which has no power of coercion.) As a result, deficient formula was still on sale at retail outlets month later. This was too much for Laskin and Pilot. They went to the media and to the politicians. By November 1979 Congressional hearings were underway,[77] legislation to provide some sort of protection was being drafted, and FORMULA, a non-profit parent-support group, had been formed. (They were to receive more than 60,000 queries as a result of the publicity they engendered.)

The major outcome of these latest errors (and Laskin and Pilot's work) was the passage of the Infant Formula Act of 1980,[78] setting nutrient standards (the 1976 ones, temporarily) and requiring routine testing by manufacturers, as well as immediate notification of any further problems that might present a health risk. A US Congressional subcommittee asked the Justice Department to prosecute the company, Syntex Laboratories, for their tardy and ineffective recall. (Investigations by a reporter uncovered not only Syntex products but also many out-of-date cans of formula, some dating back to 1972, still on store shelves.)[79] This was not done.[80]

But much of the power of the 1980 Act depended on regulations that were yet to be formulated when Reagan took office. Manufacturers agreed in principle, but disagreed in practice when the FDA drafted fairly stringent recall procedures. They were able to get the support of their long-standing allies, the organised medical profession. The American Medical Association (AMA) saw no need for legislation or regulation because – familiar theme – industry could and should regulate itself.[81] The Justice Department argued that criminal prosecution was not necessary to prevent similar incidents in future, as though this was the only point of such prosecutions. (Would they fail to convict an arrested burglar who had since been injured and in future could not steal?) The American Academy of Pediatrics (AAP) "displayed a passive attitude toward the FDA infant formula activities and the progress of legislation".[82] Later, the AAP was to come out in support of industry's opposition to the regulations because they might make formula unaffordable and reduce the number of specialised formulae available to doctors.[83] These are debatable points when the industry makes so much profit and spends so much of it on free dinners and services to doctors. Since, according to one member of the Congressional subcommittee, industry refused to divulge the costs involved in better quality control, it is impossible to judge the validity of their case.[84] Did they tell the pediatricians the details or did they take it on trust? And who won in the end? A 1983 conference was told that the US Congress gave the FDA power to regulate infant formula recalls... only after the company had decided on the recall.[85] How reassuring! Like most parents, I should prefer to pay more for safety and less for promotion. I see no reason why a product that is recommended as the sole source of nutrition for a child at its most vulnerable age should not have to meet at least the requirements that non-prescription drugs must meet before they are freely available. After all, formula is currently so expensive that an independent cost analysis would be very interesting reading. Are present prices related to the fact that these products no longer compete directly with evaporated and condensed milks in developing countries, because the whole force of the medical profession has swung behind recommending only formula – or its 'equivalent', breastmilk – for babies? Can such prices be justified? Is it true that profit margins on infant formula (for the company, not the retailer) are greater than other pharmaceuticals? If I lived in America, I know I would want answers about many infant formula issues.

It has been no surprise to read Laskin and Pilot's 1982 criticism that the AAP "has displayed no interest whatever in pursuing any research or coordinating any efforts which might stimulate any collection of new and useful information about this subject. This lack of cooperation on the AAP's part has hampered our efforts to inform pediatricians of the seriousness of the children's problems."[86] (Or of their devastating wider impact: psychological and marital breakdown, bankruptcy because of medical costs, agency charges of child abuse, long-term demands for special therapy and education.)

What happened to the FDA regulations? Well, as both the industry and the medical authorities opposed them, the outcome was predictable after Reagan came to power. As reported in the trade journal, *Food Chemical News*, "FDA got the message recently from the Department of Health and Human Services in no uncertain terms to discontinue tough regulation writing...the HHS admonition was aimed at career FDA officials who had not yet gotten the message from the new administration. FDA was to take back the proposal and rewrite it shorter and in a more general fashion. Objection was made to the many details involved in the recalls and the tough reporting requirements."[87] So the drafts continued over the next year, becoming ever weaker. As a result, there were no regulations when the next major mishap[88] occurred, years later.

In March 1982, a month after cans had gone on sale, FDA issued a public warning that Wyeth was recalling all half-million cans of its Nursoy Concentrate and Ready-to-Feed, as they lacked vitamin B6 and had twice the recommended amount of vitamin B_1. (B_6 is essential; deficiency could cause "serious health effects such as irritability and in more serious instances convulsions." Did every paediatrician attending babies with convulsions think of this as a possible cause?) A week later, another half-million cans were recalled, this time of SMA,[89] after some debate between FDA and Wyeth as to whether this was necessary. This came as a shock to people who had assumed that all the talk about infant formula safety must have created a fool-proof system. The *Washington Post* asked Wyeth why it still did not pre-test its formula to ensure content and quality. Wyeth replied that it was not required by law to do so.[90] This episode was reported in Malaysian papers as ultimately causing 2.3 million cans to be recalled.[91]

This provided further impetus toward regulation, especially as evidence of the permanent neurological damage done by B_6 deficiency was available in the US after the 1952-54 formula accident.[92] Interestingly, the FDA recall made no mention of any such horrific possibilities[93] – they too have no desire to alarm the general public or to weaken public confidence in infant formula, because like everyone else they accept it as an inescapable part of the American social fabric. (As of course it is, but need not be in future.) In April 1982 the FDA published its quality control regulation, which would become effective in July 1982. The trade press headlined this as "Flexibility foremost feature of final infant formula quality control rule",[94] which sounded ominous enough. Naturally the document was a compromise between the original tough regulations proposed and the criticisms of the companies and other vested interests. Key issues not addressed include:

• Whether exemptions can be granted to products that presently do not meet the nutrient guidelines. (The Act and regulations cover only 'infant formula', which medical/industry groups interpret as meaning "standard formulas for normal infants"[95]. According to them, other products, including that most rapidly-growing segment of the market, the so-called low-allergy formulas, ought to be exempt from the Act's provisions, both of nutrient composition AND quality control. FDA officials held to a stricter definition of formula, and notified companies that products like Nutramigen were not 'exempt formulas'. What happened? "In the future, FDA will be proposing regulations... to deal with this situation. In the interim, FDA will not take regulatory action provided the manufacturer substantiates to our satisfaction that a deviation... is necessary." FDA uses 'independent' consultants to help in this process. One such consultant on aspects of quality control was Dr D. L. Heuring, formerly of Mead Johnson, and "the principal author of Mead Johnson's comments objecting to the proposed regulations."[96] This underlines a major problem arising from the dominance of industry in research – truly independent expert consultants are not easy to find!

- Whether full-scale recalls (class 1) are necessary for particular problems.[97] Recalls are not all total or widely publicised. Class 1 recalls necessitate recall down to the consumer level, with enormous publicity. A mother need never know about recalls from distributors or retailers, and the specials she stocked up on might all be dangerous.

- Whether industry can rely on data bases about milk products[98] (i.e. presume that certain ingredients are present in the right quantity because in theory they should be).

What this stratagem amounted to was really "business as usual, folks, and we'll argue about the details when we write them later, once the heat is off in Congress!"

FORMULA and other parent groups were not impressed by the new regulations, and filed a lawsuit charging that the Reagan Administration had violated the Infant Formula Act of 1980 by leaving the specifics of quality control up to the manufacturers.[99] (Manufacturers were not required to test any pre-mixes they bought from suppliers, and manufacturers increasingly used such pre-mixes, for instance.) Lynn Pilot commented that the supposedly explicit regulations did not even rise to the level of FDA's rules for cold remedies, yet were dealing with an infant's sole source of nutrition. By October 1983 the US District Court Judge had denied both sides a summary judgment, and the matter went to to trial. The judge's order indicated "some skepticism that the final regulations reflect the intent of Congress in enacting the Infant Formula Act." Congress clearly intended "that henceforth no nutrient-deficient (or, for that matter, otherwise defective) infant formula should be accessible to potential consumers at all." And the judge wondered how "the analysis of a single newly-processed batch of formula at random every three months is calculated to give assurance that those produced in the interim are not flawed".[100] [101]Well might he wonder. Wyeth's B_6-deficient formula (more than a million cans) was produced in just over two weeks.

And these were the world's strictest standards for quality control... We in Australia certainly do not pre-test imported formula. CHO-Free was used for premature infants in Australia. Syntex attempted to export its defective batches;[102] it is unknown whether they succeeded in selling any overseas, as is common for goods too dangerous for the US public.[103] US export and labelling standards also remained to be set. Yet here in Australia our government in 1998 is pushing to have national regulatory agencies accept as safe whatever has been approved by bodies such as the FDA overseas... We should all feel really reassured about the safety of infant formula, knowing that!

US infant formula activists in 1998 would do well to see what the outcomes have been, and to actively participate in the current revision of Infant Formula standards now ongoing. It is at this political level that the important decisions are made: in

Australia, for example, it was the definition of "infant" in our Food Laws which enabled us to ban advertising of follow-on formulae in 1991. It would be a major benefit to the world breastfeeding movement if US breastfeeding advocates were able to create in the US a series of very high quality control standards: one only has to look at how influential high US standards have been in other consumer areas. But only US activist groups can do such work: it would be a pity if their focus on non-US companies such as Nestlé meant that they overlooked the real and obvious needs, which only Americans can take responsibility for, in these areas, and in fact helped US infant formula companies protect their markets to boot!

Additional results of the 1979 US disaster included the analysis of other current infant formulae; there were some surprises, and other formulae were hastily altered. Among concerned US professionals, awareness of the hazards of bottle-feeding has risen dramatically. On 17 June 1981 an historic document was filed by Public Advocates Inc., a legal firm representing a wide-ranging coalition of concerned professional, parent and ethnic groups. This *Petition to alleviate domestic infant formula misuse and provide informed infant feeding choice*[104] represented the first major public attempt to state that problems with formula and bottle-feeding were widespread within America itself. It ranged right across the problem, detailing trends in breastfeeding among specific groups, medical harms associated with formula use, factors that discouraged breastfeeding (including hospital practices, professional attitudes, and company promotional practices); institutional role models (successful breastfeeding promotion measures); and suggestions for change. Extensive bibliography and appendices were also included. Those interested in infant feeding should read this document – and then pause to consider whether things are any different (apart from a greater degree of ignorance and inertia) in their country.

The industry reacted to this document very strongly indeed[105] for it attacked the basic assumptions about infant formula that had for so long gone unexamined: assumptions about the safety of formula in America, about the beneficial nature of industry/medical interaction, about the need for formula, whether women were truly informed before making decisions about feeding, and so on. Some of the questions raised were to be tackled in what seemed like a more impartial way by a special Task Force on the Assessment of the Scientific Evidence Relating to Infant Feeding Practices and Infant Health.[106] Theirs is an important document, which raises more questions than it answers, but the value of human milk emerges clearly – as does the pro-formula bias of certain chapter authors. Perhaps the most blatant example of this is a key summary chapter, which was a plagiarised FDA report of 1979, improperly acknowledged, updated to 1984 by the inclusion of all possible breastmilk problems, but without a similar updating for all the American infant formula problems, that emerged in that period. When in Washington at the FDA I spoke to one of the authors and asked her why this was so. Initially she said that there had been no problems with US infant formula in that period. I expressed surprise and told her I was about to publish a book, with at least half a dozen recalls sourced from the FDA: was she unaware of the problems her colleagues had told me about? Her reply: "Oh, you know about those!" "Yes, I do." "Well, you have to understand the situation here. After the

CHO-Free disaster in the late 70s, American parents were really scared about infant formula. We had to reassure them that formula was safe, because American society depends on bottle-feeding." God forbid the FDA should do something so subversive as suggest American women use their own mammary glands![107] And God forbid anyone should assume without proof that even senior bureaucrats are any more objective than the society they live in. I responded in the most dulcet tones, "So you're saying that the chapter's defects and omissions are because of its political motivation, which was to reassure parents?" This dear lady was most offended, and became quite irrational and emotional as she accused me of being as emotive as Dick Jelliffe on this subject. (What a compliment!) Yet what else was she saying? How is misleading the public about the danger of formula "because American society depends on bottle-feeding" not a politically-motivated act?

In the 1980-81 atmosphere of widespread global concern about infant feeding having been spearheaded from the US, the Reaganite decision not to endorse the WHO Code, and the American Academy of Pediatrics support for that decision, seemed all the more outrageous. Yet in some ways this was the best thing America could have done: it ensured that those parts of the developing world where anti-American feeling is a real force should take the Code seriously, and it made headlines around the world. While adoption of the Code was rightly regarded as a great victory by those concerned with infant health, many consumer groups regarded it as far from adequate. As the Director-General of Health for Western Samoa put it, "The Code has such great loopholes in it that any unscrupulous manufacturer could drive a herd of milk cows through it." But it was the best that was possible given the tactics of vested interest groups. (Commercial firms and governments of milk-exporting nations have no desire to see their markets dwindle.) And of course the Code was only a beginning: once it was accepted it would always be possible to develop these concerns further by WHA resolutions and WHO actions. While it is true that WHA resolutions will not alter the International Code per se, and Code advocates should not argue that they have, resolutions have as much moral force as the Code itself for those governments whose representatives voted for them. However, advocates should not muddy the waters of international debate by alleging that infant formula companies are automatically bound by agreements entered into by their national governments: it is a separate and necessary stage of negotiation to get any company to support a WHA resolution, and governments need to approach their national industry (and WHO to approach the major industry group, IFM, the Infant Formula Manufacturers' association, which succeeded ICIFI) to elicit such support every time there is a new resolution.

Any WHA resolution should have great moral force, and we can hope that any formula company will adopt them. But it seems to me unreasonable to expect groups not involved in their development or adoption to give instant or automatic consent to them. Breastfeeding advocates never feel bound by industry Agreements to which they were not party. We should not expect people in industry to act any differently. And even breastfeeding advocacy groups may not give full assent to some poorly worded WHA resolutions: none is a sacred document commanding the uncritical belief of the faithful. WHA resolutions are not the Ten Commandments and we are not the children of Moses, however much those who draft such resolutions may wish us to assent to the words written if we agree with the *intent* of the resolution. Words are words and have precise meanings, to which other meanings can be given in different circumstances. Activists and industry alike need to remember that WHA resolutions, while having considerable moral force (and more if not badly worded), are recommendations to be interpreted in the light of national circumstances. This is explicitly stated by WHO and WHA: national pride would prevent most countries accepting as a mandatory instruction something which other nations attempt to impose. So readers need to be very clear that whatever is agreed in international forums such as the World Health Assembly, it is still up to governments to implement the Code, in conformity with local circumstances. And it is up to concerned citizens in every country – among them infant formula manufacturers – to see that governments get on with that task among the myriad others they face. In my view the place for action is in one's own country. How much better the world would be if US activists had persuaded the US government to control the activities of US companies world-wide, and Japanese and Swiss and Dutch and German and French activists likewise! Controlling industry in importing countries would be much easier if industry was subject to control in exporting nations. America still allows the export of infant formula not saleable in the US, for example!

The WHO Code has often been grossly misrepresented. It **did not**:
• ban the use of formula, or its sale to the public; prohibit industry from informing health professionals about their products, or providing supplies for legitimate research purposes;
• apply only to poor countries;
• contravene national sovereignty or restrict the 'rights' and democratic freedoms of free-enterprise industries.[108] This was the US excuse for opposing it, later rejected by the Justice Department, which ruled that the Code was not 'unconstitutional';
• restrict women's right to choose how to feed their babies.

What the WHO Code **did** do was to call on governments:
• To halt the advertising and promotion of breast milk substitutes, bottles and teats, to the public.
• To halt the free distribution of samples, directly or indirectly, to pregnant women, mothers, or members of their families. This does not prevent institutions from providing needy families with supplies so long as they "take steps to ensure that supplies are continued as long as the infants concerned need them." (Article 6.7)
• To prohibit mothercraft nurses, or any other manufacturing personnel, from contacting pregnant women and mothers. No facility of a health care system may be used to promote breastmilk substitutes – no display of products, placards or posters, or "educational" material other than materials requested and approved by governments which do not refer to any proprietary product and which meet stringent rules about content.
• To restrict industry gifts to health workers, which might range from free products for their children to an annual all-expenses-paid trip with spouse. Research grants, study tours, conferences, etc., paid for by companies were to be publicly disclosed by both company and recipient. (Shortly before the American Academy of Pediatrics

refused to endorse the WHO Code because of legal, not medical, reservations, Ross Laboratories gave them a $1 million renewable grant.) Such 'gifts' are eventually paid for by the mother who buys the formula and often dilutes it because of its high cost. Remember that the AAP opposed quality control regulations – but not gifts to them – that will raise the cost of formula!!

• To require improved labelling, emphasising the superiority of breastfeeding and the hazards of inappropriate preparation; omitting misleading terms that imply close-ness to human milk, and pictures of infants or pictures idealising the use of infant formula.

Other labelling provisions include such pertinent facts as ingredients composition/ analysis, storage conditions, batch number and use-by date, "taking into account the climate and storage conditions of the country concerned", which should mean "how long might this last when sold from the open-air shops of Asia". Given US concerns about the effects of heat and storage on nutritional quality, and the 'elegance prob-lems' that cause vomiting and diarrhoea (referred to earlier in this chapter), these are serious issues. After all, "Liquid infant formulas are fat and protein emulsions that will separate with time... resulting in an objectionable appearance or clogged nipples... the rate of separation and deterioration of nutritional quality increases at higher tempera-tures."[109] Omission of these key labelling features by any country will mean that if more salmonella-contaminated formula were exported, recalls of the relevant batches would be difficult; if children develop allergies, no one will know what formula ingre-dients they were consuming; if the shopkeeper doesn't rotate his stock, poor mothers may buy nutrient-altered and maybe defective formula which they cannot afford to throw away or replace; and so on. This really would be a cynical exercise in exploita-tion. It could also prove very costly to the dairy industry of the country involved.

None of that seems unreasonable to any sane person. Because the Code was a recommendation to governments, the key to its success was obviously what governments did about it. Most manufacturers were happy to endorse the WHO Code, fully aware that they would be consulted before any national codes got off the ground. In most cases they have written national codes, or at least heavily influenced them; often because where artificial feeding was concerned, they were the most knowledgeable or powerful players at key national meetings.

A summary record of what the world's nations had done about the Code to 1991 is available from the Nutrition Section of WHO Geneva (1211 Geneva 27, Switzerland); so too are excellent biennial reports of activities from 1983 to 1993. (Regrettably, the biennial WHO reports on Code implementation have become much less informative after controversy over one report.) The drawback of many of these reports is that of course they represent – and must – what governments have told WHO, which only rarely includes an accurate account of national deficiencies or problems. Equally, IBFAN-linked reports for the period tend to focus on the reverse side of the coin: what has not yet been achieved. There is a crying need for independent scrutiny and academic analysis in this area of history as any other. But here as elsewhere in contemporary history, independent writing is a risky enterprise: anyone foolhardy enough to criticise the actions of industry *and* its critics can expect to be anathematised by extremists from both groups. C'est la vie. The work of chronicling must still be done if future advocates are to be empowered to work productively, and not to repeat the mistakes of the past for want of knowledge of what has occurred. However, for me to write the full history of this decade from a global perspective is not possible at present. It is in fact another book rather than a chapter, and as crucial events are still ongoing I prefer to leave that global history for now. Instead, the next section of this chapter details events in Australia, 1981-97, as an example of one relatively successful local response, now beginning to be undermined by broader global forces and a less active government response to Code issues.

2 – "Act Local": Implementing the WHO Code and other breast-feeding initiatives in Australia 1981-1998

Australia is a huge continent with a small population, now about 18 million, united under a complex federal-state-local government structure that ensures more politicians per capita than most countries. Its present government is conservative and their poli-cies have been likened to Margaret Thatcher's. Policies perversely labelled "economic rationalism" (historians may deem this satirical) had increasingly dominated political debate in Australia through the 1980s, and despite differences in social service safety-nets (Labor being more generous than the conservatives) both major political parties have been keen to sell public assets, cut back public services, allow 'market forces' mysteriously to regulate themselves, enshrine the shibboleth of 'Free Trade' and gen-erally de-regulate wherever possible to allow these market forces to work their magic of creating wealth and through it a fairer society.[110] Competition has been enshrined as an unquestionable good, and monopoly is intrinsically bad, even where common sense suggests this to be a nonsense. Those raised to consider social justice and democracy and the quality of ordinary people's lives important values have been struggling to affect policy. This is not the nanny state any more, but rather the bully-boys' paradise, where a horse named Might and Power winning the Melbourne Cup in 1997 was wide-ly seen by social commentators as a fitting metaphor for the country. In short, we live in unfavourable times: not the best of climates for unpaid volunteers to be challenging the marketing strategies common to multi-national companies the world over. So any gains have been hard-won, and those of us fighting for them have had to accept certain non-negotiable realities in the struggle to achieve them.

I believe that this is why the achievements of Australia in implementing the Inter-national Code make more encouraging reading than the global history to date. What is more, these achievements give the lie to arguments so often heard by (and sometimes from) breastfeeding advocates in countries like Canada, USA, Germany, New Zea-land, and other so-called "advanced" Western democracies, that a federal national government cannot act to implement the Code without the full support of the various states or jurisdictions; or that women's freedom and rights cannot be protected if the Code is implemented. Australia has been integrating the Code into existing national systems in a way that has not been seriously opposed, because it meets all the reasonable objections of those less convinced of the importance of breastfeeding. As one of the dedicated team of long-term unpaid advocates from NMAA and ALCA and the Australian College of Midwives, I am very conscious that we in Australia have much more to do, and that times are tougher than ever: but we are getting somewhere. In fact, comparisons of hospitals or shops or parents' journals from the US, the UK, Malaysia, Germany or NZ show that we have achieved a good deal.

Yet when Australia is reported on internationally by some breastfeeding activists, the positives are rarely mentioned. The Code is not Law in Australia, they say, it is a Self-Regulatory Scheme, as though that says everything. In my view such selective negative reporting is not only a breach of the solidarity we Australian breastfeeding advocates should be able to expect from our fellow-IBFANers. It is also a great help to industry, as it keeps IBFANers everywhere locked into dogmatic thinking (Law is Good, we must insist on the Code as Law) that does not help Code advocates attract wider support or strategise in the unfavourable political and economic environments of many western communities. It ensures that the battles and confrontation continue, with power-brokers seeing IBFANers as marginal and industry as part of the mainstream. So IBFAN centres seek financial support from the compassionate in society to keep battling on, and industry keeps advertising – in England, in Switzerland, in USA, in Malaysia, despite more charitable resources and paid staff in each of those countries addressing these issues in a year than we have ever had in Australia over decades.

It is my hope that this chapter will allow some re-evaluation of national approaches to complex issues. Were it the 1960s in Australia, law might have been the right way to go, and in future it may be once again be the rational way to proceed in Australia; if it should be, I for one will go back to street demonstrations, embarrassing tactics at conferences, and other general rabble rousing. This would only be necessary should industry or government decide to abandon the agenda of negotiation for ongoing change. Already we in Australia use existing common law as an important part of implementing the Code, and much of the Code is enshrined in Australian law. Law is critically important. But to legislate The Code in toto as a special act leaves it vulnerable to repeal, and creates sympathy for the industry being 'picked on'. Look how long it's taken for us to create laws against smoking, an obvious detrimental invasion of others' rights. How many people in Australia could be persuaded that infant formula is such a dangerous product that company marketing must be regulated specifically? Legislating the Code in toto may be the right approach in some countries today. But it isn't here and now in Australia. The moral of this chapter, if there is one, is that national breastfeeding advocates may need international support, but not international pressure to pursue approaches that will not work in their national context. And international published ratings of national achievement ought in justice to be more objective, more complex and less dogmatic than some current ones, if those responsible for those published ratings wish to retain any international credibility. It's a joke to rate progress lower in a country where a voluntary scheme is achieving something, and higher in a country which has a law that is not, and cannot be, implemented, just because some group has determined that the Code should made law. In democracies, how many laws without community support are enforced?

Australia and the International Code, 1981-1996

A conservative coalition government was in power in Australia in 1981, and endorsed the Code. The Commonwealth Health Department took the line that industry is responsible and should be self-regulating; that legislation or strict regulations would be undemocratic and unnecessary. Few bureaucrats in the Health Department then seemed to realise the value of involving the community in decision-making processes: in the early 1980s a most undesirable atmosphere of secrecy prevailed. The Department of Primary Industry set up a 10-person committee, including four industry representatives, but no consumer advocates, despite repeated requests from the Australian Consumers' Association.[111] Consultations were between the Australian Dairy Board, the Commonwealth Departments of Health and Primary Industry, and the five leading formula manufacturers.[112] The initial outcome was thus predictable. The 'Code' that resulted allowed Australian manufacturers to do business as usual. True, direct advertising of formula to the public was forbidden – but bottles and teats were not, and instantly advertisements for both were again being published in the women's magazines, even if these were careful not to include references to formula, and some promoted breastmilk feeding by bottle. Perhaps the reasoning was: "bottles are used for water and juices, therefore they're not promoting infant formula". But note that the WHO Code did cover feeding bottles and teats, and breastmilk substitutes were *any food marketed or otherwise represented as a partial or total replacement for breast milk, whether or not suitable for that purpose.* Using babies in advertisements implies that the product is suitable for use by infants. As any complementary feeding, or solids, decreases breast milk intake, orange juice or even water is similarly not to be encouraged. And of course, some of the advertisements of the early 1980s quite clearly did promote formula feeding. One even had the gall to depict a svelte, immaculate mum in glamorous scanty negligee, smiling serenely, offering her laughing child a bottle of white liquid, presumably formula, the clock behind showing 2.45. The wording: "If it were any simpler he'd do it himself".[113] (Which is just what baby does do, snuggled in beside breastfeeding mother in a warm bed.) Any picture taken at 3 am of any parent staggering about carrying a baby and preparing a bottle would bear no resemblance to this image; and what parent offers juice or water at 3 am? Yet this was supposedly not advertising formula – only the bottle? In 1996 we still see advertisements for bottles and teats that are supposed to prevent colic and orthodontic problems in infants. This is a most remarkable feat, when so many babies have colic due to the contents of the bottle,[114] or facial deformities as the result of the teat, but how misleading for gullible new mothers. Why is the Trade Practices Act, with its $10 million-dollar penalties, rarely invoked for such fraudulent and dishonest advertising?[115]

But this 1983 Australian industry Code differed from the WHO Code in many other ways. Manufacturers could use far more initiative in providing 'informational' material within the health care system; the material could refer to proprietary products; point-of-sale promotion was allowed; almost all of the stringent control of educational literature was gone, even the requirement for inclusion of a 'clear explanation of the hazards of improper use'. Manufacturers could provide samples indirectly (a significant piece of article 5.2 that was omitted) to pregnant women and mothers. The moral responsibility of ensuring long-term supplies for people given samples (article 6.7) was also deleted.

In Australia, no breastfeeding advocate was able to obtain a copy of this 1983 Industry Code prior to its signing by a newly elected Labor Government Health Minister, who was presented with the Industry Code as a virtual fait accompli in May 1983, as the World Health Assembly was due to begin and Australia had to report its progress. However, the new Minister asked the NH&MRC (National Health and Medical Research Council) to set up a working party to examine the implementation in Australia of the Code. This was also to respond to submissions from NMAA (the Nursing Mothers' Association of Australia) and myself alleging that healthworkers and hospital practices were responsible for much breastfeeding failure. The NH&MRC approved Healthworker guidelines in 1984 (see below, p. 261) and in 1985 recommended the setting up of a formal monitoring committee. A monitoring committee, with limited consumer input, was set up briefly in 1985 but achieved nothing, partly because the Department rejected any consumer representative with knowledge of the issue or IBFAN links, such as myself or Yong Sook Kwok, who succeeded Dr. Kate Short at ACA. ACA, the Australian Consumers' Association, had given IBFAN financial and logistic support during the Nestlé Boycott. While Kate was working on the issue she had been a crucial figurehead and leader in this debate, pressuring government, organising groups around Australia to support the Boycott and, unlike many other consumer activists, continuing to work on infant feeding issues after the Boycott was lifted in 1984. It was Kate who organised the IBFAN protest at the 1984 International Confederation of Midwives conference in Sydney. However, Kate's relationship with the Health Department was unavoidably adversarial; this created some problems and eventually Kate moved on to help create the excellent Toxic and Hazardous Environmental Chemicals Centre, working on pesticide issues, and has played no part in infant feeding issues for most of the last decade. Her successor at ACA, Yong Sook Kwok, had many other duties and was to play a less prominent role in the events that followed, although she was for a time active in the Australian Coalition for Optimal Infant Feeding, and was the IBFAN representative for the South Pacific region until 1991, when maternity leave took her off the active workforce. (After that, Jan Mangleson, a former NMAA Board member, became the IBFAN South Pacific representative.[116]) In fact throughout the mid-to-late-1980s it was Janey Christopherson, of the NZ Coalition for Trade and Development, who was the most active IBFAN representative in the region,[117] and NZ initially achieved more than Australia, only to lose momentum by the early 1990s,[118] while Australia then began to reap the harvest of the work put in.

Australian breastfeeding advocates' discontent with the status quo, and with the Commonwealth Health Department, steadily increased over the 1980s. The 'industry' code was amended in 1986, again without consumer knowledge of the process: while the Minister's office had become more open to consumers, the mindset of the Department seemed to observers to have changed little by then, and this was an administrative procedure. Again breastfeeding advocates protested; and continued to demand an active monitoring committee to assess industry compliance. Consumer activism against the infant formula industry, led initially by ACA as noted, together with Glenyss and Graham Romanes at CAA (Community Aid Abroad) had steadily declined after the ending of the Nestlé Boycott in 1984. This was no doubt due in part to the many crises an international group such as CAA had constantly to respond to through the 1980s. And of course if the problem has been defined or perceived narrowly (and inaccurately) as that wicked Nestlé breaching the Code, then a commitment by Nestlé to do better may seem like a victory, the conclusion of a struggle. From the perspective of the committed breastfeeding advocate, it sometimes seemed as though the broader, more difficult issues related to infant feeding in Australia were too complex, or the consumer movement too divided in its responses to infant feeding issues at home, for certain types of consumer activism to continue once that negative anti-multinational focus was gone. The supporters of the breastfeeding advocacy cause are generally not intrinsically opposed to multinational capitalism, only to those of its behaviours damaging to infant health.

The Nestlé Boycott was once again revived in 1987 by the North American group which had declared it ended in 1984.[119] Despite requests from IBFAN Penang to join the Boycott, no experienced Australian breastfeeding group or individual saw a renewed boycott as a useful strategy, for reasons which will emerge as this narrative continues. It was not until 1991 that the newly-formed 'BabyFood Action Group' members were trained in Penang to undertake the launch of a boycott of infant formula manufacturers in Australia. BFAG eventually became part of the INBC, or International Nestlé Boycott Committee. While it advocated action against *all* formula companies, most of its public emphasis centred on Nestlé and Wyeth, not then the most aggressive Australian marketers. Initially this increase in consumer activism was welcomed and supported by other breastfeeding advocates, who saw it as a positive awareness-raising force on the fringe of the broader movement. This was despite the fact that neither NMAA nor ALCA could endorse the Nestlé boycott without jeopardising their own credibility with those healthworkers well-aware of the much less Code-compliant behaviour of other companies in Australia.

With the 1987 founding of ALCA, the Australian Lactation Consultants' Association Inc., a new focus for healthworker conscientisation came into existence, and leadership of the struggle to control industry began to be assumed by this new health professional group, which from the beginning was prepared to go beyond NMAA's focus on breastfeeding (but not artificial feeding), yet worked hand-in-glove with NMAA. Indeed, NMAA set up the first meetings that led to the formation of ALCA. ALCA was the first professional organisation in the world to include support for the International Code as part of its Constitution, and as a pre-condition for election as office-bearer.[120] ALCA, NMAA and individuals working for these organisations and independently, were the key change agents in what was to follow in Australia. Over the 1980s, NMAA had gradually moved towards a more active political role, and was documenting Code violations, having established a computer database for that purpose in 1989. Other breastfeeding organisations encouraged their members to send violations to NMAA, as there was no point in duplicating the work being done by a valued colleague in the struggle. Through education, ALCA actively sought to persuade healthworkers to use the power they possessed to influence the situation. A key factor assisting the development of this educational mission was the development of the International Board of Lactation Consultant Examiners and its annual Examination: see below.

The Trades Practices Commission and the Code

By late 1988, after Health Department bureaucrats had been widely quoted as saying that the problem in implementing the International Code was that "anti-competitive" actions such as restricting advertising were impossible due to Australia's Trade Practices Act, the Trades Practices Commission in the Attorney General's Department was asked to look into the matter and replace such generalities with a considered detailed report. The Trades Practices Commission then realised that the previous infant formula Industry Codes (as they were then called) were illegal, a breach of the Trades Practices Act, which could be authorised only if substantial public benefit could be shown which outweighed the presumed public detriment of restricting competition. In 1989 meetings were held separately with all the parties concerned, and the process of working towards the full implementation of the International Code really began. ALCA's submission in 1989 was to be the virtual blueprint for what followed.

ACOIF (Australian Coalition for Optimal Infant Feeding)

ABC Television consulted with key breastfeeding advocates, including Yong Sook Kwok of ACA, and myself, when making *The Formula Fix*, a documentary showing that babies were still dying for want of breastmilk. After this was screened, the key players in the breastfeeding field were strengthened by a new awareness on the part of aid and development agencies, some of whom declared that they had thought the problem solved in 1984. Greg Thompson, of World Vision Australia, and Margaret Bailey of Freedom from Hunger, called a meeting in Canberra in June 1990, where representatives of a wide variety of organisations were briefed about infant feeding issues, the Code and the current Australian situation. The decision was taken to form ACOIF, the Australian Coalition for Optimal Infant Feeding, to act as a peak lobbying body. This was enormously important: it demonstrated to government that wide cross-sections of the community, including many health professionals, were united in seeking change, and that there was a responsible agency with whom to liaise, not a series of disparate groups with different agendas. Greg Thompson became chair of ACOIF, and his input over the next few years was invaluable. The Industry Agreement's rapid achievement was ACOIF's first success.

Regrettably however, despite everyone's best efforts, the different emphasis and style of the BabyFood Action Group (BFAG) helped create tensions within the breastfeeding lobby, tensions which by late 1993 had developed to the point where ACOIF was unable to develop a united policy or agree on a representative to meetings, and some organisations were no longer sending representatives to ACOIF meetings. Collaboration on important projects has been impeded by debate over doctrinaire points and the accuracy of reportage. As a long-term participant in the process, it seems obvious to me that this tension slowed the pace of national advocacy from 1993 to 1996. Prior to this, ACOIF had been an informal group that was able to achieve genuine consensus and rapid action. In an attempt to overcome this creeping paralysis, in 1995 moves to create a formal democratic and accountable structure for ACOIF began with near-unanimous support from ACOIF members. ACOIF has since become incorporated nationally as a peak body for national organisations concerned about infant feeding issues (although enthusiastic individuals are welcome to contribute at any level they wish). Once a proper structure was in place, disagreement could be handled democratically. The continuing core members of ACOIF, the permanent breastfeeding advocacy groups such as NMAA and ALCA, continued to liaise and collaborate both on a Constitution for ACOIF'S incorporation, and on a joint response to ongoing issues such as the consultation on the Marketing of Bottles and Teats (see below). Meanwhile, in the last couple of years before its demise in mid-1996[121] BFAG increasingly went its own way. Three ad hoc meetings about implementing WHA Resolution 47.5, on the issue of free and low-cost supplies, were set up by the ACTU in October and November 1994 and then in August 1996 (see below p. 261), with a re-named Baby Food Action[122] as secretariat. Fortunately this association of a key infant feeding issue with the trade union movement at this late date, when a conservative Coalition government is again in power, has not damaged the cause. In itself this is a tribute to the widespread support created over the previous decade for breastfeeding as the Australian norm: NMAA has friends and colleagues in power everywhere in Australia, despite some hostility from powerful women who chose or were forced by circumstances to feed artificially.

The 1991 Formula Industry Agreement

In 1990 that was still to come. ACOIF meetings led to the development of ALCA's 1989 TPC Submission into an ACOIF submission, which basically argued for the implementation of the International Code and the establishment of a credible monitoring body, with consumer and industry representatives and an independent chair. Nestlé Australia's submission made it clear that one of Australia's largest infant formula manufacturers supported this basic concept, and none of the other companies explicitly opposed it in writing. The Federal Bureau of Consumer Affairs convened a meeting in June 1991 of all the various interest groups covered by the Code, and allowed each to express their views in open forum, with the government representatives stating plainly that *their Minister's instructions were to implement the Code in conformity with Australian law.* It immediately became obvious that only the infant formula companies (as distinct from, eg, bottle and teat or weaning food interests) were then willing to negotiate an agreement restricting their marketing practices, perhaps due to the greater controversy surrounding their product in past years. It was also obvious that if breastfeeding advocates insisted on negotiating the whole Code at once, and waited until all interests were aware of the issues and willing to deal, nothing would be achieved in Australia for many years. A policy of implementing the Code piece by piece was formulated and agreed by breastfeeding advocates and government bureaucrats alike. The Federal Bureau of Consumer Affairs therefore called a smaller working meeting in November 1991 to negotiate an Agreement on the Marketing in Australia of Infant Formula. Despite a BFAG vigil seen by many as inflammatory, this meeting went ahead, but only after some very plain speaking about the need for responsible behaviour by industry's critics as well as by industry. The FBCA chairperson, Garry Johnson, said that the role of street demonstrations is to get issues on to the public agenda; but once issues are on the agenda, demonstrations run the risk of inflaming tempers so that issues cannot be resolved. (A point of view breastfeeding advocates should heed, I suspect.) This particular demonstration had inadvertently offered a wonderful pretext for a boycott or walkout by any company not really ready to negotiate, and that possibility was canvassed both before and at the meeting by some angry industry delegates. However, there was clear commitment from both breastfeeding advocates and some companies (notably Sharpe Laboratories and Nestlé) to achieve an agreement, which was stated as being the only way to end such actions. The negotiating skills of those present were able to deal with this unintended threat to the negotiations, and the meeting finished ahead of schedule, and successfully, with the words agreed. Again, this was largely due to two things: the fact that the FBCA Chair had a clear mandate from the government to implement the Code in conformity with Australian law; and the prior development by FBCA of a useful working document. This listed by article number the Code, the 1986 Australian Industry Code, and legal advice in three parallel columns. Negotiation was simple: where there was no valid reason under Australian law to change the International Code, its provisions stood. Where Australian law made the Code illegal, the Code was altered.

At the Minister's direction, the Industry Agreement developed could not include any practice illegal in Australia.[123] Under the Trades Practices Act, retail price-fixing is illegal, and punishable with fines of up to $10 million. Hence some minor items such as point-of-sale displays had to be allowed.[124] The huge benefit in this approach of working within **Australian** law was the fact that in Australian law an infant is a person up to the age of 12 months; thus the term "infant formula" automatically includes follow-on formulas, specialised formulas, and the rest. Australia was thus the first western country to deal effectively with the problem that had haunted Code advocates since the companies invented so-called 'follow-on formulas'.[125]

Such formulas did not exist in 1981 when the Code was passed, so that the Code spoke of infants up to the age of 4-6 months only, since at that stage this was seen as 'prolonged breastfeeding' by many Europeans and Americans. At that time, most western babies were off breast or formula alike by six months, and on to family foods and animal milks. Regrettably, industry's likely response was not foreseen by consumer advocates. By the end of the 1980s nutritionists, following industry's lead, were advocating a continuation of both breast and formula feeding to 12 months of age. (Formula is quite unnecessary where infants are eating good family food, but that's another chapter!) The US companies in Australia in 1991 seemed well aware of the significance of this "four to six months" figure and the need to protect their ability to market follow-on products. Mead Johnson had suddenly advertised its follow-on formula Enfapro in parents' magazines in the period leading up to the negotiation, despite universal industry condemnation of an action unknown in Australia since 1978. (In 1998 some of these same companies seem to be hoping NZ would agree that infants are persons up to 4-6 months and follow-ons are not infant formulas: NZ has permitted advertising of follow-on formulas. It seems a sadly missed opportunity in an English speaking country where "infant" is usually defined in the dictionaries as it is in Australia, rather than as it is in the context of "infant formula" in the Code.)

This 1991 Industry Agreement had to be submitted to and authorised by the Trades Practices Commission before it was legal. By May 1992 this had been done and the Agreement was signed; in September the first Chairperson of APMAIF, the Advisory Panel on the Marketing in Australia of Infant Formulas, was appointed. This was Professor Kerin O'Dea, of Deakin University; unfortunately she was to resign in early 1993 due to pressure of other work. The second Chairperson, Dr. Wendy Holmes, was not appointed until later that year. Two very able and experienced representatives, Michael Sharpe for industry and Ros Escott for consumers,[126] were appointed to make up a Panel of three, directly responsible to the Ministers and working with a secretariat within the Federal Bureau of Consumer Affairs. The task of APMAIF was to monitor the observance of the Industry Agreement. Regrettably, thanks to staff crises and changes of personnel, and re-organisation within the FBCA, it took until October 1994 for the Panel to produce its first report, naming the documented Code breaches. Wyeth (20) and Mead Johnson (17) headed the table of those who were reported as violating the Industry Agreement. Douglas Pharmaceuticals (Karicare) had one violation. A second report, *Keeping an Eye on the Market*, was produced in August 1995. In the period August 1994 to June 1995 only Wyeth was stated to have breached the Agreement, by claiming that its formula's fatty acid profile "closely matches that of breastmilk." Scientific evidence was sought: this is neither scientific nor factual information and hence a breach.

A third APMAIF report, aptly titled *Room for Improvement*, became available in 1996, covering the period July 1995 to August 1996. (The conservative coalition came into government in March 1996). This was the last Report for which Dr. Holmes had responsibility, and it sounds a warning: Mead Johnson had breached the Agreement 5 times, Wyeth twice, Douglas Pharmaceuticals and HJ Heinz (free samples) both once. Mead Johnson's objectionable battery-powered singing cards offering a chance to win a free video display unit, were never going to be seen as "scientific and factual" material designed to educate healthworkers. Nor were its claim about its fat blend "closely mirror[ing]" breastmilk, or the statement that all babies needed iron-fortified formula after six months. Emphatically not "scientific and factual", these claims were ipso facto "false and misleading" and so arguably a breach of the Trades Practices Act. It seemed to ACOIF members that industry was feeling more adventurous with the new government in power, that these violations were by companies which by now knew the APMAIF interpretations and should be complying with the Agreement. ACOIF therefore warned that in future, in addition to lodging complaints with APMAIF, it might seek criminal prosecutions under the Trades Practices Act, which applies even-handedly to all commercial interests, preventing them from making false and misleading or fraudulent claims about products. Hence when in 1997 Mead Johnson launched their new thickened infant formula, Enfalac AR, ACOIF lodged a formal complaint with the Australian Competition and Consumer Commission, which administers the Trades Practices Act, alleging that the law had been broken.

After considering the complaint, the ACCC basically replied that since this advertising was directed at health professionals, who were all knowledgeable about infant feeding and reflux, it was not misleading. As the advertising was clearly intended to reach parents[127], and as there is no evidence to suggest that all health professionals are omniscient about infant feeding, ACOIF will continue to contest this.

If found guilty under this Act, Mead Johnson would face serious penalties. There is no community sympathy for any company which misleads the public: infant formula manufacturers are being treated no differently from any company which bends the truth in an effort to sell its products. Singling them out for special treatment and alleging that their product needs unique controls meets with reflexive opposition; whereas saying that they, like other companies, should not mislead consumers, does not.

There is a good deal of scope for Code advocates to establish that infant formula advertisements are untruthful and misleading, and then see the companies prosecuted, wherever consumer protection laws exist. It is the responsibility of the authorities to investigate claims that the law has been broken and to prosecute criminals. I cannot understand that there have been no such prosecutions in North America, having seen grossly untruthful and misleading advertisements for so long there. As for the UK, how did those Wyeth "nucleotides" advertisements that suggested they now provided the immunity breastmilk does, ever get past truth in advertising laws? Of course, Code advocates must learn the science, or secure the evidence from those who have it, which shows that these advertisements are deceiving by omission and/or commission: what they leave out as well as what they say. Government regulators probably believe the claims being made just as so many healthworkers do. But the Mead Johnson Peter Rabbit formula label could not survive five minutes in Australia: it idealises artificial feeding by showing Peter Rabbit standing by while his mother feeds his sibling a bottle. Cows' milk formula would kill a baby rabbit. (Well, perhaps that is an appropriate label picture...) ACOIF sought an undertaking, and were given it, that Mead Johnson would not attempt to introduce that label in Australia, even before APMAIF determinations made it clear that it would be utterly unacceptable.

Obnoxious too, but legal and not a Code breach, is the move into formula-feeding of lactating women. For quite some time Mead Johnson has been advertising a cows' milk-based product for pregnant and lactating women. This undermines breastfeeding in both subtle and obvious ways. For the covert message that is read into the advertising of such products by women conscious of the imperfections of their diet, is that breastfeeding is draining, exhausting, a strain on mothers; that special foods are needed to make good milk; that a mother who does not eat the right foods will suffer, or else her child might. How often have healthworkers dealt with women convinced that of course breast is best, but that their own milk could not possibly be right for their baby because they drink coffee or smoke or eat chocolate or love spicy food or don't eat enough vegetables and fruit or don't eat fish or hate milk or...? Such products are unnecessary in a country where good food abounds; and they are expensive for no good reason. What is more, they increase a woman's intake of cows' milk, in a community where infant reactivity to bovine milk in the mother's diet is quite common, thanks to earlier generations' feeding practices. Yet products such as this are not covered by the Code, and provide a vehicle for infant formula interests to undermine breastfeeding and present themselves as caring people who provide solutions to breastfeeding problems. (Oh yes, and formula too.)

The exceptions in Australia remained Abbott, Nestlé, and Sharpe Labs: no breaches again in 1995-1996, or in 1996-7. In the 1997 APMAIF Report, Wyeth and Douglas were found to have breached, and concerns about Enfalac AR were recorded; Amcal was noted as having done things which were breaches before it signed the Agreement (and in fact since, in the view of those monitoring, since the objectionable materials can still be found in pharmacies despite the promise of recall.) Heinz were not recorded as having breached, which can only mean that some of their advertising materials were not submitted for consideration by the Panel, an omission which will be remedied.

Copies of all APMAIF Reports are available on request from APMAIF, c/o Dept of Industry, Science and Tourism, GPO Box 9839, Canberra ACT 2601. However, the very limited budget means that only 1000 copies (of which 400 are for Federal Parliament) have been commissioned by APMAIF. ALCA therefore paid for an additional 2000 copies which it made available with *ALCA Galaxy*'s December 1997 mailout, and subsequently via ALCA branches and at ALCA conferences. (It is to be hoped that APMAIF's budget allows a much larger print run in 1998.) It is to be hoped that health professionals who know the companies' scores by reading the APMAIF reports, and who pay attention to the quality of the literature they receive from companies, will use this to guide their suggestions when asked by parents about which brands of formula to select. I believe that companies which behave worse than others, so undermining breastfeeding and infant health, should lose market share as a result. We do not want Code compliance to be associated with loss of market share, which to date has been the Nestlé experience in Australia. This is one of the reasons why I cannot support any Nestlé Boycott in this country. (For more on this, cf. "Supping with the Devil?" at the end of the book.)

Deterioration in infant formula industry compliance, 1996-1998

Thanks largely to social changes beyond industry's control, and despite the restrictions on advertising, the formula market here is growing steadily if slowly, and with it the companies' presence, and even the number of companies. In 1995 Heinz launched new products on the market, and soon after a whole series of dreadful booklets aimed directly at parents; Amcal, a major buying chain of pharmaceutical retailers, has recently launched its own brand, using Snow's Victorian factory as its supplier, and with that launch sent out the worst and most misleading comparative tables to be left on display in pharmacies everywhere, informing consumers by omission that breastmilk lacked many of the wonderful nutrients in infant formulas. What is worse, Amcal refused to sign the Agreement until April 1997 after being heavily pressured by the new government, and in late 1997 was reported as distributing free formula at baby shows. Similarly Nutricia, now the world's largest infant formula marketer, has bought Karicare, failed to sign the Agreement to date, and its marketing is of concern.

The new manufacturers' apparent disregard for the APMAIF Agreement has not gone unanswered by companies previously not offending so blatantly. Australia is now experiencing major new marketing initiatives to provide materials aimed directly at parents. This had been outlawed by the Agreement, and had not happened for years. But now we have Wyeth booklets for parents and special ones for fathers; and Mead Johnson materials "teaching" parents about reflux, a problem for 50% of babies!

Is this provision of so-called 'educational' materials for parents advertising and a breach of the Industry Agreement? Of course it is. Commonsense is all you need to assess that. But if proof you need: one simple acid test is this – does industry claim the cost of these materials as tax-deductible? If so, in the very critical judgment of the Australian Tax Office, the official agent of the Australian government, these materials are designed directly to promote the product, to make profit for the business, and are advertising. If they are not, they are not tax-deductible expenses, and the millions companies have spent on them over the years should not have been claimed as deductions. (Perhaps they weren't??) In fact, all these 'educational' materials will be paid for from the company's marketing/advertising/promotional budget. The materials are not the result of industry workers taking up charitable collections in the street so as to commission some educator to help parents with problems. They are slick expensive productions full of cute images and designed to promote the product and the company alike. In the case of Mead Johnson, they have been backed up with television advertising that carefully avoids any mention of the words infant formula, but tells parents of babies with reflux to ask their doctor about a "new option" from "Mead Johnson Nutritionals". In addition, these materials are as fully educational as one might expect given their provenance. Let's look at some recent starters.

Take the Heinz Baby Programme book, distributed direct to mothers via the Bounty bags: it gives advice about breastfeeding that is full of subtle negatives, undermining language, and painful problems, with badly positioned babies, embarrassingly-exposed large sagging breasts, sombre-faced breastfeeding women without wedding rings: and the converse: reassurance that there is no need to worry or feel guilty if you bottle feed, no problems to deal with (well, not one problem is mentioned, though lots of breastfeeding ones are) so long as you follow instructions, smiling mother with highly visible wedding ring and dads can share the feeding (as of course we know they all do, night in and night out), and everyone can achieve "the special closeness normally associated with breastfeeding" just by holding the baby close and looking at him. Incredible! The writer seems ignorant about hormonal effects of breastfeeding on the infant and mother, as of much else: the booklet equates breastmilk and formula as far as weaning recommendations are concerned, for example. False, misleading, unscientific, not factual; a breach of Australian advertising law, a breach of the Code and of the MAIF Agreement? This booklet is a classic example of why industry should not write about breastfeeding. Nor should dietitians with vested interests and without breastfeeding expertise: a book[128] co-authored by the possible author of these Heinz booklets actually states that "Bottle-feeding should not be regarded as a poor or second-rate alternative". Why not, when it is second-rate nutritionally, endocrinologically, immunologically, metabolically? Is it ethical for an author who writes such stuff not to disclose prominently on the book cover the fact that she has long worked for an infant formula company? (In a recent Melbourne *Age* article this person was quoted as though representing the Australian Nutrition Foundation when talking negatively about organic food: once again, no mention of the company connexions.)

Or let's look at Wyeth's latest production: a whole packet of "Advice on baby care and feeding for parents who have chosen to bottle feed". In this, Wyeth tells parents about everything from infant development to immunization, with lots of advice about things that are none of an infant formula maker's business, all decorated with Looney Tunes Lovables™. The material contains much that is unexceptionable, but also gems like those below:

• "Having made the decision to bottle feed you must be mindful that infant formula is the only product suitable for use until your baby is 12 months old." Curious how babies have survived so well on well-chosen family foods, whether including some mammalian milk or not, and water. And that included almost all babies before follow-on formulas were invented.

• "feeding times vary from baby to baby, so it is best to work out your own schedule. [Schedule??] Usually babies are fed every 3-4 hours, in order to establish a good milk supply." What does that suggest to the young mother whose baby is feeding 10-15 times a day and doing very nicely? Or feeding every 2 hours? or 3hrs in the morning and two in the evening?

• "Most experts agree that weaning should start at around 4-6 months." [Not if a baby is breastfed and thriving, they don't. Especially when "weaning" can be taken as getting baby off the breast.]

Part of this package is "How to survive becoming a father: a collection of handy hints." It suggests fathers get a doctor if a baby "has more than 2 runny smelly motions" or "vomits more than once". Many young breastfed babies whose mothers have a bountiful supply could be seeing doctors needlessly if this is taken seriously. And it tells fathers to "take the baby out by yourself for the first time as soon as possible. The longer you leave it the harder it is." What a lot of codswallop. Why should it be harder for a dad to deal independently with a sturdy 4 month-old with head control and reasonable feeding intervals, than a floppy four-day old baby who may need to feed frequently? How subtly undermining this is of the mammalian norm, the deeply-attached breastfeeding mother who is reluctant to let anyone take her baby out of her sight, sometimes for months after the birth. I suppose we in Australia should be grateful not to be seeing the NZ version, which prominently asserts that breastfeeding takes as much energy as coal-mining (!!), an attractive analogy designed no doubt to encourage mothers to feel they are doing something worthwhile...or was that dirty, difficult and exhausting?? Far from breastfeeding tiring mothers, it actually improves the quality of their sleep, and lactation hormones help buffer the mother against the stresses inevitable while caring for a child.

Again, *it is simply not the business of formula companies to write this sort of literature,* which has been one of the key factors in the illogical western belief that feeding problems are universal and normal. They are universal and normal if you give babies artificial substitutes for breastmilk. They are less common but occurring if you observe babies being breastfed by mothers previously artificially-fed themselves. They are rare to non-existent in exclusively-breastfed babies of mothers well-breastfed as infants.[129] And remember, *this extensive giveaway literature can only be tax-deductible if it contributes to greater sales and profits: as indeed it does.*

The infant formula industry should not be educating parents about infant feeding, much less normal developmental progress, immunisation, mothering and fathering. Full stop. The Code says it; the MAIF Agreement says it. Nestlé and Sharpe are not doing it in Australia. Let's make sure that those companies that have once again begun to produce this nonsense are not benefiting from breaking the rules. If you are a healthworker, tell their reps what you think of this; tell them that other companies will get your support until they clean up their act. Complain to APMAIF. Write to the Minister and ask him to intervene. Why should industry be permitted to use the healthcare system to undermine breastfeeding, whether by bad information or subtle positioning of themselves, not as commercial vested interests that gain from every breastfeeding failure, but as philanthropists? If they are feeling generous and want to help make parent literature available, as they say, then let them contribute more to the blind trust that has been set up to support APMAIF, and let APMAIF commission independent literature from real experts with no industry connexions and nothing to gain from pretending infant formula is the same as breastmilk. APMAIF has an industry representative, so there is little possibility of 'corporation-haters' distorting the facts.

In my considered opinion there is no doubt that some of the companies have been getting bolder in Australia since the Howard government was elected in 1996. The development of consumer "information lines" began before that date, and there is no problem if these are genuine consumer complaint lines: purchasers must have access to that sort of information for every product. But how many hardware or food or computer firms hand out their customer complaint contact numbers so freely, providing then as cute fridge magnets or tear-offs in ever shop? How many seek 'complaints' and incessantly offer to be of help about the general field they are in, rather than their specific products? APMAIF ruled in 1996 that these numbers should be promoted only to health professionals and parents already using the product, as on tin labels; that these lines should offer only information about the brand formula and not infant feeding generally; and that nothing should idealise infant formula. Wyeth bought the right to a Looney-Tunes (again, how apt) 'Lovable' baby Bugs Bunny, who sits in nappies clutching a carrot toy, above a free-call number for their 'Infant formula help line.' Not "Wyeth products help-line."

The fact is, a few years ago this blatant advertising to parents was inconceivable. No doubt these companies are trying to exploit the fact that the MAIF Agreement, like the WHO Code, theoretically allows for educational materials to be created by companies, and distributed according to government guidelines. This provision exists so companies can educate about the use of *their products*, some of which are quite specialised, not to set themselves up as teachers on the subject of infant feeding and family life generally. That would be like the Dairy Board lobby running classes on the use of olive oil, or the Meat and Livestock Council telling us about the virtues of chicken: a clear and obvious conflict of interest exists and the information provided is bound to be slanted to suit the provider.[130] The MAIF Agreement says categorically, "manufacturers and importers of infant formula should not advertise or in any other way promote infant formulas to the general public." Up until the 1997 Report there has been no discussion of this because industry had not been caught circulating these 'educational' materials. Quite clearly industry feels that with the new APMAIF, the new Government, and the new de-regulatory climate in Australia, they can go for broke now and try to push through the barriers that have prevented them reaching parents directly. Add to this the widespread advertising of their so-called 'help-lines' (well, they help the company) and it seems to me that they are positioning themselves to replace health professionals as the main source of information about infant feeding, whatever lip service they pay to the idea that parents should talk to such professionals. Will a free-market government give away our babies into the care of the companies?

There are worrying signs. The 1997 APMAIF Report called for "research into a range of issues surrounding the impact of infant formula marketing practices on breastfeeding and women's decisions to cease breastfeeding. This kind of research is considered to be essential to provide a current factual basis for various clauses of the MAIF Agreement and interpretations of it." Sounds great until you read it closely, and then I start to worry, because it is in keeping with the way industry sets up straw men to be demolished by 'objective' research, which then justifies advertising. Just imagine a few questions:

• Did advertising influence your choice of feeding/time of weaning? [What woman would say yes…]

• Was access to comparative information about infant formula helpful to you? Would you like more detailed information about infant formula brands? [What western consumer would say no…]

There is a great deal of infant feeding research done which is abysmal, in Australia as elsewhere. There are only a very few research centres of sufficient excellence in this country to handle a complex investigation of this nature. Suppression of unacceptable bits of research findings is not unknown. Is this government really going to sponsor research that could be confrontational for the infant formula industry? Or is it, as I suspect, industry which is demanding this research so as to enable it to do in Australia what it does elsewhere with impunity?

No one aware of the infant feeding literature or with any brains would assume that there is any simple linear or causal relationship between advertising and women's decisions to breastfeed or not, or to wean. (Yet this is what seems explicit in the APMAIF call for research as it is currently worded.) Advertising influences are far more subtle, and serve different purposes in different societies. Infant formula is entrenched in Australia. Most advertisers do not have to create a market, merely to maintain one. Advertising by established marketers is about legitimising and normalising artificial feeding, and making it socially acceptable; and then only secondarily about persuading parents to choose brand A rather than brand B. If this were not so, advertisers would engage in cut-throat advertising, pointing out the obvious hazards of competitors' products, of which they are all well aware. Real competitive brand advertising is something all advertisers agree is A Bad Thing as it undermines public confidence in the product in general to see that any brand can be flawed. The research that needs to be done is of what parents and health professionals believe about infant formula and breastmilk, and how close this is to the scientific literature on the subject. If either parents or professionals believe breastmilk and formula to be nearly equivalent, it becomes 'reasonable' for them to choose either, or to wean early. Investigation could also be of how close the specific infant feeding beliefs of health professionals and parents are to advertising campaigns and infomercial literature by industry in the last decades. In my decade of teaching healthworkers about infant feeding, I have noted time after time that professionals believe the content of company literature (on the naive "they wouldn't be allowed to say it if it wasn't true" principle) and are amazed to discover that what they think they know is not what science says about infant feeding. The ACCC may believe doctors cannot be misled (see p.246), but educators know they already have been.

At the time of writing there were few signs that government will enforce the Agreement strictly, or put into writing that signing the Agreement is a condition for marketing infant formula in Australia, even if in practice it has been pushed as such. What will happen to APMAIF? The Independent Chair knows less about the issue and plays a less active role now; the industry rep seems far less aware of the health consequences than his predecessor; the bureaucracy is once again losing experienced assistance: what kind of APMAIF will 1998 bring? The infant formula market is now worth over $100 million annually. Most of this growth is happening at the expense of breastfeeding duration. Yet the current Health Minister, Michael Woolridge, seems genuinely concerned to protect promote and support breastfeeding. I will await his response to these matters with interest. ACOIF is considering a proposal to publish its own Annual Report on company behaviour and APMAIF and Ministerial performance in 1998. Concerned readers can keep up to date on these issues by subscribing to *ALCA Galaxy* and watching for relevant reports. And readers can help us keep abreast of developments: the price of freedom from bottlefeeding as the social norm, à la the USA, is eternal vigilance. All the achievements of the last decade could be lost in a matter of a year or two if ACOIF does not continue and strengthen its advocacy role, or if APMAIF is co-opted by industry. Constant ongoing committed advocacy is needed, not flash-in-the-pan heroics. We can never congratulate ourselves that the struggle is over and we can relax: the profit imperative drives each new generation of marketers. Those of us who care about babies and their mothers need to be just as persistent.

Bottles and Teats

But the formula companies were only one of the series of interlocking interests covered by the Code which, as stated above, Australia is implementing piecemeal.

Bottles and teats are widely advertised here, and represent the most visible aspect of artificial feeding promotion. After the June 1991 meeting, the companies involved in the import and distribution of these objects formed a Baby Products Association, and at the request of the FBCA, produced a draft voluntary Code. In later 1993 this was sent out for comment from concerned groups. ALCA's submission, made jointly with the then IBFAN South Pacific representative,[131] was a highly detailed critique of the draft BPA Code, with a request that the FBCA facilitate a negotiation on these issues similar to the November 1991 meeting. Some of the key figures in the Baby Products Association have stated their willingness to abide by any Agreement negotiated by government and policed by APMAIF. Another draft Agreement was circulated in September 1995, and then again in December 1995. This latest is in the useful tripartite form used to negotiate the Formula agreement. Departmental re-organisation has slowed the matter, but a meeting in March 1996 went ahead despite the change of government. A subsequent working meeting between BPA executives and ACOIF representatives achieved substantial further progress, but the subsequent draft has not yet been sent by BPA to ACOIF for critical evaluation.

The Baby Products industry is not willing to consider giving up the possibility of marketing directly to families, seeing this as the only way to protect a brand name market and prevent all competition being based on price, thus encouraging a further flood of junk products, teats and bottles made to Third World standards rather than of food grade materials. This seems a legitimate concern, but of course it could be addressed by making a Standard for Australian Bottles and teats and policing that standard, so that poor quality product was excluded as hazardous. Apparently only the UK has a Standard for these products. Discussions are ongoing, and ACOIF has decided to adopt a higher public profile on this issue in 1998 if progress is not immediate.

Breastfeeding advocates do not anticipate that there should be any serious problem with the present Coalition government, as the protection of babies' health and the negotiation of industry codes of conduct are hardly party-political matters, and it was a conservative federal Coalition government which originally voted to support the International Code in 1981. Moreover, this new federal Government has allocated $2 million for the promotion of breastfeeding. However, the recent serious cutbacks and erosion of support services for mothers and babies in Victoria by a State coalition government has left some breastfeeding advocates concerned. Breastfeeding certainly does need promotion in some niche markets, such as poor families and young and immigrant mothers. But mostly in Australia, breastfeeding needs protection and support, not simply promotion. Unless, of course, that promotion includes a comprehensive catalogue of the dangers of artificial feeding – which I doubt it will.

The Baby Friendly Hospital Initiative has been a catalyst in this matter of bottles and teats, raising awareness of the need to alter marketing to pregnant women, for example, via agencies such as Bounty, a group that makes up sample bags for hospital patients. This group has recently made a commitment to end all provision of teats in their sample bags, and to omit discussion of bottle-feeding in the pregnancy booklet they produce. Full marks to them for this, even if they have a way to go with advertisements for teats in other publications. Whether this commitment will survive the sale of the Bounty Australia business to the parent group from the UK remains to be seen. ACOIF will be lobbying them to ensure that they do honour previous commitments such as this, and readers might like to write to the magazine's new owners.

Free and low-cost supplies of breastmilk substitutes

The issue of free and low-cost supplies of breastmilk substitutes within the healthcare system has largely been resolved in practice, though not in theory. In 1986 Australia had voted for WHA resolution 39.28, which urged an end to these in "maternity wards and hospitals". This wording was unfortunate as it allowed a semantic debate to develop over whether WHA 39.28 covered all hospitals or merely maternity hospitals. Literalist governments and bureaucracies interpreted this as meaning just that – maternity wards and hospitals, not *all* healthcare facilities (such as clinics surgeries). They were technically accurate in this legalistic stance, but advocates stated that it meant all healthcare facilities even if it didn't say so in so many words. (This conflict could have been avoided if the Resolution had been better worded in the first place.) At the November 1991 negotiation of the Industry agreement, all parties, including ALCA, BFAG, and NMAA, agreed that this issue of free and low-cost supplies was not ready for negotiation and could not be allowed to delay the Agreement covering those items in the Code per se, not later resolutions: the Minister's instruction was to implement the Code, not all related WHA resolutions. But with continued pressure from ACOIF and Nestlé Australia, and reminders that Australia did indeed vote for 39.28, the government began a process of consultation. The federal Health Department convened a meeting in November 1993 at which it was clearly stated that the question was not *whether* Australia would end the practice of free and low-cost supplies in maternity facilities, but how this would be achieved and what were the obstacles to doing so. There was considerable discussion of what healthcare facilities were included under 39.28, with breastfeeding groups arguing for the Australian government to adopt a wide interpretation, including community private practice healthworkers. Thankfully, WHA Resolution 47.5 in May 1994 was to render this obsolete by making it clear that all healthcare facilities were included. However, industry did not immediately signify its assent to this clarification of the original purpose of the 1981 Code and WHA 39.28, and if we are to be just we must acknowledge that their assent cannot be presumed without consultation, any more than the assent of breastfeeding advocates can be taken for granted if they are not involved in the process of negotiation. Australia is not a dictatorship, but a democracy, after all. The Commonwealth Government agreed to consult the States and Territories on the issue, since they, not the Commonwealth, have control of public hospitals and some other healthcare facilities. A report was subsequently published of both the meeting and the replies received. It was immediately obvious that the situation around Australia is very varied, and some States are much more amenable than others, so that advocates will need to work at state level. This issue was complicated by the Attorney General's written advice that it would be illegal to ask companies to set any minimum price on their product, as this constitutes pricefixing. Australia voted for WHA Resolution 47.5 in May 1994, and so stated that government policy is to end all such supplies within the healthcare system. The matter was then raised again between the Commonwealth and the States in October 1994. The companies have been reluctant to take action as no one wanted to go it alone, and so lose market share if any of their competitors continue. Unilateral action is likely to result in poorer profits, and managements and Boards of Directors have been sacked for less. ACOIF wrote to each of the companies to ascertain their intention in this area, and shared the replies with all its constituent members. Nestlé Australia was the only company to make any written commitment to ending all free and low-cost supplies everywhere in the healthcare system, and to give a date, revised now to take account of delay.

Other means were subsequently tried. In May 1994, as part of a series of meetings arranged by the ACTU with key industries, Nestlé Australia asked Martin Ferguson, then head of the Australian Council of Trade Unions (ACTU) to use his influence to resolve the free supplies issue, the one outstanding matter that Nestlé needed settled in order to be completely Code-compliant in Australia, in the widest interpretation of the Code. Nestlé had earlier stated its willingness to end free supplies by the end of 1992, on the assumption that the government would co-ordinate this so that there would be no gain to any company. They were subsequently accused of bad faith for not ending free supplies unilaterally, and this was part of the reasoning given to justify the resumption in Australia of the boycott, in which some unions were involved. Yet despite its commitment to social justice, the trade union movement might reasonably be reluctant to campaign against a large Australian employer, since such a campaign, if successful, could result in more lost jobs for Australian workers. The ACTU was reported to have given Nestlé a fair hearing and promised to expedite matters. Subsequently the ACTU asked BFAG (at this point still a part of CAA, Community Aid Abroad, which was then an ACOIF member) to organise a meeting in October 1994 to address this issue of free supplies. ALCA was not permitted to attend this meeting; nor was ACOIF invited, although the ACOIF correspondence with the companies over supplies was cited. The proposal re the supplies issue noted in the written record of that first meeting was clearly unacceptable to breastfeeding advocates: that the government provide money to purchase formula presently being 'donated'. This potentially both maximises industry's profits and legitimises their product, and should be considered only when truly necessary for child health, with strict income limits for recipients. Breastfeeding advocates were clear that the small amount of formula truly needed could be purchased out of existing budgets. The second meeting a month later, which I attended with the formal support of the ALCA Council as ALCA's Code spokesperson, was a good deal more productive. A widening of the powers of APMAIF was called for, along with support for the Baby-Friendly Hospital Initiative (see below).

It was clear from comments in that second (November 1994) meeting that at least some union representatives appreciated the commercial folly of any company acting unilaterally and advantaging its rivals, and also appreciated the difficulties inherent in legislation in the Australian context. It is unlikely enough that a law could pass in this climate of deregulation; even less likely that any court would enforce it; and counter-productive for consumer critics for this to be our avenue of complaint, since we can never match the money and influence of industry, and could not even criticise matters which become sub judice. However, the collective bargaining power of the ACTU meant that a meeting with the then Labour Federal Health Minister resulted in May 1995. The Minister reiterated that any continuing problems were at state level and there was a limit to what the Commonwealth Government could mandate in a federal democracy. The issue was again raised in the meeting of Health Ministers nationally. There certain State governments, notably Victoria, scuttled the idea of ending free and low-cost supplies. Agitation is needed at the State level, not the Federal. Indeed, the Commonwealth's refusal not to throw money at the problem is to be commended in this instance: it would not help breastfeeding for the Commonwealth to subsidise artificial feeding any further than it already does.

What is the situation as I write in early 1998? Nestlé remains the only company to commit itself to ending all free and low-cost supplies everywhere in the healthcare system, with the exception of truly charitable supplies, which they notify in writing to APMAIF. Douglas Pharmaceuticals (Karicare) say quite openly that they need to and will provide these supplies anywhere they are wanted, to gain market share. Mead Johnson and Wyeth say that they will not provide subsidised supplies to hospitals, but are silent on every other aspect of the healthcare system, and are reported as giving product to such persons as doctors and dietitians, getting them to sign for the supplies even when the initiative to leave product came from the reps. Heinz is still said to be handing out free supplies. Amcal is certainly giving the stuff to parents at baby shows, but I do not know of it being accepted in any hospital to date. Polls of healthworkers in teaching seminars indicate that almost all companies are still actively offering free or low-cost products to healthworkers, with – I hate to say it, as doing so causes me to be thought partisan, but truth should be told – markedly fewer reports of Abbott, Nestlé Australia or Sharpe Labs doing so. Sharpe's formula brands have been bought by Nutricia, which has not signed the Agreement and which is providing advertising material to parents. In short, very little has been achieved in this area of free supplies at the level of government or industry, except to confirm to industry that they can ignore the matter with impunity, and that taking it seriously leads to market share losses, as it has for Nestlé. How long Nestle will continue to comply is thus uncertain.

What are Australian hospitals doing about free and low-cost supplies? We don't know the complete answer. The Commonwealth Health Department paid BabyFood Action to undertake a survey in 1996, to see what hospitals officially claim to be the present situation in relation to free supplies. The survey caused some controversy. ACOIF was not informed of it, so that prior scrutiny of the questionnaire was not possible. Its wording made very clear what the desired reply should be. The names of a number of organisations were cited in the correspondence to hospitals without their prior knowledge, in some cases despite their clear statement that they were not part of any formal coalition other than ACOIF. The survey results also were hard to interpret: 243 hospitals responded, but what percentage this is of those surveyed is not stated and could not be ascertained from BFA in the subsequent meeting at which it was discussed. However, there was some good news: 75% of those (self-reporting, remember, to a survey which made the 'right' answers extremely obvious) stated that their policy was to end subsidised supplies. This group was said to cover roughly 60% of all births. Yet over 500 maternity units exist in Australia. One might also guess that respondents had a more positive attitude to the survey. So without knowing response rate, or characteristics of responding/not-responding units, and with no independent validation of self-reported compliance, it is unclear whether half of Australia's maternity units have followed the government's urgings (since 1993) on this issue. Astonishingly, the Health Department, which subsidised this survey, has apparently not been able to obtain the original data so no further analysis has been possible.

Powerful medical groups are opposed to any increase in hospital costs, and also ignorant of how much subsidised supplies cost hospitals, families and the taxpayer in increased ill-health. The current Chair of APMAIF, a doctor from a Women's Hospitals' Association hospital, has opposed ending such supplies, though this is APMAIF policy. The WHA themselves went on record in late 1994 to "Support the maintenance of free and subsidised supplies of breastmilk substitutes, or financial subsidies for such supplies, to hospitals for appropriate use," on the basis that "Claims that free and subsidised infant formula to obstetric hospitals increases bottle feeding are not supported by the current experience of member hospitals", after another self-report survey of nine member hospitals (not completed by those most knowledgeable about breastfeeding). Oddly, this vested interest, which apparently does not support either BFHI or the Code, has very recently become part of the Reference Group of the consortium for developing national standards for Maternal and Infant Care (see p 271-3). Despite this, this latter group is expected to strongly endorse BFHI (with its ban on free supplies) as part of the two national hospital accreditation processes, thanks to the government's clear support for BFHI as a unique international evidence-based quality assurance programme, akin to the globally-accepted "universal precautions".

The issue of ending free and low-cost supplies of formula is a publicist's nightmare. It can very readily be misrepresented as breastfeeding fanatics punishing poor families, causing bottle-fed babies to go hungry, and/or giving greater profits to industry. Some aboriginal women, strong advocates of breastfeeding, have said that it would be disastrous in some aboriginal communities to end the practice of providing free infant formula: parents would simply revert to using the Sunshine full-cream powdered milk they themselves were fed on as infants. And after all, why shouldn't industry give charitable supplies? say the unthinking. In fact, breastfeeding advocates want to stop unethical marketing, not charity. The Code and subsequent WHA resolutions did not ban company provision of truly charitable supplies, where enough is given for the period of need. Companies can indeed give truly charitable supplies under tightly controlled circumstances. No one wants to see babies go hungry. But the wasteful distribution of endless samples, small quantities to healthworkers designed to get from them to a variety of families, not only undermines breastfeeding, but probably causes some of that hunger by jacking up the cost of infant formula at the retail level, where poor families must buy it after the few free cans run out. Free supplies are not free, any more than any other industry gift to healthworkers. 'Free' supplies are paid for by the families who buy formula. Why should these families, in Australia among the lowest socioeconomic groups, subsidise wealthy health institutions, even private ones? Why should those institutions go on wasting any product, even one they do not attempt to audit because it is free or cheap? Once they have paid the company for the formula, healthcare institutions can indeed choose to give it to poor families: supplies paid for can be given away. But maternity hospitals should not do so when breastfeeding is still a possibility, and will not be accredited as baby-friendly if they are misusing formula. Controls on the use of infant formula in healthcare institutions need to be as strict as those of any other potentially lethal product. What other substance do healthworkers blithely give babies, without parental consent, without recording its administration, when that substance can not only lead to decreased milk production in the mother, but dramatically transform infant gut flora, leaving babies more susceptible to infectious, allergic and inflammatory disease? How many deaths from necrotising enterocolitis have been the result of needless formula-feeding? How long before someone sues?

The ACTU's laudable 1994 efforts on the matter of free supplies were resumed after a break of two years, with a third meeting of what was being loosely referred to as a coalition to end subsidised supplies, in August 1996. The personnel of what had been BFAG[132] acted as the secretariat. This meeting, with a few new players and many absentees from the previous list,[133] decided to seek an interview with the new Federal Health Minister. Other groups have not had a report of this meeting to date. The situation with supplies remains largely unchanged, and it is BFHI and professional education which is having a positive effect on this (see below p. 261)

For there is some good news on this issue of free supplies. It is clear that there are many hospitals which no longer accept subsidised supplies; which use much less formula now than ever before; which find that they are saving money by doing so; which advise mothers who choose to bottle feed to bring the brand of their choice with them. These mothers are being taught how to make that brand of formula and are practising doing so under supervision in hospital: all of which reduces some of the risks of artificial feeding. Ready-to-feed bottles have disappeared except in paediatric units. Even those hospitals which give formula free to mothers – often private patients get very angry at the idea that they should pay for infant formula – are paying for it as they do for the food the mother eats. No hospital has been reported as giving breastfeeding mothers formula cans or samples to take home any more.

If a national survey ascertains that almost all Australian hospitals follow such policies, Australia would have achieved much of what the ending of free supplies is designed to achieve: the end of the hospital's financial dependence on the infant formula industry and the use of the hospital as a marketing agent for brands of formula, together with the undermining of breastfeeding mothers by 'gifts' of formula not paid for by the hospital. That achievement would not have been the result of regulatory government action at state or national level, or even of our political pressure and lobbying of government, but of breastfeeding advocates' work to educate healthworkers, and the federal consultative processes that resulted in the APMAIF position on free supplies. Reasonable people will usually agree to reasonable proposals if a forum for discussion is created. And then it takes time for change to filter through complex healthwork systems. BFHI is accelerating that process, not creating it, in most cases. Breastfeeding advocates have been instrumental in all these processes, even though we cannot in truth point to any one event whereby we forced industry to agree to end subsidised supplies, or the government to regulate this matter. It would be untruthful in the extreme for breastfeeding advocates not to acknowledge that by 1996 it suited all the major companies in Australia to end subsidised hospital supplies, and that in the end they went ahead and did so, although our best efforts never got the government to order them to. And no one has stopped Karicare (now owned by Nutricia) or Heinz from doing as they please with free formula; nor will they until it suits them, unless some sanctions are applied. I for one have stopped buying all company products other than Nestle until the companies act more ethically. Secondary boycott laws prevent me from urging concerned readers to do the same. But if it should happen that you feel incensed by any aspect of what you see in practice, remember that you do have power both to act, and to inform the relevant company of your decision to act.

Before I leave the supplies issue, I would like to stress again the point that education of the people responsible for accepting and using free supplies proved more effective than overt lobbying to have the government enforce a no subsidised supplies policy in a top-down way (though we did that too, and the fact of the previous Health Minister's stated commitment was crucial to persuasion at other levels). Local transformation is the goal of breastfeeding advocacy, which aims to reinstate a breastfeeding culture, where breastfeeding is something everyone knows about and takes for granted. Government decrees cannot achieve this, though government funding can certainly be of considerable assistance, and government leadership is crucial: and both money and power should be expended more readily on this vital health issue by any rational government. But ultimately, the factors which influence each mother's infant feeding choices are specific to her, and depend largely on whether the people around her understand the issues and can give her the support she needs to breastfeed. Politicking is indispensable, but can take many forms and work in many ways: education and support at the local level is a form of activism and advocacy, just as is lobbying at the federal level. We cannot all do the latter, but we can surely do the former.

Other Code issues

Other Code issues still to be acted upon by the Australian government are Guidelines for Retailers, which both ACOIF and APMAIF have worked on; and a Code for those making babyfoods and drinks. Another area of concern is the role of pharmacy in promoting artificial feeding inadvertently or otherwise, and the role of healthworkers. More anon.

The initial APMAIF draft retail guidelines did allow for price promotion of formula, as required by the Trades Practices Act. This means it is OK to state that Product X is selling at \$Y (but not to show a pack-shot), and to allow enough stock to be present for likely demand. There are differences in the way companies respond to these retail guidelines: I have seen very highly-visible promotion for Wyeth, Mead Johnson, and Karicare products. If the cans are less boring, more decorative and more obviously for babies, the sheer weight of visibility will serve to promote the normalcy of artificial feeding, and APMAIF may have to review its guidelines allowing such retail displays. Now that Wyeth has switched from pharmacy only to supermarket sales, the retail area has become highly competitive. (Although oddly, still not very price-competitive.)

Readers should be warned that in 1998 industry is still pushing to be allowed to use pack shots in advertising in retail catalogues, now that can labels look prettier. Should this be allowed, APMAIF's credibility with breastfeeding advocates will be destroyed. Experienced consumer representative Ros Escott, trained by WHO on Code issues, has recently retired and been replaced by Dr. Patricia McVeagh, a long-standing breast-feeding advocate who has no public national record on Code issues. How APMAIF will perform in 1998 and beyond will depend a great deal on her ability to identify, consult with, and represent the national groups which have real experience of Code issues nationally and internationally, especially (but not limited to) ACOIF. While Dr. McVeagh must be given every support as she undertakes this job, it was disappointing to see that yet again the government feels that only medical *doctors* can represent the interests of *consumers* in the area of infant feeding – the NMAA/ALCA/ACOIF nominee for the position was a Breastfeeding Counsellor with great experience of the Code and of consumer needs and concerns.

Another new initiative is in the area of working mothers. Both government and the unions have been active here. In 1996, after consulting NMAA, the ACTU published a Mother-Friendly Workplace booklet, as an extension of its 'family-friendly' policies. Although the first list of resources at the back is seriously defective (consult NMAA or ALCA for overlooked local contacts) the booklet is a useful resource. For a copy write to the ACTU or contact your local union rep. And in 1998 the Commonwealth govern-ment has allocated some part of its $2million grant for the provision of information in this area: as yet unseen and so unable to be evaluated. But these schemes are tinkering around the edges of the problem of employed mothers of young children. What would help here would be far more serious re-arrangements of social priorities: adherence to ILO conventions allowing breastfeeding breaks for working women; shorter hours of work for parents as in Sweden; and major reforms such as reasonable periods of paid maternity leave: a minimum of six months paid and preferably another 6-18 months unpaid leave as well. Even better would be to allow women at home to receive the substantial amounts of money the government will pay for their children if put into other people's care. And I would suggest that any government which runs 'work for the dole' schemes should immediately classify as 'working for the dole' all low-income mothers who have young children under the age of three, especially (if being a mother is not considered sufficient work) those who train and serve as NMAA peer counsellors.

Other Interests and the Code

The work of breastfeeding advocacy never ends. All sorts of vested interests can act in ways that are inimical to breastfeeding, for their own reasons, and the same small batch of volunteers has to respond. Late in 1997 NMAA has been involved in protesting to groups as different as Amcal re their provision of infant formula at baby shows, and Greenpeace over an irresponsible fund-raising campaign in which, in order to generate concern about environmental issues, they labelled a breast with poisonous contaminants and talked of Dutch women filtering their breastmilk (!!). Yet Greenpeace supports breastfeeding in theory, though they seem ignorant of the risks of the alternatives they promote by denigrating breastmilk. Or is it just that this ad campaign was so successful at raising money in Europe that it seemed like a good idea to try it here? I have to hope it failed, that all those who support Greenpeace were outraged by this unscrupulous nonsense. Unintelligent, poorly informed, and divisive breastfeeding 'advocates' are harmful to the cause of breastfeeding in any country, just like the powerful vested interests which are so often blamed for breastfeeding failure.[134] And there are many groups besides infant formula companies which seek to use infant feeding as a way of achieving other aims, sometimes to the detriment of infant health.

But as the rest of this book should make clear, what commercial interests do is not the sole or even major reason why Australian women are having difficulty succeeding at breastfeeding. And here we should stop to acknowledge the Commonwealth Health Department's greatest achievement to date in this area: the formulation and passage in 1984 by the NH&MRC of guidelines to promote breastfeeding and implement the WHO Code. By concentrating on the whole range of practices impinging on the breastfeeding mother, and emphasising the need for improved education of health workers, these guidelines have done more to help Australian women than would any control of industry practice (though the latter is also necessary). In many ways these guidelines justified the revision and improvement of postnatal practice that was the hallmark of the 1980s in Australia, preceding the BFHI by some years. Again, they arose from direct consumer pressure. In 1981 NMAA and I had recommended in substantial written submissions that the NH&MRC or some designated body should "formulate and circulate rational policies of hospital ante-natal education and hospital management of the new baby, as well as a programme to educate medical professionals". The response was these 1984 Guidelines, which were well ahead of their time, but naturally have dated. In 1994 a process of revising these began, which culminated in revised Infant Feeding Guidelines for Health Workers being published in late 1996, and the launch in 1997 of a companion document, *Naturally: the facts about breastfeeding*. Yet again the process of consumer consultation by these health channels was far from adequate, the committee was heavily dominated by healthworkers, and NMAA was not represented. As a result some criticisms of the final Guidelines are justified. (Its medical approach to and disproportionate emphasis on gastric reflux, for example, could not have been more timely for Mead Johnson!) Still, the overall effect has been very positive, and revision of details is always possible in due course. Copies of both books are available from any Australian Government Printing Services bookstore or from AGPS, PO Box 84, Canberra ACT 2601. NH&MRC materials can be obtained by writing to the NH&MRC, P. O. Box 100, Woden, A.C.T. 2606, Australia.

The Baby Friendly Hospital Initiative

Another major boost to the promotion of breastfeeding world-wide was the development of the Baby Friendly Hospital Initiative. At the UNICEF-convened meeting in New York in February 1991 which led to the formation of WABA (World Alliance for Breastfeeding Action)[135], the suggestion was made of formal recognition for hospitals which provide appropriate care for breastfeeding women and babies. James Grant, then UNICEF's Executive Director, announced in May 1991 that UNICEF planned to recognise hospitals which were "Baby-Friendly" because they followed the Ten Steps to Successful Breastfeeding first enunciated in the Joint WHO/UNICEF Statement of 1989, *Protecting, Promoting and Supporting Breastfeeding*. The idea had been spelt out; a programme had to follow. Dedicated work followed, by the Wellstart[136] team in San Diego, together with WHO Geneva input and that of an international team[137] created by Helen Armstrong, an American UNICEF New York consultant working from Tufts University Nutrition faculty in Boston, who had been one of the founding mothers of the influential Kenyan Breastfeeding Information Group. Thanks to Grant's commitment and UNICEF funding, and building on earlier Wellstart work, Global Assessment Criteria and evaluation tools were ready by February 1992, when hospitals in the first 12 lead nations were assessed, after receiving significant UNICEF funds to enable them to prepare for this process. I was fortunate enough to be asked to go to Nigeria – at ten days notice! – to assess hospitals there, and so had access to these global documents hot off a Lagos fax machine. Not surprisingly given the haste involved in their drafting, these first documents, while generally very sound indeed as a basic programme, had some minor problems both of content and of tone. After returning from Nigeria with the BFHI documents and this experience of national hospital assessment, I approached Margaret Peters, then President of the UNICEF Committee of Australia, and a Taskforce was set up to investigate the feasibility of BFHI implementation in Australia. This consisted of representatives of the Association of Directors of Nursing Inc., the Australian College of Midwives, the Australian College of Paediatrics, the Australian Lactation Consultants Association, the Royal Australian College of Obstetrics and Gynaecology, the Australian College of Hospital Administrators, the Private Hospitals Association, the Nursing Mothers Association of Australia, and the Maternal and Child Health Section of the Victorian Health Department.

Its first task was to evaluate and then revise the Global documents, making them suitable for an industrialised democracy where women are free to make even the wrong choice. There was a need to distinguish clearly between the hospital's responsibility and the mother's prerogative to decide, even if the staff or BFHI assessors wished she had decided differently. This was more a matter of language than of content: indeed the Australian version of BFHI was strengthened by including some additional aspects overlooked or not then deemed relevant in the developing country context, such as the staff's use of nipple shields, and an explicit investigation of the free and low-cost supplies issue.

This process took most of 1992, as committed professionals met to examine all the UNICEF documents in great detail and re-write passages that would be counter-productive in the Australian context. Until her departure for the USA, Dr. Pat Lewis worked closely with me on this project, together with representatives of the Australian College of Midwives (Lorraine Wilson), Royal Australian College of Obstetrics and Gynecology (Christine Tippett), the Association of Directors of Nursing (Netta McArthur) and the Victorian Department of Health and Community Services (Liz Scott). By early 1993 it was decided to hold a two-day workshop to introduce key national professional organisations to BFHI. Together with Jan Edwards (Geelong Hospital) and Neil Campbell (Director of Neonatology at the Royal Children's Hospital) I updated this group about the importance and management of early lactation, and introduced them in detail to the BFHI documents and process. The group agreed that the process and programme, Australia's first independent postpartum Quality Assurance Programme, was worthwhile. The Australian BFHI Steering Group, the national authority for BFHI was then set up. This was convened by Margaret Peters, then the immediate Past President of UNICEF Committee of Australia and still on the UNICEF Australia Board of Directors. It included the previous representatives and new nominations from the Royal Australian College of General Practitioners, as well as the Australian Association of Paediatric Teaching Centres, the Public Health Association, the Australian Nursing Federation, and Community Aid Abroad. The Royal Australian College of Obstetrics and Gynaecology was no longer represented, however, though it had been on the Taskforce, where Dr. Christine Tippett had made a valuable contribution. Given the impact of obstetric practice on breastfeeding difficulties, this is a serious omission.

The National Steering Group's task was to oversee the further development and continuing administration of BFHI in Australia, setting up State Administrative Bodies and creating guidelines for their operation and all aspects of the BFHI process. (Core groups that may always be represented in the State Administrative Groups were NMAA, ALCA and ACMI.) The National Steering Group worked as a largely independent group reporting to UNICEF Australia but developing its own programme and funding. UNICEF support for the first printing of the revised documents came via the far-sighted Regional Representative, Anwarul Choudhury, who visited Melbourne and was impressed with the structured manner in which the NSG was proceeding; this grant was later repaid, and indeed in 1994 some profits were remitted to UNICEF New York. The programme was a matter of considerable interest to overseas groups for whom large ongoing UNICEF or government grants were needed to achieve a less integrated programme.

An assessment programme requires trained assessors. In November 1992 the first assessors' workshop was organised in Melbourne. Under the conditions set by the National Steering Group, those who wish to organise these UNICEF-approved 10-hour workshops must agree to the terms of a contract covering content and financial obligations, such as the substantial levy per registrant to support the National BFHI. Those conducting other educational courses were encouraged to ask for a copy of the contract to consider, though until a member of their team had completed an accredited 10-hour course groups were unable to offer the official 10-hour programme. This was because those who are educators themselves need to have considered all the possible subtleties of interpretation and understand the spirit underlying the documentation. Where education about BFHI takes place by those without such understanding, negativity towards the programme is likely to be the result, and hospitals will not be attracted to consider it. This chain also means that the BFHI national authority can rapidly amend and update any information or documents being distributed, as the educators talking about BFHI in the community will all be on file. And of course it means that BFHI benefits from its own intellectual property, the documents UNICEF New York spent thousands of dollars creating and the National Taskforce many hours adapting for Australia. Here in Australia, BFHI was created by the Taskforce and the NSG to be a self-supporting programme, and only approved educators were to be given all the official documents for use in approved 10-hour workshops, all of whose graduates will be eligible to be considered as assessors. This did not prevent shorter or more informal information sessions being conducted, but attending these did not qualify anyone for consideration as an assessor, or provide anything like the depth of understanding of BFHI needed for implementation.

Hospital assessments began in 1993. A team of four donated their time and expertise to conduct a pilot assessment programme at the Royal Women's Hospital in Melbourne over two days in late July. This tested the workability of the documents and agreed procedures. Not until 1994, however, were any hospitals formally assessed and accredited as Baby-Friendly. Mitcham Private Hospital in Melbourne, in March, and the Royal Women's Hospital in September, both attained this distinction. Around Australia, scores of other hospitals are working towards this assessment, and many are almost ready to apply. Perhaps BFHI's greatest impact has been through getting hospitals to consider submitting to an external assessment: no one wants to lose face by failing, and so strenuous efforts have gone into re-thinking attitudes and practices, arranging in-service, and so on. BFHI has lent credibility and authority to those many voices calling for change from within: it has empowered midwives and breastfeeding mothers alike. Without the existence of the assessment process it would be very easy to ignore those voices.

The Baby-Friendly Paediatric Unit

Work in late 1993 resulted in Guidelines being developed for the Baby-Friendly Paediatric Unit. These 11 Steps to Optimal Infant feeding in the Paediatric Unit were approved by the National Steering Group in April 1994, and key paediatric units are now testing the concept. Christine Minogue, at the Royal Children's Hospital in Parkville, was Chair of the sub-committee developing these. Since by 1996 UNICEF New York had not evaluated these for global distribution, they have been published in *Breastfeeding Review*, and so made available globally. A quick reading will show that a complete assessment programme could be constructed from these for very little outlay, but in the absence of UNICEF interest or any financial support this seems unlikely. The BFPU Guidelines are included in chapter 8 (see page 180).

Another BFHI sub-committee, ably headed by Dr. Lisa Amir, BFHI representative of the RACGP (Royal Australian College of General Practice) on both the National Steering Group 1993-1995 (and National Advisory Council 1995-7) set up a most successful August 1995 International Scientific Conference designed to introduce doctors to the benefits and management of breastfeeding. This was combined with an ALCA-Vic Branch initiative: a 2-day national conference on human milk banking, fractionation, and use for small sick infants. The $25,000 profits from this 1995 conference were being used to support the BFHI in 1997, as UNICEF's promised matching grants had not been received by ACMI.

Of course all this voluntary activity required some national co-ordination. In 1992, Andrea McGinlay, an education officer working for UNICEF Victoria, was given the task of assisting the Taskforce, and did so ably and enthusiastically until her contract expired. The part-time position of National Co-ordinator was then advertised, and Lisa Donohue was appointed in September 1993. A research-based midwife with experience in family planning and other women's issues, Lisa was doing research at the Centre for the Study of Mothers' and Children's Health, and represented the Public Health Association on the National Steering Group; she proved to be an ideal choice. Her commitment and willingness to work long hours were to be tested to the limits by the full-time demands of a part-time job, but she succeeded not only in holding together a national initiative with state-based administrative groups, but in making it profitable, so that UNICEF New York received some thousands of Australian dollars as a result of the BFHI work here in Australia. Lisa's skills were recognised globally when she was asked to fly to China to assist in that country's implementation of BFHI. To her surprise she found that Australia's Paediatric Guidelines preceded her; it was not at all surprising that they were highly esteemed! Unfortunately her contract was not renewed at the end of 1994, and the absence of any National Co-ordinator allowed failures of communication with the States to develop throughout 1995.

What Australia had done about BFHI to the end of 1994 was truly remarkable. A small group of unpaid representatives of national associations, meeting monthly, shaped a national strategy and structure such that BFHI was proceeding in every State of Australia. With no handouts or grants, these volunteers had done more than has been achieved in some other countries with much more money.

Yet even though BFHI had been largely self-funding, within UNICEF Committee of Australia's Executive Board there had always been ambivalence re a 'domestic' project which promotes breastfeeding in a culture where bottle-feeding is not a death sentence. This curious attitude has been reflected in the language used by some UNICEF employees around the world, and in the way breastfeeding is presented in UNICEF appeals: as late as 1997 in Australia, the only mention of breastfeeding in one appeal was as a reason for greater need for food supplementation in women. Breastfeeding is not as obviously and immediately urgent as child prostitution or sanitation or iodine deficiency... Such ignorance is perhaps understandable among those chosen by UNICEF for their expertise in public relations or management or other areas than breastfeeding. But surely some education of all UNICEF staff and volunteer committees would be in order, when over a million babies die every year for want of breastmilk, and breastfeeding advocates worldwide recognise that the elites in poorer countries take much more notice of what we in rich countries DO than of what we say. The best way Australia could encourage breastfeeding in less affluent nations where

UNICEF devotes resources, would be to model a breastfeeding society to those coun-tries. By omitting positive images of breastfeeding women from their myriad cards, calendars, and other visual and written depictions of women, UNICEF says unwitting-ly that *breastfeeding is not a central or valuable female or human activity.* By saying that the BFHI is not their business in rich countries, UNICEF is unwittingly saying that elites in poor countries can ignore it: it's just for poor people. 'Poor people' don't like being patronised, and can smell a double standard a mile away: in Nigeria a wonderful market woman challenged me in front of others at the MCH clinic as to whether breastfeeding was promoted so heavily in my country, or whether doctors were just trying to make Nigerian women breastfeed because they couldn't afford formula. I was glad to be able to say that I had breastfed all my children for years, the youngest for almost four years: she was more impressed by that than anything else she'd heard. Breastfeeding is an issue about which there can be no double standards. By accepting earlier industry propaganda that "it doesn't matter that much what we do in Australia, but of course poor women should breastfeed" we are in fact acting as global promoters of artificial feeding. So 'domestic' breastfeeding promotion is in fact international action for the one world of which we are an integral part, and it's about time UNICEF Australia, and America, realised that. (And of course every year thousands of white affluent babies die for want of breastmilk.)

Stasis in BFHI 1994-6

UNICEF, quite properly as an auspicing body, had not intervened in any way in the creation of the BFHI National Steering Group. The national role of the National Steer-ing Group and its thrifty self-funding policies were apparently not understood by some state-based BFHI workers, who wanted (NSG-paid-for) State representation on the na-tional committee. Despite the fact that only national groups were represented, without such state-based representation the NSG was not seen as national by them. Obviously the NSG could not spend money on paying for airfares, and had taken the rational course of asking for fully-supported representatives from the national organisations which wanted to be involved in BFHI. Naturally this meant that the organisation was centred upon one state, where national organisations chose representatives who cost them very little. That state was Victoria, where core groups NMAA, ALCA, and ACMI all had their national offices and where Margaret Peters was located. The NSG unanimously agreed that BFHI money should not be spent on interstate representation, although of course any organisation could choose its representative from any state and pay their costs. Monthly NSG meetings thus cost nothing except the time of volunteers and their expenses, absorbed personally or by their organisation.

It became clear that a few key NSW midwives were not happy with being unable to attend NSG meetings, and this was (and still is) discussed in language that suggested interstate rivalry was alive and well. This misunderstanding must be seen as a failure of communication by representatives within the organisations concerned, as well as a failure of the NSG to take such concerns as seriously as its many other BFHI tasks. (To be fair to the NSG, most feedback it received from around the nation to the end of 1994 did not reflect any such concerns, but was focussed on BFHI work. And to be fair to the organisational representatives, people may not listen if the communication is not what they want to hear!) Partly due to lobbying of NSW-based UNICEF Board members and expressions of dissatisfaction with the NSG within NSW, the issue of UNICEF Australia's involvement with BFHI in this country was again discussed at UNICEF Australia's November 1994 Board meeting. An options paper was commissioned. There were some surprising omissions in the consultative process: the Sydney-based consultant interviewed members of the NSG, and just two other persons in NSW who had expressed dissatisfaction; and she interviewed the National Co-ordinator, Lisa Donohue, only very late in the process. UNICEF did not permit the NSG to continue key aspects of its work over this time of review. New restrictions kept on being communicated verbally via the Chair, some of these (such as the decision that no further accreditation be conducted) months after a UNICEF Australia decision. UNICEF never consulted the NSG before taking such decisions. A number of proposed or ongoing NSG projects (e.g., the breastfeeding teaching doll; distinctive Australian artwork for the Award; the Baby Friendly Paediatric Unit project) were shelved as the NSG waited for UNICEF Australia's decision after the review. Most have not been revived as yet, although in August 1997 the proposal to go back to a prominent Australian artist, Louis Kahan, and ask for the use of one of his artworks as the national BFHI symbol was approved.

In April 1995, UNICEF Australia agreed to provide some funding ($5000) towards making the initiative an independent incorporated body, as well as providing a small matching grant ($10,000 for two years). This was exactly what members of the NSG had proposed in writing and had begun work towards. Groups represented on the NSG were asked to ascertain the willingness of their organisations to commit themselves to an equal share of the needed matching $10,000, and a collaborative bid was envisaged and discussed by all active members of the NSG. It was minuted that NMAA, ALCA, and two other groups had formally expressed willingness to meet their fair share of the matching grant from UNICEF, and the NSG was led to believe that ACMI would be an equal partner; the NSG also assumed that, via the usual lines of communication, this bid would be communicated to UNICEF *on behalf of the NSG.*

At this stage it was generally thought that there would be little money in BFHI other than that contributed by professional organisations and grant bodies or governments. All that changed in late May 1995 when Bounty Australia approached the NSG with an offer of at least $10,000 for at least two years, provided it could be linked with BFHI.[138] The NSG talked with Bounty, and outlined their concerns about that company's links with bottle and teat advertising as well as the content of its sample bags to hospitals, in relation to the International Code of Marketing of Breastmilk Substitutes. The NSG acknowledged that Bounty had made some significant changes (e.g., had decided not to allow bottle and teat advertising in their booklet for pregnant women) and were grateful that Bounty expressed its willingness to consider others if the NSG would consider the sponsorship offer. The NSG therefore advised that it would recommend that the incoming BFHI authority would consider this matter of sponsorship generally, and create guidelines applicable to all sponsors. This was because the incoming BFHI body would be responsible for dealing with any adverse publicity such commercialisation of BFHI might generate, and would need to write the terms of the agreement with Bounty very carefully. It was explicitly stated in NSG Minutes that this would be dependent on Bounty's willingness to further consider its position in the advertising of bottles and teats.[139] Naturally representatives on any committee making such a serious decision would have to be authorised by their association to do so in its name. NSG members had believed in May 1995 that UNICEF would soon create an incorporated successor body, and so the NSG might not be in existence long enough to get such feedback before making the decision. NSG members would not allow any hasty decision as some still had grave reservations. None of these were insuperable, and the reservations did not arise simply because Bounty Australia was involved: there was a prior policy decision to be made as to whether any commercial interest should be allowed to link its name to BFHI, and if so, on what terms.

Bounty clearly believed that "UNICEF Australia's requirements of the successor body meant it was possible to establish a sponsorship relationship". This was news to some NSG members. Bounty's firm position that they would not go beyond "reasonable levels in the matter of bottles and teats" clearly needed to be explored: what is reasonable to breastfeeding advocates is the International Code, accepted globally. NSG members knew that Bounty had not considered this reasonable in the past, and was still a strong proponent of advertising of bottles and teats. Indeed, Bounty person Arthur Bateman was the founding President of the BPA, and one of the most vocal in meetings on this issue, although he made no baby products but instead gained revenue from those who did and wanted them advertised. So the issue was two-fold: commercial sponsorship generally, and then Bounty Australia in particular. I would stress that it was perfectly proper and appropriate for Bounty to make this offer on their terms; it was necessary for BFHI partners to consider their response collectively and carefully.

I was coming to the end of a full term on ALCA's National Council, and ceased to be ALCA's BFHI representative in late May 1995.[140] At the very next meeting, June 1995, the NSG, which had been expected to continue "in place until the successor body is formed," was persuaded that its meetings "should be put into abeyance" as from June 30, 1995.[141] Some NSG members at the time felt they had little choice but to agree to this, although a protest by key member groups might have averted this shutdown. However, ALCA was not even aware of what had happened, as its South Australia-based representative did not attend this crucial meeting. Apparently no one was too concerned (except about the unnecessary delay) because the NSG had been repeatedly assured that it was to be succeeded by an independent incorporated collaborative body[142] and all NSG members assumed not only that their collective matching bid had been faithfully communicated to UNICEF, but that UNICEF would see the value of continuing with the democratic collaborative cost-effective approach already pioneered by the NSG.

There is no doubt that UNICEF Australia's ambivalence, its review process, and its failure to maintain the role of the National Co-ordinator after December 1994, had slowed momentum since the second half of 1994 and confused and discouraged many people. It did not help that a Melbourne-based committee was being administered from

Sydney from January 1995, by individuals who seemed at pains to tell BFHI enquirers that they had more important things to do. Materials taken to Sydney without the knowledge of the former NSG seem to have been completely mislaid, for example. Finally in August 1995, on the very eve of the scientific conference that the NSG conference sub-committee had gone on producing, UNICEF announced that BFHI would continue in future under the auspices of the Australian College of Midwives Inc. (ACMI). This was devastating to all other NSG members. After all, they had been requested by the midwife chair of the NSG to seek collaborative matching funding from their organisations to set up an incorporated body. ACMI had been reluctant to commit itself publicly to any financial support of BFHI.[143] It was only with this UNICEF announcement that other ex-NSG members discovered that apparently after June 21, 1995 (when the NSG was closed down) ACMI decided to tender separately for total control of BFHI nationally, without informing its partners. It remains unclear whether UNICEF ever was made aware of the NSG collaborative bid, other than via the Minutes of NSG meetings. It is also unclear what if anything the NSG Chair knew of the College's internal processes, as she was not the ACMI representative. Breastfeeding advocacy organisations which had committed to the collaborative bid felt great concern about such behind-the scenes manoeuvres without consultation of other BFHI partners. Such concerns were in part allayed when former NSG members were assured in August 1995 that ACMI intended to set up an autonomous national body of the various interest groups willing to contribute time, money and expertise to the furtherance of BFHI in Australia. This has not happened. The reality since is that ACMI has taken complete control of the Initiative, insisting (despite the advice of at least one BFHI state group) on the title of "governing body" as if to underline that point. It has not set up an autonomous national body, but a National Advisory Council which is responsible for *advising* on BFHI policy and content, but not for the Project Officer, or decisions about money, staffing, budgeting, or other key aspects of autonomy. What is more, policy advice can be and is ignored if ACMI chooses to do so. And by 1998 there was no dedicated Project Officer in place to further the Initiative nationally.

So from August 1995 UNICEF Australia devolved responsibility for BFHI in Australia into the hands of the Australian College of Midwives Inc., in a process that from the point of view of BFHI stakeholders has been far from ideal. The reported loss of many records, for example, has been said to have hampered ACMI's ability to manage the initiative and created needless work. Former NSG members have spent time on re-creating records that should never have been lost. And the failure to make public the UNICEF-ACMI agreement whereby responsibility for BFHI has been transferred has caused concern. It is difficult to advise when basic terms of reference are unknown.

Also of great concern to some in December 1995 was the reported willingness of ACMI to accept Bounty sponsorship money for BFHI and for midwifery scholarships, thus making a far-reaching policy decision before creating the promised independent body, or formally consulting its putative BFHI partners, State Administrative Bodies, or even adequately consulting ACMI Branches, some of whom objected strongly to the idea of a Bounty-sponsored BFHI. Although the Bounty decision was evidently reversed, and no Bounty money has been taken for BFHI, the failure to consult again undermined confidence in the process. This was an apt symbol for much to come.

New beginnings BFHI 1995-7

However, in late 1995 the Australian College of Midwives did invite some groups to nominate a representative for a policy-making body to advise the College.[144] NMAA, ALCA, and RACGP accepted the invitation, despite some concerns about the structure, powers, and finances of this new entity, concerns shared by some State BFHI groups. This new National Advisory Council was then first convened in late August 1996, it met again in February 1997, April and August 1997, and May 1998. It consisted initially of representatives of ACMI (Chair and one other), ALCA, NMAA, RACGP, and State delegates (almost all midwives, and some ACMI office-bearers).[145] Some state committees have been unable to attend meetings because of travel costs. Representation from the Australian College of Paediatrics has been added, and some other were also invited to join in late 1997. All members of the National Advisory Council are committed to getting national progress underway after this hiatus, and have worked very hard to review and create all the necessary new documentation for the Initiative nationally. The Initiative was administered 1996-7 by a Brisbane-based National Project Officer, Rowena Chapman, employed by ACMI. In December 1997 it reverted to being controlled by ACMI National Office.

For all those who care about breastfeeding, it has been very hard to watch BFHI development slow nationally in the period 1994-1997. Yet enthusiasm and progress at the state and grassroots levels continues unabated. Much positive work has continued at the State level, using the guidelines written for these groups, set up by the outgoing National Steering Group, and the BFHI materials developed for Australia by the NSG. Those breastfeeding advocates in Australia, mostly midwives and mothers, who have given so much to BFHI cannot know what the future holds, but can be proud of what has been independently achieved at state and national levels. But I believe that the processes of decision-making by UNICEF and ACMI must be more transparent and collaborative than they were in the period 1994-7, or support of other breastfeeding advocacy groups for BFHI at state or national level may not be maintained. ALCA for one has invested literally thousands of dollars into BFHI at state and national levels, and to discover in April 1997 that UNICEF Australia has still not paid its matching $20,000 is somewhat disillusioning, to say the least.

From what is said above it is evident that I believe that UNICEF Australia has little to be proud of in the way it has auspiced BFHI in this country. A legacy of disillusion has undermined support for UNICEF among breastfeeding advocates. This should be said publicly, because for UNICEF globally to similarly dissociate itself from the BFHI project would be catastrophic for its own credibility, for the process of change it has set going so widely, and for its ability again ever to harness volunteer support for UNICEF breastfeeding projects. Indeed, the fear that UNICEF might not support the project long-term was a real one for many Australian volunteers initially, and some put their credibility on the line by assuring others that of course UNICEF realised that this was not a flash-in-the-pan project, but a sustained long-term educational process.

Similarly, of course, the Australian College of Midwives has some repair work to do on relationships with breastfeeding organisations, and must build trust in its ability to work transparently, democratically, and accountably. It cannot take co-operation for granted on any terms it sets as the self-styled "governing body". Only the commitment of other groups to the Global BFHI process kept them working with the College after the events of 1995-1996. Most breastfeeding advocates and BFHI State Committees would still like to see BFHI set up as an autonomous group, rather than persist with a structure they never approved, which has led to many tensions over accountability and access to information. .It seems likely that few would have qualms about breaking with ACMI and acting to implement the Global BFHI standard, as has happened in the USA, if it should ever seem that ACMI Council is not actively protecting, promoting and supporting Global standards. In 1998 ACMI has been part of a national group set up by QIC, which accepted a large grant from the Government's breastfeeding funds, intended to develop national standards of maternal/infant care and to complement BFHI. The latest draft is unacceptable to the National Advisory Council. If these standards do not affirm BFHI as a necessary minimum evidence-based standard, the NAC may dissociate itself from them, despite ACMI's involvement. It has already made it clear that the NAC itself has not approved any draft or elected a representative to meetings of the Consortium or its Reference Group (see p. 257, 273). The Reference Group for the project included many with no specialised qualifications in infant feeding, BFHI, or other WHO initiatives, although the intent as stated in the contract was to write Standards that would support breastfeeding and complement BFHI.

Yet to be fair to the College, some of the earlier events were outside its control. And it should also be said that in fact ACMI at many levels has played a very important part in breastfeeding advocacy in this period. The 1984 ICM Declaration on Breastfeeding was the beginning of a decade of increased awareness among midwives that breastfeeding did matter, and that they needed skilling in this field. It may have been largely ALCA and NMAA which were bringing the radically new knowledge to midwives' notice, but this translated into support by ACMI for virtually all breastfeeding initiatives. ACMI did respond to members' criticism of infant formula advertising in its journals by banning such advertising. And in 1991 ACMI became the first Australian professional group after ALCA to write a policy about formula sponsorship of its conferences, strengthened in 1995. Midwives have been the spearhead for much of the change discussed in this chapter, particularly that within hospitals. For that matter, it is mostly midwives who go on to become lactation consultants, and around 55% of the ALCA Council are midwives! Critical evaluation of certain actions of an organisation is occasionally needed (and any *truthful* record must be critical) but that does not detract from the achievements of that organisation elsewhere, whether we are talking of ACMI, ALCA, UNICEF or IBFAN.

To end this section on BFHI on a positive note: before 1997 had ended assessments were once again proceeding, and now 12 more Australian hospitals have been declared "Baby-Friendly." Wangaratta and District Base Hospital in Victoria was the first rural Australian hospital to achieve this status. Since then in Melbourne, the Angliss Hospital, Knox Private Hospital and the Bays Hospital Group (Mornington), John Flynn Maternity Hospital at Tugun near Coolangatta in Queensland, along with the Queen Elizabeth and Crystal Brook District Hospitals in SA, St. John of God Hospital, Geelong, Bairnsdale Regional Health Service and Mildura and Kyneton District Hospitals in country Victoria, and Forbes District Hospital in NSW, have all attained the global standard. They are accredited for a period of three years and join the two existing baby-friendly hospitals (Mitcham Private and the Royal Women's Hospital in Melbourne). Geelong Hospital is to undergo assessment very soon. There is a backlog of hospitals to assess in most states, and Australia should soon see many more hospitals, large and small, receiving the award, and so proving that they are both Mother and Baby-friendly, providing evidence-based, quality postpartum care for all women. By now any hospital not accredited or at least actively working to become Baby-Friendly should be viewed with deep suspicion by women wanting the best care postpartum, as it reveals substantial ignorance of world's best practice.

BFHI and the Code, including the Subsidised Supplies Issue

As stated earlier, the Baby-Friendly Hospital Initiative has been quietly having a very positive effect in this issue of free and low-cost supplies. A question was written into the 1992 Australian version of the Global documents, although the original Global BFHI Assessment tools did not formally include it, and so the National Steering Group felt it could not make rejection of free and low-cost supplies mandatory for BFHI accreditation. However, the NSG immediately re-defined "low-cost" supplies. The UNICEF definition was "less than 80% of retail", which effectively forced hospitals to pay full market price and guaranteed huge company profits. The NSG decided to adopt usual commercial practice for guaranteed sales to a reliable customer. BFHI is not in the business of maximising industry profit, and some competition is essential to keep prices down. I have been told of a company representative charging a hospital full retail and saying that BFHI has mandated this, creating ill-will towards BFHI quite unjustly, while maximising profits. Caveat emptor: in Australia the definition of low-cost supplies is less than 80% of WHOLESALE, if any institution wants to be recognised as Baby-Friendly. To say hospitals cannot afford to pay this price is simply silly.

When in 1997 hospital assessments began again, one of the gaps immediately identified by experienced assessors was this issue of free and low-cost supplies. While the question is asked in the Global and Australian programmes – does the hospital accept free or low-cost supplies? – there is no formal outline of what this means for hospitals, or how this is assessed. The CEO and Supply Officer must state that the hospital pays for its stores, but there should also be a detailed visual and verbal check that the many other areas of the hospital (paediatric wards, dietitian, NICUs, antenatal and many more) are not quietly being serviced by reps who drop off cans and materials as they like in some hospitals. Assessments to date have shown that some hospitals have no idea who industry reps are talking to, much less where they leave samples. Senior staff have been astonished that what they thought was hospital policy, that no such supplies be accepted, was routinely breached by staff unaware that to accept such gifts was a breach of the hospital's policy and professional ethics. This finding casts further doubt on the accuracy of answers to the BFA 1996 survey (see p.256-7). In 1998 ACOIF will be proposing to the BFHI NAC a formal protocol re "supplies".

It should of course be noted that ending free and low-cost supplies is in the interests of industry, which had found this policy an increasing financial burden in many markets. Achieving cessation of free supplies is one of the easier tasks once companies have judged them ineffective as a marketing tool, and wish to spend funds on doctors. I am very conscious that the voluntary end of free supplies was inevitable once midwives in Australia were better educated and therefore supplies were not being misused as they were in the 1970s, and so were not a useful marketing tool, though they still are to community doctors and centres in some places, where ignorance persists. Health professional education and consciousness-raising achieves many ends.

Other Governmental Initiatives.

Each state of Australia could list a variety of initiatives in relation to breastfeeding, but very few have spent serious money over this period to protect, promote or support breastfeeding. Some notable policies have emerged that are worth mentioning briefly: NSW's official policy that no child should be given a so-called "complementary" feed without the mother's written consent; WA's insistence that industry representatives may not call on clinic sisters in work hours; the Victorian government's breastfeeding guidelines; and the NT government's holistic strategy document.

The Queensland Government has given substantial assistance to BFHI, with funding to hospitals to create change, and the employment of a co-ordinator for a period of a year. To date in this country, they are the only government to give any money to BFHI, although the previous Commonwealth Health Minister provided some financial support for the BFHI conference in August 1995, and Dr. Wooldridge, the 1998 Health Minister, has said that in funding the Consortium (see p. 271) consisting originally of the ACHS (Australian Council for Hospital Standards), ACMI, and QIC he was lending support to the incorporation of the BFHI standards in all Australian hospitals. Dr. Wooldridge supports BFHI and the International Code, and his government has never repudiated its obligations under the Code and WHA resolutions such as those about free supplies. Nor would citizens expect any Australian government to!

Among other initiatives of Australia's Commonwealth government was the 1983 multi-lingual breastfeeding pamphlet; the 1989 circulation of 5000 copies of the Royal College of Midwives' *Successful Breastfeeding* (the first modern breastfeeding guide for health professionals, which generously acknowledged and incorporated the new clinical information from *Breastfeeding Matters*). Australia's 1982 Dietary Guidelines included "Promote Breast Feeding"; regrettably, in the 1992 revision, this first Dietary Guideline was placed number nine on the list, on the peculiar basis that it applied only to a small segment of Australia's population. (Since we were all infants once, from one perspective this was the only truly universal and primary dietary guideline!) Dietary Guidelines for Children were also developed and passed by the NH&MRC in June 1995; "Encourage and support breastfeeding" was naturally the first. And in 1988 the official *Health for All Australians* report set a goal for the year 2000 of 80% of all infants breastfeeding at 3 months: a goal we are unlikely to reach without drastic social change or serious government action to halt the erosion of breastfeeding.

Commonwealth reviews of the Australian implementation of the International Code have also occurred, as part of Australia's responsibilities to the World Health Organisation. In 1991 a Committee was set up "to assess actions taken in Australia to give effect to the aims and principles" of the International Code, based upon the WHO Common Review and Evaluation Framework sent out to selected countries. Being composed largely of healthworkers with epidemiological skills,[146] this Committee was dissatisfied with the WHO CREF as it then stood, and developed a number of strategic questionnaires as part of its task, reporting in 1993. Subsequently WHO went on to commission Ros Escott, the APMAIF Community Representative, to develop the CREF utilising responses from the countries involved in this first pilot project, and the WHO published in 1996 *The International Code of Marketing of Breastmilk Substitutes: A Common Review and Evaluation Framework*[147] which now provides an epidemiologically credible way of assessing national compliance with the International Code. National monitoring using this WHO technique will not attract the criticism that less "scientific" consumer monitoring inevitably does, and so is more likely to convince policy-makers that a country has a problem it should attend to. Just as both qualitative and quantitative research techniques are valid but different, there is room for both types of surveys and reports: one hopes that the consumer advocacy movement will read carefully and then promote this extremely useful WHO tool, as well as continue to submit its own research protocols to such careful epidemiological scrutiny. In my view, to ignore or denigrate this WHO document is show oneself to be unaware of the *realpolitik* of healthworkers and politicians in 'advanced' countries where science has been deified. And to use bad research tools is counter-productive.

Important too in Australia in this period has been the review of standards for infant formula. Until 1991 the NH&MRC (National Health and Medical Research Council) had responsibility for Infant Formula standards. In 1986 the NH&MRC adopted Standard R7 for Australian Infant Formula, subsequently revised so that it closely paralleled the Codex Alimentarius standard and also attempted to incorporate the labelling requirements of the Code. (These requirements were made mandatory on relevant exports from Australia in 1985.) Consumers strongly criticised the mandatory labelling of any infant formula as "Suitable from birth" but this was not listened to at the time, when so many of those involved in the revisions had no problem about lending their credibility to the preposterous statement that any artificial substitute is "suitable" for all infants from birth, despite the evidence that it leads to allergy, diabetes, colitis, even anaphylaxis in some infants. Times change: it seems likely that in the next revision of Australian formula standards no such guarantee of suitability will be given; the formula will simply be labelled "may be used from birth" or "…from six months", though I believe the latter should be labelled "not safe for infants under 6 months", since that is the problem we now face! Professor Roger Short's proposal for mandatory health warnings on labels seems quote appropriate and indeed overdue.

So-called 'special infant formulas' were covered by the Therapeutic Goods Administration throughout the 1980s. With the changes in the TGA, including changes in the definition of what constituted food, and the process for establishing that a therapeutic claim could be made about a product, these special infant formulas needed to have a food standard developed for them. In August 1991 the National Food Authority (NFA) had been established, and it was given responsibility for this. A review was commissioned which recommended that before any standards could be set for 'special infant formulas', it would be important to revise the 1986 standard for regular infant formula. The process has been ongoing since. In late 1996-early 1997 significant progress was being made, then cutbacks, the re-organisation of the NFA into the ANZFA (the Australian and New Zealand Food Authority) as from July 1996, and the loss of the expert staff person involved with the process, have delayed matters until more urgent issues were dealt with. It is anticipated that 1998 will see a further process of consultation in both Australia and New Zealand, and a joint food standard for infant formula set for both countries. Although at present a great deal of money has been made available for contracting out to private sources tasks such as this, ANZFA rightly retained this crucial task for its own diminished staff. There can be no more important or sensitive food standard: infant formula is the sole source of nutrients for the most vulnerable class of human beings for a long period of time, a time of maximal brain growth and physical development. To be solely reliant on a single food violates the usual fundamental principles of dietary safety: diversity and moderation (which breastmilk, with its amazing complexities, can supply but formula cannot). If infant formula provides too much or too little of any nutrient, an infant has no way of balancing that ingredient from other components in its diet. Hence ANZFA staff are working carefully and consulting the best scientific authorities for the latest research to determine an acceptable standard for both countries. And that national standard must be scientifically defensible, as countries can be accused before the World Trade Organisation of a breach of the GATT (General Agreement on Trade and Tariffs) if they set a standard higher than the lowest-common-denominator, industry-dominated Codex Alimentarius world standard for infant formula (currently also in the process of revision) and then refuse to allow the import of products which breach the ANZ standard but meet the Codex one. There is probably little real risk of this, for two basic reasons: the enormous publicity and questioning of the safety of infant formula which could be generated by a vigilant watchdog group such as ACOIF if Australia were to be told that its standards were too high; and secondly, the fact that standards are usually written around the parameters of existing formula, since almost all the major formula-exporting companies have huge influence on the development of standards in every country. Only the naïve believe that regulatory agencies can lightly disregard powerful vested interests and tell them to re-formulate. Consumers' natural desire to trust in all such agencies needs to be tempered by realism.

ANZFA, like every other government instrumentality, has been put on notice that it is to reduce rather than increase regulation of the food industry. There is no time to go into this in detail, but I strongly suggest that readers interested in the quality of Australian food keep a careful eye on developments. The ANZFA Website is excellent; look for it at **<http://www.anzfa.gov.au>**. ANZFA has a highly professional (but cut-back) staff and so crucial issues like infant formula have not been outsourced, but it is almost morally certain that in a country with such a small population and industry base, some food reviews will be being conducted by those with direct links to the industry involved: that is where the expertise is. Consumer input will be more needed than ever before, as industry pressure is intense.

The overall effect of many other national and state government policies has not been supportive of breastfeeding. Women forced back into the workforce by economic necessity are less likely to feed their babies for the WHO recommended period, although if they were allowed to claim from government for the full period of lactation the amount available as childcare subsidy if they were to leave their babies in care, many might. One thoroughly positive development has been a number of complaints by women discriminated against for breastfeeding in public: under Equal Opportunity laws forbidding sexual or racial or other discrimination, this is now considered a cause for complaint and remedy. There will always be antediluvian restaurateurs who oppose such freedoms for women and their children, and they can always count on mobilising some support if they are noisy or obnoxious enough, but these fly in the face of intelligent social opinion. To keep each generation comfortable with seeing breastfeeding in public and so to maintain such freedoms, women need to exercise them, so I actively encourage brazen breastfeeding. Ignore the baby rooms (except for change purposes) and liberate a lobby! It is good to see that Victoria's Equal Opportunity agency has published a poster informing women of their right to breastfeed under the law.

Lactation Consultancy

In this last decade, Australia has benefited from the uniquely American concept of Lactation Consultancy. In the early 1980s, largely as the result of far-sightedness on the part of LLLI and key professionals such as Chele Marmet and Ellen Shell, Ruth Lawrence, Audrey Naylor and Ruth Wester, America pioneered the concept of professional education about lactation and breastfeeding. The creation of the International Board of Lactation Consultant Examiners (IBLCE) in 1985, and the increasing number of lactation consultants and training institutes are the result. ILCA (the International Lactation Consultant Association – LC usually stands for Lactation Consultant), also developed in 1985 as a professional association for International Board-Certified Lactation Consultants, or IBCLCs, and other health professionals interested in lactation. While standards of competence in this new field of professional assistance to breastfeeding women are presently very variable around the world, a great deal of useful information is beginning to be generated and recorded in professional journals. The task of reviving breastfeeding as the 'community norm' is intrinsically more difficult in the US than in Australia or Britain, but there is immense enthusiasm for the project in some circles. And major American initiatives, such as IBLCE and ILCA, have had enormously positive consequences in other countries.

Australia was involved with both groups from their beginnings. ALCA, the Australian Lactation Consultants' Association, was set up with support from NMAA in 1987. Nationally incorporated in 1987, its constitution differed significantly from ILCA's, in that ALCA made the IBLCE certification the definitive entry standard for member-ship. This committed ALCA to slower growth, as potential membership was obviously confined to the number of successful candidates. But in the 'British' world all the newly-forming national associations (as distinct from local or regional groups eager for sufficient members to be viable) realised that credibility as a professional associa-tion would not last long without a credible and defensible minimum entry standard. So in New Zealand, Canada, South Africa and other countries such as Israel, membership of the national professional association is limited to IBCLCs. Quality, not quantity, was the motto. Not surprisingly, in 1997 ILCA itself voted to move to an IBCLC-only voting membership structure.

ALCA has been and still is a very significant part of world development of the profession. It negotiated the right to send a representative to the IBLCE Examination Committee, in recognition both of its status as the national professional association for LCs, and the role of ALCA in encouraging candidates for the exam. Australia actually has the highest per capita ratio of International Board-Certified Lactation Consultants. This universally-recognised qualification is the only valid guarantee of a minimum standard of basic competence in lactation consultancy. Only those who do not under-stand just how expensive and difficult it is to create and maintain an independent health professional certification process in the United States would seriously propose that ALCA or any other professional body for lactation consultants should recognise any other credential for membership entry. Major midwifery bodies certainly appreciate IBLCE's standard: the Royal College of Midwives has a representative on the IBLCE Board, and was involved with the IBLCE Exam Committee for some years.

A professional association must have some legally-defensible, non-discriminatory minimum entry criteria, to provide some guarantee to the public that its members are basically competent in the field of expertise. This is not elitism, but professionalism. Obviously there are those in many countries who for a variety of reasons consider that successful completion of a local course (sometimes one they or their friends are asso-ciated with) is as good as successfully passing an international exam. ALCA allowed for future developments in its constitution by permitting membership of persons who had passed the IBLCE exam "or an equivalent assessment process approved by the ALCA Council." But as yet there is no equivalent assessment process, and the task of judging "equivalence" would be huge. ILCA's Education Committee has considered for years the problem of professionally assessing educational offerings for equivalency with one another, despite the bureaucracy, problems of confidentiality, and costs this would involve, but no one has seriously considered setting up any other examination.

Yet to accept course graduates as the equivalent of an IBCLC for membership purposes was proposed to National Council by the executive of ALCA NSW branch in 1993. ALCA put this idea to its membership, and feedback was almost universally negative. Two years later that Branch executive subsequently went on to create a new organisation in which such equivalence is given; indeed, in which any health profes-sional with an interest in lactation may be a full member. In a number of states some course graduates are now calling themselves Lactation Consultants, while recently another new organisation was set up for "qualified LCs" which does not recognise the

IBLCE qualification as the standard for membership, adding that the person must also be a "recognised" health professional or NMAA Counsellor; while any Counsellor or health professional with no lactation qualification whatever can be an "associate member". It seems to me unwise for any volunteer Breastfeeding Counsellor to be considered or to consider herself a Lactation Consultant: the volunteer NMAA Coun-sellor is explicitly forbidden to give medical advice while the Lactation Consultant is a health professional who is obliged to do so. Yet if a Counsellor or healthworker is in-troduced as a member of a "college of lactation consultants", or a "lactation college", one might expect her to be competent to give full medical advice about lactation. NMAA may well find that difficulties arise from members of the public dealing with NMAA Counsellors who are members of a self-styled college of lactation consultants. So the waters are becoming muddied indeed about who and what is or is not a Lacta-tion Consultant in Australia, as locally-powerful healthworkers sit in judgment on the worth of the IBLCE qualification as a stand-alone credential.[148]

In a field such as breastfeeding, where many of the pioneers of education were mere mothers, like myself "not even a nurse", this medical bias seems not just quaint but truly sad. It first emerged in America a decade ago among doctors and nurses, who wanted to have organisations that were "medical professionals only". Of course the territoriality is understandable, and it does simplify things to be able to presume some basic medical knowledge. As well, the elitist nature of medicine means that there are some health professionals who will not take seriously any organisation which is not exclusive, and there is no doubt that many people love discriminatory barriers that make them feel part of a special enclave, even when it is demonstrable that one does not have to be a doctor or nurse to understand lactation better than many such persons ever will. But creating ghetto organisations can also have major drawbacks. In my view it is destructive of the unity and cross-disciplinary skills needed to keep nurses and doctors in particular from medicalising breastfeeding. And the contribution of highly trained health professionals in a more catholic groups can be valuable in raising standards of knowledge generally: this is lost where such persons seek out their own rather than interact with others. So too is the unity and increased advocacy power of the profession as a whole, when it is divided into competing chunks. I look at the Academy of Breastfeeding Medicine, a doctors-only organisation, and even while I understand the culture which bred it, I lament the diversion of such resources from ILCA, which would be far more effective world-wide with it. And drug remedies are more likely to multiply where doctors discuss problems. In division lies weakness.

Australia has not escaped these tensions. A sociologist friend recently commented on the propensity for women, and nurses in particular, to weaken their own cause by not dealing with disagreements appropriately. She noted that powerful dissident fig-ures tend to form their own little splinter groups rather than work together for a single coherent powerful national body. Regrettably such a split occurred within ALCA in the period 1995-1996, for reasons that were both political and personal.[149] New local "colleges"[150] were created after ALCA dissidents were defeated in a deeply-divisive May 1995 national ballot with a very high participation rate.[151] The state-based colleges, presently led by former local ALCA office-bearers who objected to some

National Council actions and decisions, contain many excellent breastfeeding advocates, and have benefited from the past national support of ALCA, which has educated via *ALCA News* (now *ALCA Galaxy*), and subsidised national tours to all states of outstanding international speakers, etc. They are maintaining their own education programmes. Thus there is no doubt that these new groups[152] should continue to provide good education and local support for professionals interested in breastfeeding. Of course if ever there are too many non-IBCLCs in these new groups, (and in their haste to grow at least one has provided heavy financial incentives for every conference attendee to become a member) standards may eventually diverge from the globally recognised ones: the current office bearers must move on eventually and may be replaced by non-IBCLCs, or IBCLCs with no national or international connections or awareness. It is to be hoped that in the future, when tempers cool and office bearers are in charge who were not involved in the events of 1995-6, some reunification between professional LC groups will prove possible, for the sake of breastfeeding families and LCs themselves, as well as breastfeeding advocacy in Australia. After all, as of December 1997 there are only 1329 IBCLCs in Australia. For them to be split between one national organisation with branches in virtually every state, and 6 separate state organisations, seems positively farcical. As for two rival national organisations, when only one has sufficient resources to employ a national co-ordinator, and that part-time: it's hard to imagine that this is the result of either commonsense or any desire for effective national advocacy for LCs or breastfeeding. If East and West Germany can hazard reunification after decades of separate development, this hope is surely not too ambitious!

In the face of this split, widely publicised by a commercial interest,[153] with publications and membership numbers of the new groups even advertised on Lactnet,[154] ALCA has again chosen, in my view appropriately, to continue to restrict membership to IBCLCs (the only legally defensible global qualification for LCs), and in no other discriminatory or arbitrary way.[155] In December 1996 ALCA strongly reaffirmed its commitment to the IBLCE certification as the gold standard for Lactation Consultancy. NMAA found it necessary to do so at the same time.

ILCA itself has played a peripheral but generally positive role in Australia, and from the beginning ALCA has influenced the development of ILCA. There have been numerous interactions, from ILCA's re-wording of ALCA's aims and objectives to ALCA's re-working of ILCA's then Recommendations and Competencies into ALCA's Standards of Practice... which have since been re-worked into ILCA's Standards of Practice! The input has been through an exchange of people as well as ideas and documents. Australia has had a representative on ILCA's Board for most of ILCA's lifespan[156] to date. By 1997 it was surely time that New Zealand was represented, and so ALCA, jointly with NZLCA, endorsed a NZ candidate, Heather Jackson. Then ILCA President Jan Barger was a guest at ALCA's 1992 conference, Dr. Felicity Savage (another former ILCA International Delegate) at the 1994 conference in Adelaide, and the outgoing ILCA President, Karen Kerkhoff-Gromada, attended ALCA's 1996 conference in Hobart. As Australia's ILCA National Affiliate from 1989, ALCA has offered its members access to the world of Lactation

Consultants. Every year ALCA has been officially represented at the ILCA conference, an astonishing learning-fest where much is gained by networking.

Such international affiliations are important to developing the profession world-wide, even if the benefits are not immediately obvious. However, ALCA may be forced to re-consider its official ILCA affiliate status now that ILCA has lowered the standard for affiliates,[157] decided to eliminate the separate category of National Affiliate, and made a provision that at least 25% of all affiliate members must be also paid-up ILCA members. ILCA membership is expensive for Australians, many of whom have arranged for subscriptions to the ILCA *Journal of Human Lactation* to be taken out centrally, and for whom there are no other real benefits of ILCA membership. (A conference discount of a few dollars is irrelevant when travel costs thousands.) How 25% joint affiliate-ILCA membership can be achieved or monitored by national organisations such as ALCA is completely unclear. It would seem likely that ILCA will reconsider this provision, as it will certainly lose affiliates, or find itself confined to very small elite groups of affluent members. It could result in acceptance of an affiliate with 20 members, of whom 5 are ILCA members, in North America, and rejection of a group of 500, of whom 95 are ILCA members, in Australia. Yet advocacy at national and international levels requires unity, or we duplicate efforts and reinvent the wheel repeatedly. So I am informed that ALCA will continue to support ILCA, despite growing concerns about how little ILCA does for affiliates or members outside the USA. That support could continue even if ALCA decides that in future that there is little justification for spending members' money to remain an ILCA affiliate, now ILCA has apparently decided to treat a large national fully-democratic organ-isation of IBCLCs as the same as a group of diverse health professionals in a small town. In my view, applications for ILCA affiliation should always fail where group membership qualifications exclude any IBCLC, or accept the IBLCE certification as equivalent to local courses in which affiliate members have an interest.

In response to these changes of ILCA policy, in 1997 I resigned from the ILCA Professional Advisory Board, of which I had been a founding member, as I could not in conscience lend my name to an expensive US-based organisation whose policies suggest to me that it believes that it can single-handedly represent the world of LCs, and does not need to deal respectfully and collaboratively with national IBCLC-only organisations in other countries. My vision for ILCA has always been of an eventual democratic federation of world IBCLC associations, not a US-based ILCA with token non-US representation, which undermines or ignores national IBCLC organisations. I have remained an ILCA member and have no intention of giving up on that vision.

ILCA and ALCA both acknowledge that professional education is one crucial key to a better future for infants. If health professionals were truly professional in their infant feeding knowledge and skills, and vigorous in political advocacy, many more women would be breastfeeding, and industry would not be a problem. The task of community education is huge, and around Australia many groups have been tackling it with enthusiasm. Breastfeeding education in Australia is now a growth industry, ran-ging from university-based nurses-only courses to innovative free-standing and corres-pondence programmes, the most influential of which have probably been the Alma courses in Melbourne since 1986, and Australasian Lactation Courses, set up in Adelaide in 1989. Between them these two groups have educated literally thousands of healthworkers about breastfeeding. Australians are even educating overseas: a group called LIFE (Lactation and Infant Feeding Education) Inc. has pioneered team-teaching in Asia, while numerous Australian educators have taught in New Zealand and America. ALCA's own Biennial National Conferences have been enormously important in introducing to Australia major international speakers such as Dr. Mike Woolridge, Miriam Labbok, Felicity Savage King, Tony Williams, Jack Newman, Tom Hale and in 1998 Ruth Lawrence, Grø Nylander, Randa Saadeh, and Kerstin Uvnas-Moberg, to name a few of many. In every state ALCA members past and present have been key players in this task, many supported by ALCA in overseas travel and networking: ALCA Vic Branch has been outstanding in the range of topics and speakers it has showcased since 1986. So too has NMAA, via its massive International Conferences in 1988 and 1997, Health Professional workshops (many in conjunction with ALCA) and regularly via the outreach of the Lactation Resource Centre, which since 1991 has been collaborating with Alma in a 28-hour teaching programme. Membership of the LRC is strongly recommended to anyone dealing with breastfeeding families. NMAA's LRC maintains a database of courses and educational offerings around Australia, and should be the first port of call for any interested person. So too does ALCA, although not all courses provide materials to either centre.

Midwives undoubtedly have been the group most responsive to new information to date, as breastfeeding is 'their' territory if it belongs to any one professional group predominantly. The 1984 ICM statement[158] was a wonderful inspiration for this decade of change. It is to midwives and mothers that I give credit for most of the positive changes within the hospital system. Almost without exception, they have paid for their own education and set about implementing what they have learned, challenging everything from breastfeeding management to formula procurement. General practitioners are also beginning to respond, although strangely, unlike midwives, many seem to expect to be paid to learn. Quite a number have sat the IBLCE examination. Probably South Australia has the highest number of GP IBCLCs, although Victoria is not far behind. This is of course a gain, so long as GP practice can be re-structured to give women the time a proper breastfeeding consultation involves, or else GPs employ Lactation Consultants to do so for them, a practice pioneered in SA.[159] And the first course offered by the Pharmacy College in Melbourne in 1995, a spin off generated by the involvement of Simon Appel of the Pharmacy Guild on the BFHI NSG, indicates that the need for infant feeding knowledge is recognised by this professional group: over 90 pharmacists enrolled! The course has continued since and is being offered again in 1998. Work is also continuing towards a Best Practice Infant Nutrition scheme for pharmacies, recognising those that handle these issues appropriately. Draft guidelines for retail pharmacies were approved by ACOIF and are now being discussed with pharmacy interests; in late 1997 Dr. Peter Hartmann was working with some pharmacy reps in WA on this issue.

Halting the erosion of breastfeeding is more than controlling industry.

Despite all the deficiencies, a good deal that is positive has emerged, all around the world. But with so much achieved, what remains to be done? This is where the work begins, not ends. It is the major re-structuring western society has undergone and is undergoing which poses the greatest threat to breastfeeding. This is discussed in chapter 13, and will be dealt with at greater length in my next book. Industry is one part of that western social mixture which is eroding breastfeeding. Eighty years ago it was a key force in eroding breastfeeding in some communities. In others it still is.

Previous criticisms of *infant formula* may create the impression that I see all formula *manufacturers* or their employees as wicked or criminal. I do not. But nor do I see industry as altruistic philanthropists working solely to support health professionals and help children. Industry is industry, with its own legal duty to make profits for shareholders. The shareholders' appetite for profit may be boundless, and this ensures that ethical standards cannot be such as to put the company out of business, or even seriously reduce profits. I agree that industry's product is currently necessary, and I do not consider industry solely responsible for the decline in breastfeeding, much less all infant mortality and morbidity. Neither do I consider industry guiltless, as the evidence for its involvement in the complex processes leading to lactation failure past and present is simply overwhelming. I have considerable respect for industry's ability to create a need for a second-rate product by advertising their belief in a first-rate one, namely breast milk. The formula industry's marketing strategies have been among the smartest known. Industry's ability to create diversions, whether by labelling their opponents Marxists or opposed to free choice for women, is really amazing, as is the way they have become an accepted adjunct (a partner, even) to the medical profession. That most rewarding of liaisons has a very long history by now, and it can be difficult for professionals to step back, view themselves dispassionately, and accept that such a liaison has shaped their assumptions, attitudes and beliefs, as well as their clinical practice, and that they will need to re-think much that seems normal after long acquaintance with industry infomercials.

Can breastfeeding advocates work with industry?

Despite all that, I believe that it is both possible and necessary for health professionals such as myself[160] to shape a working relationship with industry which does not threaten the integrity of either party. At the present time some of us do have to deal constructively with industry: we can hardly ignore it while it controls most healthworker information and resources. While trying to generate additional independent information[161] it is necessary to have input into what will reach professionals from industry.

There are simple ways of reducing the real risk of co-option through association. For example, if you want to make sure written material is not harmful to breastfeeding, agree to review it on condition that:

- you will not be paid for doing so;
- your name will not be attached to it in any way, or
- if your name is attached to the material, you will have the right to edit every

version until the final print is done;
- if your name is attached a strong disclaimer is also there to say that you agreed to assist in order to help women and children and this should not be construed as endorsement of the company or any of its products.

Then add in strong information about the risks of artificial feeding if writing for a formula company; or the benefits of low-cost technology rather than high tech if dealing with breast pump literature. If they won't publish what you have written, they are not genuine about wanting to help women breastfeed and you can later publish a factual (not emotional) account of your dealings with them which makes that clear. In general they'll choose to publish and honour the terms you've set. (And not ask you again!)

If you are asked to speak at an industry-sponsored meeting, consider the target audience and likely good you can do. If it will be a waste of your time, don't accept. If you feel you can reach even a few people via practical topic that will ensure that the audience is better skilled at helping women afterwards than before, then say yes; and make sure that in developing the presentation you document some of the harms that are done by artificial feeding as a process and a product. You might like to begin with a thank you to the organisers for the invitation, and also to the artificially-feeding families who are subsidising the conference through the cost of the product they are purchasing; along with a reminder that your presence should not be taken as an endorsement of any commercial interests visibly associated with the meeting. Then or later in the presentation you may wish to go further and state that you accepted the invitation because you wished to let attendees know that independent education is available inexpensively, and ask them to think about the realities of company-sponsored meetings; that you are accepting no payment for being present, and not eating the expensive lunch usually provided, but donating your time and bringing lunch, so as to minimise the cost of your own presence, since it is poor families who bottle-feed and you feel uncomfortable with the idea that companies over-charge for a product in order to have an advertising budget that allows healthworkers, not the poorest people in any society, to enjoy lavish lunches and subsidised education. The adage that "there is no such thing as a free lunch" is familiar and effective.

I can live with those whose principles will not permit them "to sup with the devil", even so circumspectly as this. To stay clean and undefiled by commerce with industry is one understandable way out of major dilemmas. But I think that babies will be worse off if **everyone** adopts that policy of "purity" and isolationism, and it is babies (and their mothers) we are working for. Too often those with such principles cannot talk without judgmental outbursts about those of us with more pragmatic views of working with industry. I know that holier-than-thou attitudes on this issue of industry liaison are NOT persuasive to the unconverted, who are the audience we need to reach. Like them, it makes me angry to have it insinuated that I am a simpleton who is unaware of the risks of co-option, or to hear others tell me what they think is ethical in ways that are profoundly disrespectful, often while those same people behave in divisive or aggressive ways which I think grossly unethical. I know it makes industry reps very angry to be insulted and stereotyped, and that this discredits our cause. So does assuming venal motives for the involvement of healthworkers with industry:

many provide their services for free, and out of concern for babies. Ranting about the evils of formula salespersons is just tacky and stupid. They are people and deserve courtesy and respect (and education about infant feeding, which can have some remarkable results).

Health professionals are becoming far more conscious of their interaction with industry. It is heartening to see that in 1997 the Australian College of Paediatrics has developed an excellent draft statement on industry sponsorship of research. Copies are available from Dr. Karen Simmer, Flinders Medical Centre, Adelaide. It is to be hoped that the College adopts it and goes on to strengthen its stance on these issues, and that other reputable organisations follow suit.

Of course in this regard I have been addressing questions of interaction with vested interests who profit from breastfeeding failure. Healthworkers also need to interact with those who seek to help breastfeeding succeed, whether by supplying pumps or nipple devices or other paraphernalia for breastfeeding. Here the dilemmas are less severe. If a product helps mothers and keeps babies breastfeeding, it is useful. It may be over-priced: let's say so. It may be untested: let's say so. It may be a good idea but a bad item, made of unsafe materials or poorly designed: let's say so. It may work for some mothers and not others: let's say so. (Indeed, let's try to identify those for whom it is likely to work and recommend it discriminatingly.) But let's not fall into silly Luddite denunciations of all technology or gizmos or creams as automatically wicked because they make money out of lactation, or are not scientifically proven. For goodness' sake, doctors, nurses, lactation consultants, midwives, and the rest make money out of breastfeeding, and they are not considered ipso facto to be wicked! And as for treatments needing to be scientifically proven: yes, this would be good, but if doctors or midwives only did that which has been proven to be safe and effective, there would be no call for the development of evidence-based medicine. Every day medicine acts on the basis of experience and empirical beliefs, not just randomised double blind controlled trials... And for my money, if NMAA tests a product and gets positive feedback from intelligent breastfeeding mothers who say they liked it or it was helpful, that seems a reasonable basis for giving any product a go if its design does not offend basic principles of safety or science. Common sense at times seems a most uncommon virtue in the breastfeeding world. People who make breast pumps are commercial entrepreneurs, just as are people who make infant formula, but there are serious differences between the two. If there is a baby to be fed, the one is useless once lactation ceases; the other benefits when it does.

Controlling artificial feeding industry marketing practices is necessary, and important in efforts to prevent further erosion of breastfeeding in this country, but will not fix all our infant feeding problems. Breastfeeding rates will not rise simply because industry stops advertising. History will discredit us if we say that it will. This is not a simple issue. Simplistic solutions create problems and do not always have the desired result, which is better health for babies. To value one's perceived purity (yes, the word is even used by some) over what helps women and children seems to me narcissistic, self-indulgent and foolish. So what if a few people misrepresent or misunderstand things? Anyone doing anything worthwhile will be criticised by someone. The only way not to be criticised for one's actions is to do nothing, to make no waves, to upset no cosy vested interest. Our life's work will not be judged by who we worked with, or what rude names we were sometimes called, or by whom, but by what positive improvements we were able to bring about for the world's families. We should not be buffaloed by purists, but by all means take care to avoid co-option: by refusing payment, insisting on full control, and so on as outlined earlier; working only on our terms, not those either of industry or industry's critics.

The next chapter: what?

We are all writing the next chapter of change in infant feeding history. Only if our analysis of the real problems in our particular situation is correct, based on solid information, and our strategies well thought out, can we hope to protect promote and support breastfeeding effectively. Frankly, I think our advocacy strategy remains behind the times, as it always has been. Industry is not the only key element in Australia. And hospital-based healthworkers are better than ever at supporting breastfeeding. Yet breastfeeding rates are no better and in some places worse. Why?

What we are doing about industry and hospitals is good, is useful, is necessary to stem the tide: but is less and less effective as the century rolls on. Look at our society. Look at the social structures changing. Westpac Bank gives women 6 weeks maternity leave: write those women off as breastfeeders. The ACTU has negotiated just three months' paid leave: formula company profits will grow as mothers get their babies established on the bottle before going back to work they are now afraid to give up. Six months unpaid leave would have been less harmful to breastfeeding, but the ACTU was not advised by people who know about breastfeeding, it would seem. Case-mix formulas derived from America throw women out of hospital on day two or three or four after birth: watch the rates of mastitis and early weaning increase as unsupported women struggle to manage their milk supply. (We are already reading of "breastfeeding malnutrition" in *Pediatrics*.) A 'conservative' (actually "radically destructive") government privatises MCH services in Victoria: watch the development of commercial services for women who can afford them, while breastfeeding slowly declines despite those hospital improvements and much greater community awareness of its importance than ever before. It is in this context that formula companies are beginning to make hay by direct advertising to parents: a need is being created that they will fill. (Badly.)

The evidence of a reaction against breastfeeding promotion is everywhere in the media, because breastfeeding does not fit into the lives women are being forced to lead by our ad hoc social restructuring, in which breastfeeding or babies are simply not a consideration. So we now see more and more destructive articles and books by good feminists and failed breastfeeders who go on to blame breastfeeding advocates for making them feel bad, rather than understand the causes of their failure[162] and deal with both their feelings and the objective social circumstances that make breastfeeding failure almost inevitable. We have two mutually exclusive choices here: we can say, "Breastfeeding is often impossible in society as we have it [true], so we must not make too much of it or we upset those women who truly cannot breastfeed, and a choice not to try is rational." Or we can say, "Breastfeeding is often impossible in society as we have it, and breastfeeding is so important – to babies, to women, to families, to nations, to the environment, to humanity – that it is society which MUST be changed to make it possible." Too many people are wimping out on the latter clear and evidence-based stance just because it seems too hard.

Only if we can weld concerned parents and professionals into an effective political lobby to halt the changes most detrimental to women and children can we expect to improve breastfeeding rates. It is pointless telling a mother to breastfeed when her employment demands that she is back on the job six weeks after birth and there is no on-site childcare. Yes, some women manage quite well in this situation. Some women can succeed regardless of anything. But many women will not. Many will soon be feeding their babies bottles of formula. This is already the norm for three month old babies, not breastfeeding. Breastfeeding can't be delegated (until the re-birth of wet-nursing as a paid profession, anyway). And breastfeeding is so important to women that it should not be delegated, any more than intercourse and orgasms should be given up just because IVF is a modern option for the wealthy. Anthropologists are right to emphasize that women's infant feeding actions are determined by their sociocultural context, and that telling them what to do or how to manage breastfeeding is pointless where breastfeeding cannot fit into the context of their lives. Women frequently have no choice. And as chapter 1 makes clear, the cost of failure to breastfeed is high, for families and society.

Breastfeeding advocates need to be united in re-structuring Australia according to a blueprint that includes breastfeeding as central. We need to write a charter for breast-feeding women that empowers them to breastfeed, not tells them to. Decades ago we allowed companies to alter the market, and noticed only decades later. We allowed healthworkers to enshrine authoritarian practices, and unravelled them decades later. Will we now allow Australia to be re-structured on the American model, without support for women at home as well as work, and then decades later wonder why breastfeeding has become a forgotten art, a quaint minority activity, faintly disgusting or embarrassing to most, as it is in America?

Sadly, despite all the hard work of so many, despite all that has been achieved in Australia, we are still at the beginning. Artificial feeding fits well with a society that has disempowered women, that defines women as objects of sexual desire and docile workers needing to be separated from their infants, that sees them and their infants primarily as consumers, as units to be exploited – milked? – for economic benefit, that denies an infant's need for frequent physical closeness and considers institutionalising babies in creches to be acceptable care, despite the increased sickness and sorrow such babies manifest. Breastfeeding is always going to be a struggle in societies where women of reproductive age cannot expect a living unless actively participating in the extra-domestic labour market, where mortgages demand two incomes, where those who are no longer sexually attractive are discriminated against in employment, so that taking time out to mother children may make a woman less employable. When women cannot choose between working and staying at home, women have won, not freedom, but another emotionally and physically exhausting form of servitude. It is astonishing that so many intelligent women have been sucked into slavery of this kind, although it is heartening to see that many are now realising the costs.[163] And so many in this past and present generation of wage slaves have believed they must sacrifice breastfeeding. Progress??? Feminists need to see infant feeding as a paradigm of what patriarchy had done to women: disempowered them, convinced them that they are readily replaceable, that they have no unique value as women, that men can perform any of their tasks as well as they can. No one who has experienced breastfeeding as the incredible experience it can be would ever believe such nonsense. Breastfeeding mothers are utterly unique, the wellspring and centre of their child's life, and if they are like my now-breastfeeding daughter, they know it in their bones. No wonder inadequate or deprived men feel jealous, left out. But they are not mothers, they are fathers, and should take on their own responsibilities as such.

Sacrificing breastfeeding to the demands of the workplace is bad policy, bad economics, bad psychology. If this trend to employ young mothers continues and reaches critical mass, eventually our Australian consumer protection and health agencies will also be busy reassuring parents that "formula is safe because Australian society depends on bottle feeding" as the US FDA, and an Irish consumer magazine, and so many more supposedly independent groups with consumer interests at heart, routinely do. Our consumer protection authorities will be cosily confiding to industry that

> It is incumbent on all of us, industry, academia and government, to do the best possible job in providing consumers with the most up-to-date, advanced infant formula known to promote infant growth and development. Whenever a recall is initiated, whenever a problem is identified, the FDA, and industry in particular, are recipients of consumer criticism, and consumer confidence in the product and the system is lost. **It is our responsibility to restore this confidence so that parents throughout the US will not be wondering, as they are now, if the product they are feeding their infants is indeed complete and wholesome.**[164]

And there I was, silly me, believing that it was incumbent on industry, academia and government to protect promote and support breastfeeding, and to educate parents about the real risks of not breastfeeding so that they could make informed choices, not to reassure them about the safety of an always fallible product! For it is unwarranted blind confidence in a fallible product that means it is often suspected too little and too late, so that infants are needlessly harmed...

These are political problems. They demand political solutions. It is impossible to be apolitical when you care about women and children. Not party political necessarily: but policies advantaging women and their babies need to be at the forefront of every party's policy thinking. It will not happen easily. Chief among those policies must be generous family support and child care payments and policies that allow women-who-want-to (a hugely important qualification) to stay at home (without starving or being homeless) while their babies need breastfeeding. If Norway can do it on a population base of just 3 million people and a far smaller resource base, so can we. No female person is a feminist who denies this right of women to know what is best for baby feeding, and to determine how their children should be fed or cared-for: in my view that female person is a patronising matriarchalist of the worst order.

What can you do? Will you keep silent while strident voices accuse breastfeeding activists of being fanatical "lacto-nazis", of not caring about women, of restricting the god Free Trade, and all the rest of that inimitable bulldust? Or will each of you urge your organisation, whatever it is (church, community, overseas development, environment, feminist, professional) to join a national coalition such as ACOIF or NABA[165] and work actively for OPTIMAL infant feeding in your country? Help us to help families: support NMAA and ALCA, get active in ACOIF or Maternity Coalition, report Code breaches to APMAIF, talk to people about breastfeeding, brazenly breastfeed in public and congratulate mothers who do, whatever. You can know exactly what is happening in these "political" matters: subscribe to *ALCA Galaxy* (formerly *ALCA News*) and the NMAA Newsletter, as these two magazines are committed to letting you know all that is going on in Australian infant feeding circles. Join ALCA if you are an IBCLC; join your local college of lactation consultants and work towards reunification of professional breastfeeding advocacy. And look to see where support for breastfeeding is needed in your organisation, community, workplace, church, school, home... None of us can do everything, but we can all do something. Lao Tse was right to say that "The journey of a thousand miles begins with a single step".

NOTES
CHAPTER 10: THE HISTORY AND POLITICS OF INFANT FEEDING
[1] Hardyment. C., *Dream Babies* (Jonathon Cape, 1983, OUP paperback). This is the perfect baby present for any new mother
[2] Fildes. V., *Breasts, Bottles and Babies*. (Edinburgh University Press, 1986); *Wet Nursing* (Basil Blackwell, 1988). See also "The age of weaning in Britain, 1500-1800", *J. Biosoc. Sci.* (1982) 14, 223-240; "The early history of the infant feeding bottle", *Nurs. Times* (1981) 77, 3, 128-9; 77, 4, 168-170. Other references can be found in these articles.
[3] Pandora Press, London 1988. Palmer has personally acknowledged her debt to *Breastfeeding Matters*, so similarities between her book and mine are not surprising.
[4] Smith, F. B., *The People's Health, 1830-1910*. (A.N.U. Press, Canberra, 1979), p. 91.
[5] Ashby, H. T., *Infant Mortality* (Cambridge, 1922), 24-25.]
[6] Radhill, S. X., "Infant Feeding Through The Ages", *Clin. Pediatr.* (1981)20, 10, p.615
[7] Hanson L.A., "Breastfeeding stimulates the infant immune system", *Sci. Med.* (1997) 4: 12-21.
[8] The Report of the ACC Sub-committee on Nutrition's Consultative Group on Maternal and Young Child Nutrition (Nov 1979) put in order of priority for failed lactation in developing countries –
(a)   Re-establishment of lactation.
(b)   Breastfeeding by surrogate.
(c)   Feeding non-human milk as a milk product.
(d)   Feeding a cereal/other staple gruel augmented by milk/other protein sources.
[9] Fildes, V., *The English wet-nurse and her role in infant care, 1538-1800* (Thesis)
[10] Quoted in Digby, I; Mathias, B., *The Joy of the Baby* (L. Frewin, London, 1969), p. 38.
[11] Wood, C.; Walker-Smith, J., *MacKeith's Infant Feeding and Feeding Difficulties*. (Churchill Livingstone, 6th edition, 1981), p. 71,75.

[12] Saint, L.; Smith, M.; Hartmann, P. E., "The yield and nutrient content of colostrum and milk of women from giving birth on one month post-partum", *Br. J. Nutr.* (1984) 104, 187-194.

[13] Quoted in Hardyment, op. cit., p. 5

[14] Stone, L., *The Family, Sex and Marriage in England* (Penguin, 1979), p. 272.

[15] Hardyment, op. cit., p. 18.

[16] ibid., p. 10.

[17] ibid., p. 3.

[18] Cone, T. E., *History of American Pediatrics.* (Little, Brown and Co. 1979). p. 57.

[19] op. cit., p. 71-3.

[20] Short, R. V., "The biological basis for the contraceptive effects of breastfeeding" in Jelliffe, D. B. & Jelliffe, E. F. P., (ed). *Advances in International Maternal and Child Health*, v.3. (O.U.P. 1983), p. 37

[21] Hardyment, op. cit., p. 94.

[22] Cone, op. cit., p. 131.

[23] Mrs Panton, "perhaps the most outspoken of the anti-breastfeeding-school", Hardyment, op. cit., p. 95.

[24] Possibly it did for some, because of the intake of alcohol suggested as useful for keeping up the supply of milk.

[25] ibid., p. 4.

[26] ibid., p. 49.

[27] ibid., p. 47.

[28] Radbill, op. cit., p. 613.

[29] Jellet, H., *A Short Practice of Midwifery for Nurses* (6th edition, J. & A. Churchill, 1922), p. 349-50.

[30] Hardyment, op. cit., p. 53.

[31] Gathorne-Hardy, J., *Rise and Fall of the British Nanny* (Hodder, London 1972)

[32] Smith, op. cit., p. 93-9.

[33] Schlebaum, A., "From zygotes to zombies? – a critical look at our children's brave new world of chemical abuse", in (ed) *Man, Drugs & Society* 181-7.

[34] Anderson, S. A., Chinn, H., Fisher, K. D. "History and current status of infant formulas", *Am. J. Clin. Nutr.* (1982) 35, 381-397.

[35] Apple, R. D., "'To be used only under the direction of a physician' – commercial infant feeding and medical practice, 1870-1940", *Bull. Hist. Med.* (1980) 54, 3.

[36] ibid., p. 406.

[37] ibid., p. 404.

[38] Hambraeus, L. "Food and growth in children with special reference to breastfeeding versus formula feeding", *J. Food. Nutr. (*1982) 39: 1-12.

[39] Apple, op. cit., p. 411, Cone, op. cit.

[40] ibid., p. 412.

[41] ibid. cf. also Levenstein, H., "'Best for babies' or 'preventable infanticide'? The controversy over artificial feeding of infants in America, 1880-1920", *J. Am. Hist.* (1983) 70, 1, 75-95.

[42] "Confronting the U.S. Infant Formula Giants", *The Corporate Examiner* 1982, II, 7-8. Available from the Interfaith Centre on Corporate Responsibility, 475 Riverside Drive, (RM.566) New York, N.Y. 10115.

[43] Post, J., Statement to the Sub-committee on oversight and investigations of the Committee on Energy & Commerce, House of Representatives, U.S. Congress, June 17 1981. (U.S. Government Printing Office, Washington 1981, serial 97-73)

[44] Lewis, M., "The Problem of Infant Feeding: the Australian experience from the mid 19th century to the 1920s", *J. Hist. Med,* (1980) April, p. 174-187.

[45] "WHO Press release: Don't withhold food from children with diarrhoea", *Aust. Nurses' J.* (1983) 12, 8, 35. See also Minchin, M., *Food for Thought* Alma/Allen Unwin 1983) ch. II, 7; Ciba Foundation Symposium, new series, no. 42: *Acute Diarrhoea in childhood* (Elsevier/Excerpta Medica 1976), pp. 171-80.

[46] Armstrong, D. *Political Anatomy of the Body: medical knowledge in Britain in the 20th century*, (Cambridge University Press 1983) p.14.

[47] *The Glaxo Baby Book*, (Glaxo, 1918, 11th edition), p. 25.

[48] The body of well-intentioned ladies from which Britain's system of Health Visitors derived.

[49] Armstrong, op. cit., p. 15.

[50] Lewis, M., (1980), p. 177-8.

[51] Sir Arthur Newsholme, "On the child mortality at the ages 0-5 years, in England and Wales", *J. Hygiene*, Cambridge, (1917) 16, 69-71.

[52] *Australian Medical Gazette.* (1894) 13, 60-61.The diet of infants deprived of breast milk.

[53] Lewis, M., *Populate or perish* – Thesis held at Australian National University, Canberra. One Sydney campaign between 1905 and 1911 raised the percentage of wholly breastfed infants from 72.2 to 94.2% but there is no record of duration of breastfeeding. Interestingly, this campaign used visitors rather than asked mothers to come to clinics.

[54] Jelliffe, D. B. & Jelliffe, E. F. P., *Human Milk in the Modern World* (O.U.P., 1979), p. 274 letter to Pediatrics, (1979).

[55] Cone, op. cit., p. 253.

[56] Such figures conceal huge geographical, class, and ethnic differences – Boston breastfeeding rates had reached this point by 1958. For a good discussion of available data and its limitations, see Hendershot, G. "Trends in breastfeeding", *Report of the Task Force on the Assessment of the Scientific Evidence Relating to Infant Feeding Practices and Infant Health*. Supplement to *Pediatrics* 1984, 74, 4.

[57] Jelliffe & Jelliffe, (ed) op. cit., p. 294.

[58] ibid., p. 234.

[59] Wong, H. B., *Breastfeeding in Singapore* (Choon Kee Press, Singapore, 1971).

[60] Breastfeeding and morbidity in industrialised countries, 1900-1980: an update in Jelliffe & Jelliffe (ed) *Advances in International Maternal and Child Health* v. 1. (O.U.P. 1981). For further discussion, see the Report of The Task Force alluded to earlier.

[61] Martin, J. E., *Infant Feeding 1975: attitudes and practice in England and Wales* (London: HMSO 19778), p. 86. Only 14% of UK mothers delivered in hospital had NOT given formula within the first week after birth.

[62] Dugdale, A. E., "The effect of the type of feeding on weight gain and illness in infants", *Br. J. Nutr.* (1971) 26, 423-432. This study is criticised in the *Task Force Report* (ref. 55. More recent statements included in *Med. J. Austr.* 1981, July 25, p. 107.

[63] Yet doctors even in the last decade keep setting up daft trials that a broad-scale common-sense evaluation might suggest were risky: such as the multi-centre trial to see if high doses of immunoglobulin (such as is routinely found in breastmilk) reduced rates of necrotising enterocolitis in preterm infants. Great idea, even if the outcome (if it worked) would be enormous costs to taxpayers for such products made by a drug company, when any old mother could supply it free. The only problem was that they forgot that in adding immunoglobulin for immune purposes, they were effectively adding to the child's total protein intake, and the levels of protein being given to the infants were in excess of levels safe for normal brain development and kidney function. A nutritionist pointed out the obvious; the trial was stopped. What did it cost? in money and in infant health? why did the NH&MRC not immediately set up a trial of breastmilk, the only food that contains a wide variety of immunoglobulins and has been proven to prevent almost all NEC in prems?

[64] In Cameron, M., Hofvander, Y., *Manual on Feeding Infants and Young Children* (2nd edition, U.N. 1975), p. 103, there is a table showing cost/income ratio of formula feeding in a number of countries. This is discussed also in Jelliffe & Jelliffe (1979). And the figures are updated in the latest edition, published by Oxford University Press in 1983.

[65] Environmental issues are fashionable in the western world at long last. Babies are not. Perhaps we should emphasize less the harm done to children, and more the harm done to the Earth by bottle feeding. Let's try to persuade some environmental activists and some animal-rights groups to take up the cause of the **only** ecological option, women's milk for women's children. Our new promotional slogan might be: Breastfeed to save the Earth!

[66] For some idea of its safety and nutritional adequacy, cf. *The Other Baby Killer*, by Consumers' Association of Penang, Malaysia. (Available from CAP, 27 Kelawei Road, Penang)

[67] For an excellent overview of the infant formula controversy as it developed in the 1970s, I would recommend a tape by Kathleen Cravero, UNICEF, NY, Staffer, recorded at the 1983 LLLI Physicians' Seminar. Available from LLLI.

[68] For details of what did and what did not change, see IBFAN News, March 1984. Available from IBFAN, cf. p. 332. see also F. Clarkson, "The taming of Nestlé", *Multinational Monitor*, April 1984, 14-17. Other companies can now expect a greater scrutiny of their behaviour, long overdue.

[69] Smith, F.B. op. cit. p.93.

[70] Baer, E., "An update on the infant formula controversy", *Studies in Family Planning*, 1983. Also on U.S. Congressional Record-Senate-May 26, 1983.

[71] Nickel, H., "The Corporate haters", *Fortune*, June 16, 1980, p. 126-8, 130, 132, 134, 136. Letters, 14 July 1980, p. 172; July 28, 1980, p. 100

[72] *Food Chemical News*, April 27 1981.

[73] *Food Chemical News*, Nov. 12 1979, p. 25, 47.

[74] *Food Chemical News*, Dec. 10, 1979, p. 15.

[75] Laskin, C. R., Pilot, L. J., "Defective Infant Formula: the Neo-Mull-Soy/Cho Free Incident" in *Early Intervention Programs in Infancy* (ed) Moss, Sweet & Swift. (Haworth Press, 1982). Reprints available from C. Laskin, 2723 Devonshire Place, N.W. Washington, D C. 20008.

[76] ibid., p. 99.

[77] Reported in *Food Chemical News*, No. 5, 1979, p. 41

[78] Public Law 96-359-Sept. 26, 1980. Infant Formula Act of 1980. One FDA official then argued that the financial penalties imposed by this Act if a recall was not properly managed would possibly lead companies not to institute recalls at all (for which there is no penalty) rather than face the possibility of fines for doing it wrong. This implies a belief in the companies as capable of heinous behaviour surprising in men who then went on to allow companies wide powers of self-regulation.

[79] The Nation's Health. American Public Health Association) 1980, April, p. 4 When visiting the U.S. I was told (how truthfully I cannot assess) that outdated formula was very common in poorer areas located near manufacturers' plants.

[80] *The Nation's Health*. (Newsletter of American Public Health Association), April 1980, p. 4.

[81] *Food Chemical News*, May 14 & May 21, 1984, p. 29. Laskin & Pilot, op. cit., p. 103.

[82] ibid., p. 104.

[83] *Food Chemical News*, May 25, 1981, p. 23-4.

[84] *Food Chemical News*, March 15, 1982, p. 46.

[85] Forbes AL, Miller SA, Duy N, "FDA's perspectives on infant formula", in *Production, Regulation and Analysis of Infant Formula: Proceedings of the topical conference, May 14-16 1985*, Association of Official and Analytical Chemists, Arlington, Virginia, 1985, p. 6.

[86] Laskin & Pilot, op. cit., p. 104.

[87] *Food Chemical News*, Oct. 19, 1981, p. 29.

[88] *Food Chemical News*, March 8, 1982, p. 31.

[89] ibid., March 15, 1982, p. 46.

[90] *Washington Post*, March 11, 1982.

[91] *Star, Penang,* 14-3-1982.)

[92] Vitamin B_6 was inadvertently destroyed by heating. Medical journals in 1954 discussed the effects, some of the victims, permanently damaged, appeared on television during 1981. cf. *Food Chemical News*, Feb. 2, 1981, p. 55; March 15, 1982, p. 48.

[93] ibid., March 15, 1982, p. 48.

[94] ibid., April 26, 1982, p. 26

[95] *Food Chemical News*, May 25, 1981

[96] *Food Chemical News*, 6-12-1982, p.16.

[97] *Food Chemical News*, Jan 18, 1982, p. 11-17.

[98] *Food Chemical News* Jan. 31, 1983 p. 4

[99] *Food Chemical News* Dec. 6, 1982, p. 15

[100] ibid., Oct. 31, 1982, p. 18.

[101] The Food and Nutrition Service of the US Department of Agriculture provides a publication to WIC agencies which describes in a completely uncritical fashion all the current infant formulas and gives some background to the regulations in place at any point in time. It was instructive both for its acceptance of industry information as totally reliable, and its failure to go beyond what the companies provide by way of product information. First published in 1990, it was to be reviewed in 1992. Copies are available from WIC Formula Reference, Nutrition and Technical Services Division, Food and Nutrition Service, US Department of Agriculture, 3101 Park Center Drive, Room 607, Alexandria, VA. 22302.

[102] *ICEA News*, 1981, 20, 4, p. 2.

[103] Consumer Interpol, or Health Action International, can provide many examples of such practices.

[104] L. Salisbury; A Glover-Blackwell, *Petition to alleviate domestic formula misuse and provide informed infant feeding choice* – filed June 17 1981. Available from Public Advocates Inc., 1535 Mission Street, San Francisco, CA 94103. # (415) 431 7430

[105] *Food Chemical News*, Jan. 4. 1982, p. 18-19. The Infant Formula Council produced a massive response, available from them at 5775 Peachtree-Dunwoody Rd., Suite 500-D, Alanta Ga. 30342. A further reply and counter-reply followed, both fairly predictable and both capable of being criticised for their interpretation of data.

[106] *Supplement to Pediatrics* (1984 74, 4.)

[107] Substantially the same thing was said by senior FDA officials, in writing, in the report of the 1984 conference on infant formula hosted by AOAOC. See p. 287.

[108] This argument is fully discussed in Toll, M. A., "'Spilled Milk': a rebuttal to the U.S. vote against the International Code of Marketing of Breastmilk substitutes" *Boston University International Law Journal* (1983) vol.2: 103; 103-132.

[109] *Food Chemical News,* July 18, 1983, p. 6.

[110] Why it is assumed that this will be the result, rather than greater social division as previously in history, eludes me.

[111] Who were later to nominate me as their first choice of representative for a monitoring panel, only to have it refused by the Health Department.

[112] Minutes of these meetings are available under the Freedom of Information Act.

[113] Advertisement for Maws Simpla sterilising and feeding set, *Women's Day*, July 18, 1983, p. 70. Mind you, it does say that 'after 150 years of making baby products we've found the ideal

method of sterilizing and preparing your baby's feed.' Perhaps in another 70 years the companies will find the ideal mixture to put in it.

[114] That colic is due to the contents of the bottle was clearly established by Lothe, T. et al, "Cows' milk formula as a cause of infantile colic: a double blind study", *Pediatrics* (1982) 70, 1, 7-10, and dozens of subsequent articles, including a 1997 review.

[115] It is of interest that in Australia the NUK advertisements no longer talk of their closeness to breastfeeding, after the Trades Practices Commission in 1993 asked the distributor to justify its claims or face prosecution.

[116] Jan was a very experienced breastfeeding counsellor who had pioneered working with aboriginal women on breastfeeding; subsequently a co-founder with Grace Close and others, of ABBA, the Aboriginal Birth and Breastfeeding Association, and in 1996 President of ALCA. Her position as representative for the South Pacific region on IBCoCo was abolished after she lent IBFAN support to ALCA Inc by a joint submission re Bottles and teats. This action was one of the triggers for later overseas interference in ALCA affairs.

[117] It must be recognised that in every country where progress is made, there are usually a few key individuals who work tirelessly on the question, and if they cannot support themselves to do so, or if funding for the position dries up, progress starts to slow. In these days of economic pressure on families, it is harder than ever to find volunteers able to give the time needed. It is often not recognised that breastfeeding advocacy centres in receipt of any ongoing funding are scarce around the world: whatever funds UNICEF or WABA may have made available world-wide for this work, in Australia not a cent of overseas or government assistance has been received by ACOIF to assist in Code implementation. Of course Australians have no problem with the idea that all UNICEF funds should go to nationals of even less affluent nations, but do not consider the UK, America or Europe as such! It remains a source of irritation that WABA does not publish any accounting for the moneys received from UNICEF for world-wide breastfeeding advocacy, and that all processes relating to finance are unaccountable to the WABA membership.

[118] In 1995 there were signs that interest was again increasing in NZ and monitoring has begun again, but consumers are unhappy with the way this has been done to date. At present in mid 1996 the NZ Government is trying to develop an Industry Code, and the companies which market formula there have drafted a very weak Code. This will be quite unacceptable to Australia, and as our Food Laws are to be 'harmonised', it has caused a great deal of concern to Australian breastfeeding advocates. Interestingly, almost all of these same companies agreed in 1992 to the much tighter Australian Agreement, which had Nestlé Australia's full support: Nestlé does not market formula in New Zealand, and no formula company there has taken a comparable lead role among the industry groups.

[119] By a group which in 1996 has been declared persona non grata by IBFAN because of its links with American industry.

[120] As a founding member I wrote this in; when on the ILCA Board 1989-1991 I was able to persuade ILCA to do likewise, and NZLCA has similarly adopted this position; ILCA has since made it a pre-condition for affiliation.

[121] Although CAA agreed that BFA(G) should be wound up in 1996, pages of old BFAG material using CAA's name and affiliations continued to be listed on the web for much longer.

[122] It is not clear exactly when the word "Group" was dropped from letterhead.

[123] This is not a permanent restriction. Should the voluntary Agreement not work, consumers can press for legislative change. But the whole ethos of Australia at present makes it unlikely that without serious financial resources such a course of action is doomed to failure.

[124] This could be abused: there will still be a role for consumer criticism of companies which observe the letter of the Agreement but not its spirit.

[125] I cherish a letter from a leading IBFAN lawyer, enquiring as to how this had been achieved: did the companies not realise what they were giving away?

[126] I was appointed Consumer Alternate representative and have been actively involved with the Panel's work, although I later recommended that the position of Alternate be abolished.

[127] It included pads of 50 tear-off leaflets for patients: not something doctors paper walls with...

[128] Hillis A, Stone P *Breast Bottle Bowl: the best-fed baby book*. (Bay Books, 1993) There are many inaccuracies in this book, many of which undermine breastfeeding and promote artificial feeding. Whether this is due to ignorance or deliberate intent is irrelevant to its harmful effects.

[129] I am not aware of studies in the child development literature that are careful to identify feeding status of the baby and the mother as a child: most 'normal' and normative child developmental studies came out of the western world in the era of bottle feeding's dominance.

[130] Naively trusting that industry will serve the common good (eg by promoting breastfeeding), or being angry that it does not, both deny the profit imperative of industry.

[131] By now, as stated earlier, this was Jan Mangleson, a very experienced breastfeeding counsellor who had pioneered working with aboriginal women on breastfeeding; subsequently a co-founder with Grace Close and others, of ABBA, the Aboriginal Birth and Breastfeeding Association, and in 1996 President of ALCA.

[132] As of about the end of July 1996, Rae and Greg Perry (husband and wife) and CAA "mutually decided" to wind up BFA, and it is defunct.

[133] These absentees presumably were still supportive of the initiative, as their names were still publicly being used to lend credibility to the coalition. NMAA and ALCA have both asked that their name not be used without prior notification.

[134] It is for this reason that every country needs one good solid working coalition of breastfeeding advocates, such as we have achieved in ACOIF. But given human nature, it will probably not be long before a more radical group, one which refuses to be accountable to the wider breastfeeding community or to work together with ACOIF, develops here again.

[135] WABA began as a commendable attempt to unite breastfeeding advocacy around the world, and has largely focussed on producing materials and campaigning around World Breastfeeding Week, in August each year. Its website is interesting and informative, and should be checked out. However, WABA's failure to involve any of the world's major health professionals bodies as part of a coalition for breastfeeding advocacy has limited its impact drastically. Mothers' support groups and other grassroots breastfeeding advocacy organisations such as the NCT, national Lactation Consultant organisations, and others from developed and developing nations are also seriously under-represented in policy-making and funding. It is symptomatic that organisers of a recent WABA workshop in the Pacific region did not even invite NMAA or LLLNZ, ALCA or NZLCA, to send a representative while 8 of 51 registrants were from the USA. The old IBFAN networks were heavily represented at this workshop and in WABA generally, especially at governing levels. I believe that unless WABA can widen its support base beyond old IBFANers like me, into the institutional health professional community, it will have as much and as little global impact as the IBFAN networks have always done: it will do good work, but too slowly, and fail to speak to any but the converted (who, after all, are not the problem!). So I hope my readers will all get involved with WABA as endorsers and active participants, as I have always been. More about this in the next book...

[136] Wellstart began as the San Diego Lactation Programme in 1981 and evolved into a huge programme supported by USAID, which among other things educates selected teams of healthworkers from around the world. The vision of Dr. Audrey Naylor and her co-worker Ruth Wester have contributed greatly to the global breastfeeding revival, and they will be recognised as major pioneers in the field of improving healthworker knowledge and skills, even if Australians have had minor reservations about some aspects of that clinical teaching.

[137] I had strongly urged Australian participation in the final workshops and recommended midwife Suzanne Murray when asked for suggestions. Suzanne was thus the only Australian with direct input into the Global BFHI documents. Despite my subsequent suggestion, seconded by Dr. Pat Lewis, that Suzanne be co-opted to the BFHI Taskforce, she was not.

[138] Minutes of NSG meeting 25/5/1995

[139] ibid.

[140] Endacott to NSG Convenor date unknown, NSG convenor to Minchin 30/5/1995; Minutes June 1995 NSG meeting.

[141] Minutes June 1995 NSG meeting.

[142] NSG Convenor's letter to LIFE and other collaborative bid partners, 18/7/1995.

[143] NSG Minutes indicate that in March 1995 the Australian College of Midwives had queried the financial viability of the project; in April it had sought further information; in May and June it had yet to consider the issue. But verbal reports were being given to say that it was virtually a foregone conclusion that ACMI would join in.

[144] UNICEF Australia had originally been seen as the auspicing body and the former NSG, in which power was shared equally between a variety of organisations, had been seen as the governing body, right up until UNICEF Australia decided to set a review in place. ACMI did not even contact all former interested parties, but made its own selection of groups to be on the new Advisory Council: legitimate, but not wise. It was then very dilatory in contacting some.

[145] At the first BFHI NAC meeting 10 of 13 representatives were midwives, and of these a majority were on the ACMI National Executive or held office at State Branch level of the College. While some over-representation of midwives is inevitable given their role in relation to breastfeeding, this is hardly a hugely diverse or catholic coalition of Australian BF interests.

[146] Involved were Dr. Margaret Dean (Health Dept.), Dr. Pat Lewis (NMAA LRC), Dr. Dorothy Mackerras (Uni. Of Sydney), Margaret Miller/Yong Sook Kwok (ACA), Stephen Fox (FBCA, A-G's Dept), Denise Drane, and Cathy Meyer/Sue Jeffreson (Nutrition, Health Dept.). I also did a great deal of work on drafts of this report, although in an unofficial capacity!

[147] WHO/NUT/96.2

[148] I would be the last person in the world to maintain that passing the IBLCE exam is proof of equal competence or sensitivity or skill. IBCLCs will be as variable as doctors, nurses or any other group. But at least there is a an impartial, financially disinterested guarantee of basic competence at a given point in time, which no other process can give. The IBLCE credential is legally defensible. I am sure course attendance and performance cannot be, when the assessment process is in the hands of the paid educators. Separating education from assessment is fundamental to legally-defensible credentialling in the US.

[149] If any university department has a PhD candidate searching for a spectacular case of organisational politics and pathology, I shall be very happy to provide access to documentation of this issue, but the time for a definitive history is not yet. As in any organisational split, personalities were a large factor, but two important underlying and preceding controversies were ALCA national membership standards and policies re Code implementation. It is documented that dissidents were given active support by certain vested interests, some overseas.

[150] Being a member of a College is not usually attained by paying to attend a conference and agreeing to support Rules one has not seen. In health professional terms it usually signifies recognition of a set standard of achievement, considered to be a high one by all members.

[151] Even more regrettable was the less than professional behaviour in the setting up of some of these new organisations, e.g. gross misrepresentation to state-based ALCA members of the national situation, with no opportunity for another perspective given; breaches of branch obligations; some financial and other ALCA records not returned to the national office despite repeated requests; improper disbursement of ALCA assets, in some cases to the new breakaway

organisation; retention and use of ALCA mailing lists; heavy pressure on local members to resign from ALCA.

[152] Now organised in an informal network, which claims all members of the local groups, although none of the membership application forms for local "colleges" seen to December 1997 asks individuals if they wish to join two organisations, or spells out the rights of members of the network. Personally, I consider myself a member of only those groups I sign my name to join. Nor have I seen the network acknowledge that many of its members remain ALCA members, or state how many are IBCLC and how many are "interested healthworkers" or associates.

[153] *Birth Issues*, 1995. The role of this journal should also be part of any PhD research.

[154] But with numbers of IBCLCs not stated. Lactnet is a US-based global chat-line for health professionals. It has a policy of not allowing advertising of any kind. It can be accessed by sending a message "subscribe Lactnet" to LISTSERV@LIBRARY.UMMED.EDU.

[155] Such as a policy that a member of the present governing committee must sign every candidate's application form!

[156] Jan Edwards was ILCA South Pacific delegate 1993-1997; I served a term as International Delegate 1989-1991, resigning from the PAB to do so, at a time when the affiliate criteria and Position Paper and much more was drafted, and ILCA began to seek NGO status with the World Health Organisation (since achieved thanks to James Akré and Felicity Savage).

[157] In 1991 affiliation criteria included "a demonstrated history of co-operation with other LC groups in the region."

[158] Appropriately enough, this developed in response to an IBFAN protest at the 1984 ICM meeting, where we went around and collected advertising material from all the companies present (except Nestlé) and pinned it up under a heading "Code violations at this conference". Nestlé was not included because none of its material breached the Code: that was 1984!

[159] It is however worrying to find GPs doing more and more breastfeeding work because MCH centres are under-staffed, when the GP knows little or nothing about breastfeeding: but can claim a rebate where a community midwife visit would cost money.

[160] WHO would define someone who is paid to educate health professionals in breastfeeding management as a health professional, even if some doctor or nurse-based groups might not!

[161] As I do, inter alia via my role as ALCA-Vic seminar programme co-ordinator.

[162] Yes, it is factually a biological failure not to breastfeed one's own child adequately, just as it is a biological failure not to conceive or safely bear a child. This does not mean the woman is a failure as a mother or a person. But all biological failures do have an emotional impact that can be very important to one's sense of worth as a person, and we ignore them at our peril. Failure to breastfeed causes many women great distress and grief.

[163] Quite a number of journal and newspaper articles are now lamenting the impossible burden mothers of young children face if they return to the paid workforce.

[164] Forbes AL, Miller SA, Duy N, "FDA's perspectives on infant formula", in *Production, Regulation and Analysis of Infant Formula: Proceedings of the topical conference, May 14-16 1985*, Association of Official and Analytical Chemists, Arlington, Virginia, 1985, p. 6.

[165] National Alliance for Breastfeeding Action, 254 Conant Rd., Weston. MA02193-1756 USA fax: 1 617 893 8608.

Think about it.........
       "Taking paths of least resistance is what makes rivers – and men – crooked"
                                         Palmerston North, NZ, bookshop poster 1996

A USTRALIA: A SUMMARY

Australian politics of breastfeeding timeline, 1981-1998

1981 • Submissions to Commonwealth Health Department and NH&MRC re hospital practices and breastfeeding promotion

• *International Code of Marketing of Breastmilk Substitutes* passed by World Health Assembly: Australia votes in favour

• Health and Primary Industry Depts negotiate with industry to create "code"

1982 • *Food For Thought*: first published chronicle of western formula disasters

• Australian Dietary Guidelines formulated

1983 • Conservative Labour party forms government

• Australian industry "Code" signed; revised 1986...

1984 • ICM Congress in Sydney: ICM Declaration on breastfeeding

• End of Nestlé Boycott worldwide negotiated by US group

• NH&MRC Guidelines for Healthworkers on implementing the Code

• NMAA's 20th anniversary

1985 • *Breastfeeding Matters* published (January)

• Inaugural meeting of IBLCE in Washington (March)

• Formation of ILCA, the International Lactation Consultant Association

1986 • WHA Resolution 39.28 re free supplies; Food Standard R7

• Australian industry code revised

• First independent educational course for healthworkers on infant feeding, at Prahran College of TAFE, Melbourne (after 1991, at Monash University, with NMAA LRC)

1987 • *Successful Breastfeeding*: Royal College of Midwives

• Formation of ALCA, the Australian Lactation Consultants Association Inc.

• Nestlé plans to enter US Market; different US group revives boycott

• Australians previously involved decide not to participate in boycott

1988 • Australian Code illegal: TPC consultation process begun

• NMAA International Conference in Melbourne

• *Health for All Australians* report

1989 • ALCA submission re Marketing of Breastmilk Substitutes

- Joint WHO/UNICEF statement: *Protection, Promotion and Support of Breastfeeding: the Ten Steps to Successful Breastfeeding*
- Australasian Lactation Courses, first Australian correspondence course

1990
- Innocenti Declaration; World Summit for Children
- *Infant Feeding: the Physiological Basis* (ed. Akre, WHO) published
- TPC Report on implementation of the Code
- Creation of ACOIF (Aust. Coalition for Optimal Infant Feeding)
- Creation of *ALCA News* (renamed *ALCA Galaxy* in 1997)

1991
- Creation of National Food Authority
- WHO CREF (Code review and evaluation framework) committee

Feb. 1991 UNICEF meeting that led to formation of WABA and idea of BFHI
- *Bestfeeding* (Renfrew, Fisher & Arms) first BF book with accurate pictures

May 1991 James Grant announcement of BFHI (no programme at this stage)

Nov. 1991 ACOIF in negotiations re Australian implementation of WHO Code
- Wellstart San Diego development of BFHI assessment programme

1992
- Australian Dietary Guidelines revision
- Formation of Australian BFHI Taskforce; priorities:
  * adaptation of Global Documents
  * workshops for assessors; national database
  * development of BFHI educational resources
  * creation of administrative infra-structure

Feb. 1992 First BFHI assessments in 12 countries

May 1992 Signing of Australian Agreement, negotiated in November 1991

Nov. 1992 Creation of APMAIF: Advisory Panel on Marketing in Australia of Infant Formula

1993
- Publication of CREF committee (1991) report

Feb. 1993 National BFHI workshop for professional groups: agreed to proceed and create a national initiative with their support.
- Creation of National BFHI Steering Group

Aug. 1993 Appointment of Lisa Donohue as BFHI co-ordinator
- Pilot assessment of Royal Women's Hospital
- Availability of UNICEF 18 hour course kit
- Establishment of assessment process; criteria for assessors; call for State Administrative bodies (regional auspicing groups, responsible to a wider group in each state.) (Groups created in every state over time.)
- Establishment of Baby-Friendly Paediatric Unit working group.

Nov. 1993 Consultation on ending free and low-cost supplies.

Jan. 1994 Assessment of Mitcham Private Hospital: successful

Mar. 1994 The 11 Steps to Optimal Breastfeeding in Paediatric Units finalised by NSG and sent to UNICEF NY for comment. Mitcham Private Hospital assessed and declared Baby-Friendly

May 1994 WHA Resolution 47.5

Sept. 1994 Assessment of Royal Womens Hospital Melbourne: successful

Nov. 1994 Announcement to BFHI NSG of review process by UNICEF Australia; National Coordinator job to end at end of year; NSG action limited

1995 • Australian Dietary Guidelines for Children published

Jan 1995 Federal consultation on ending free and low-cost supplies (community)

• Nestlé reiterates they will end them, but are waiting for agreed timeline

Feb. 1995 UNICEF Executive Board proposal to be created; uncertainty re future delays further assessments and BFHI work

Mar. 1995 End of federal consultation on Guidelines for Healthworkers...

July 1995 National Steering Group comes to end of term. Still no leadership for BFHI

Aug. 1995 Breastfeeding: an International Scientific Conference, NSG's project.

• UNICEF gives BFHI responsibility to ACMI, who are to consult with NSG partners

• BabyFriendly Victoria created; runs workshop at PANCH

• Second APMAIF report: *Keeping an Eye on the Market*

• Draft 1.7 of Agreement covering bottles and teats circulated

Sept. 1995 ALCA Inc leases Canberra office

1996 • The International Code of Marketing of Breastmilk Substitutes: A Common Review and Evaluation Framework (WHO/NUT/96.2)

Mar. 1996 Conservative coalition parties win government.

• Meeting re Bottles and teats code

June 1996 Nestlé date for end to all free supplies in healthcare system

• Dr. Christine Bennett becomes chair of APMAIF

July 1996 NFA (1991) becomes ANZFA, begins work on revising R7

Aug. 1996 BFHI NAC meets for the first time

• APMAIF Report: *Room for Improvement*

• ACTU Mother-Friendly Workplace Initiative

Nov. 1996 ACOIF draft of Retail Guidelines sent to Pharmacy Guild

• John Baker replaces Michael Sharpe as industry representative on APMAIF

Jan. 1997 ANZFA consultation re Standard R7

Mar. 1997 Jack Newman National Tour for ALCA

April 1997 ALCA News critiques Enfalac AR materials and unsafe bottles on market

July 1997 ALCA Vic office moves into Queen Vic Women's Centre

Aug. 1997 BFHI Hospital assessments resume; UNICEF reneges on 1995 funding

• ACOIF complaint to ACCC re Enfalac AR

• *ALCA News* becomes *ALCA Galaxy*

Oct. 1997 NMAA International Conference in Sydney

• Commonwealth grants $2 million for breastfeeding promotion

• Discussions with pharmacy interests re Code issues inc. retail guidelines

Nov. 1997 APMAIF Report: ALCA pays for 2000 copies to circulate

Dec. 1997   BFHI National Project Officer position ended. BFHI now administered from ACMInc national office

Mar. 1998   Dr. Patricia McVeagh is appointed consumer representative on APMAIF, replacing Ros Escott

Some facets of the Australian approach

• Piecemeal and negotiated approach rather than a single legislative mandate, which works only if it can generate widespread community support. Multi-factorial problem: multi-dimensional strategy seen as imperative.

• Government commitment and leadership at federal level (resistance at some State levels) has been crucial. Ministers have mandated the implementation of the Code *in conformity with Australian law*. Thus we are limited by provisions of Australian Trades Practices Act, but not seriously, and benefit from strong Australian general consumer protection law and regulation of foods. 1997-8: in keeping with federal deregulatory policy, these safeguards are being weakened, and some companies begin to advertise directly to parents, sensing government tolerance of technical observance of Industry Agreement is all that is required, while the spirit is being breached.

• Industry co-operation was essential, and unlikely to have been achieved without Sharpe/Nestlé Australia leadership. It remains essential, and is more likely to be achieved if industry can see that Code-breaching companies are being penalised by aware healthworkers, and that this results in losses.

• Huge potential for backlash in a country where women's rights are widely seen as more important than infants' needs: hence there has been a need for skill in presentation of issues so as to avoid a "consumer" backlash. Increasing evidence of spin-doctoring aimed at generating this reaction in Australia and NZ: identical articles with names changed placed in both countries.

• Healthworkers have enormous power to influence the market, but this is rarely utilised consciously or positively to police industry behaviour. Industry has utilised that power and still does, although professionals and their associations are beginning to consider these issues.

• Awareness by breastfeeding advocates that industry issues are only a small part of the whole, and over-emphasis to the detriment of major structural issues (e.g., the terms of women's workforce participation; the destruction of free community health services and other supports) can be totally counter-productive.

• Tolerance and awareness of the need for individual consciences to be respected: ACOIF allows individual groups to undertake individual actions while providing a mainstream consensus approach.

The outcome: a society in which artificial feeding is not as "normal" and ubiquitous as in comparable western countries, and where women feel free to breastfeed to an extent that amazes some visitors. Yet limiting unethical marketing has NOT limited the growth of the infant formula market or drastically improved breastfeeding rates.

Requirements for safer infant feeding that Australia lacks in 1998

- Substantial and widespread medical appreciation of the importance of breastfeeding and the hazards of artificial feeding;
- Eminent health professionals willing publicly to challenge the assumption that artificial feeding is safe because it is accepted and customary;
- Appropriate milk banking (women's milk, that is);
- Structured federal or state support for breastfeeding women who do not want to return to paid employment;
- An up-to-date standard for infant formula, and independent quality control at all stages of the process of manufacture and distribution;
- Any standards at all for bottles, teats, or other feeding devices, and any awareness of the hazards of many freely-available products;
- Universal clean water supplies, or failing that, community-accessible information about the multiple risks of much local water used for infant feeding;
- Research knowledge as to the least unsuitable infant formula, bottles or teats;
- Education of bottle-feeding parents about the hazards of usual methods of preparation, storage and heating of infant formula;
- Detailed practical advice for bottle-feeding parents about minimising risks;
- Mechanisms monitoring rates of illness according to type of feeding in children hospitalised or consulting doctors for serious illnesses;
- Real state and federal government commitment to controlling industry marketing techniques that observe the letter of the law (perhaps) but breach its intent and spirit.

THE BUILDING BACKLASH

Fashions in infant feeding have come and gone for centuries. Breastfeeding has been adopted by many as one such fashion. Very little substantial knowledge of the new scientific evidence has filtered through into the community, even in the 1990s. Sure, it's supposed to be better for the baby, but everyone can cite one neighbour with a 'perfectly normal' bottle-fed baby and another with a sickly 'breastfed' baby. Think of all the publicity given to the fact that celebrity babies are bottlefed, with no one publicly suggesting that wealthy parents are either ignorant or irresponsible to 'choose' qualitative dysnutrition for their much-loved infants. In this last decade we saw that Princess Beatrice was deliberately bottle fed, and what a delightful baby she was according to the media (despite the frowns on most of her earliest public photos, the congested look and shadowed bags under her eyes that suggested allergy is a problem; the temper tantrums and open-mouthed adenoidal look she went on to develop). Nothing like the same coverage was given to the fact that Princess Diana's babies were breastfed, initially at least. Little Lourdes Ciccione certainly was, but have we heard anything positive about that experience? Not in Australia, anyway. It is astonishing how many wealthy women actively decide to 'combine breast and bottle feeding' so as not to be too tied down. People have not absorbed the new data about breastfeeding any more than they have begun to question the old myths about infant formula.

This is hardly surprising. There is an unwritten but widely accepted shibboleth: thou shalt not make some mothers feel anxious by informing the public about the problems of formula feeding. Breastfeeding organisations maintain an 'accentuate the positive' attitude, asserting that human milk is superior but never criticising formula. Talk of breastfeeding as best (rather than the only safe norm) may actually make some mothers feel that it is an ideal to strive for, but like all other ideals, not to be achieved in less than perfect circumstances. Where else in life can all mothers afford the best, not merely the adequate? When babies have problems bottle-feeding, there is no organisation of bottle-feeding mothers to take up the data and start asking questions about common factors. Organisations of parents of damaged or dead children naturally want explanations. But they want explanations that do not make them feel guilty about something that might have been avoided. It is a brave minority which accepts personal responsibility for doing the sub-optimal when that very probably contributed to damaging their child, and then goes on to focus on preventing that harm for other people's children. Even pro-breastfeeding literature can inadvertently pass on the message that a switch to bottle-feeding solves breastfeeding problems: this is implied by the absence of any warnings or advice about what to do if the decision to wean from the breast proves disastrous, as it sometimes does.

So what happens when breastfeeding fails? When a breastfed baby becomes ill, or dies of cot death? Because no one tries to unravel why breastfeeding in this case proved to be less protective than it's cracked up to be, women get very angry about the glowing pictures that were painted. I don't blame them. There, but for Mavis Gunther, go I. The bitterest disappointment will be felt by every woman who hoped to breastfeed and had difficulties. Disillusion and rage characterised my first three months with Philip. (And no, he didn't notice a thing: he was too busy coping with his own gut problems to tune in to my feelings.) Women who, like myself, deferred childbearing till their late twenties or thirties are probably most likely to make their rage public. We have sufficient knowledge to hope that breastfeeding will be a positive experience. And we have sufficient self-confidence, and skills, to refuse to be put down by other people's expectations.

Herein lies a problem: When women's hopes for breastfeeding are unrealised – see some of the case histories in Chapter 12 – articulate women help create a climate of opinion, a backlash, in which public breastfeeding advocacy is difficult. Such women could also influence women's and feminist networks to ignore the issues of lactation leave, nursing breaks, and so on; indeed, they could actively oppose these as discriminatory, in the absence of a strong pro-breastfeeding lobby to explain the wider social justification of such practices. Divisions among women will lead, as always, to the continuation of a status quo, handicapping all women and children.[1] Industry advocates have been quick to assert that those opposing the misuse of formula or the irresponsible advertising of products covered by the International Code are really trying to restrict women's freedom to choose[2] – as though anyone can make a free choice in the absence of true knowledge of the problems of both alternatives.

My earlier prediction that further mindless 'breast is best' publicity and promotion will trigger just such a response has since been vindicated by events. Failed, now anti-, breastfeeders are becoming more vocal. Parents' magazines bear witness to this, and their editors seem to be becoming more circumspect about breastfeeding. Books entitled *Bottle Feeding Without Feeling Guilty* have been published in America as well as Australia, in response to promotional writing that does not acknowledge the real causes of women's problems.

Although they make breastfeeding advocates fume, with their mixture of poor factual information and special pleading, these books are an important contribution to the infant feeding debate and should not be just written off and criticised for their obvious factual errors and ignorance of the scientific literature The very fact that they are written says that we breastfeeding advocates are not communicating well to women. Much of the criticism they contain of the 'fanatical' attitudes of breastfeeding supporters is based on women's experience, experience we should not ignore. And the hysterical condemnation these books[3] trigger in breastfeeding networks such as on Lactnet, does more to make the authors feel vindicated than anything else could. Of course their writing needs rebuttal. But this needs to be factual and empathetic: these are not wicked women, but sad ones, good mothers who wanted to do the best and could not for reasons beyond their control or present understanding, and who are making sense of that experience as best they can from their knowledge base and in their cultural context. I am aware that even that analysis may sound patronising and be highly infuriating in the absence of detailed substantiation: it is not meant to be. Facts are facts, and the fact is that with better help almost every single failed breastfeeder could have enjoyed successful breastfeeding. If you know how much that matters, to women and to children, of course it is sad that they did not succeed.

Whether pro- or anti-, women do not need more propaganda. The problems with breastfeeding lie elsewhere. Those who delight in media attention should know by now that confrontation between extremes is the most likely outcome of yet more exhortations to breastfeed in the absence of practical help to make that possible. Women do need real education. UNICEF had a series of excellent radio spots which are not just slogans, but very pithy comment. That would perhaps be a beginning, while we planned a national campaign, identifying the major national problems (such as economic pressures on families) and tailoring strategies around them (such as making available to all women who breastfeed and stay at home to do so, the money available to those willing to bottle-feed and leave their children in childcare). Anything less, given Western assertiveness, is quite likely to provoke great confrontation and bitterness.[4]

But women's voices, unless organised well, matter less in our society than scientific or medical voices. And both science and medicine are subject to equally dramatic reversals of opinion. Because of the difficulty of proving anything definitively in human subjects, it is always possible for scientists to hold and promulgate diametrically opposed views. Here the advantage lies with the person who defends the possibly deviant and indefensible status quo (which in this instance is the necessity and normalcy of bottle feeding). Think how long it has taken many scientists to risk ostracism by publicly denouncing smoking, or alcohol, or lead, or asbestos, as health risks. Think how much longer it has taken since then to see smoking finally outlawed in health institutions, much less public places! There are still persons ignorant enough to consider that absence of proof of harm can be confidently taken to be proof of absence of harm, despite the statistician's maxim that "absence of proof is not proof".

Thus doctors conditioned to evade controversy will fall back upon the wimpish stock excuse, "Well, there is no clearcut conclusive scientific evidence that bottle-fed babies are less healthy, less intelligent, or whatever." The public believes they are saying, "Bottlefed babies are just the same as breastfed babies" – which doctors may believe (due to monumental ignorance) or may not, but which is not what they are saying. Why the obfuscation? It's easier not to challenge the status quo, the norm, of bottle feeding as safe in our country.

Doctors whose research work depends heavily on formula companies may be able to accept their money and stay totally independent. But this sponsorship raises serious ethical problems. Working under someone's sponsorship can indeed subtly alter perspectives. A commissioned writer has mental boundaries pre-set by what would not be acceptable to the sponsors.[5] It takes awareness and conscious action for this not to affect what is written. Of course it can be done, but it is an effort, and one has to weigh every word.

In academic research, sponsorship may not often alter the facts and figures, but it can influence the questions asked and the conclusions drawn from figures. I received a letter from a person who had done all the interviewing, compiled the statistics, and so on for a study on one aspect of infant mortality. She concluded: "Although I did the work, the final writing-up was not by me, so of course a different emphasis has emerged." From her detailed interviews, she saw infant feeding as having been a very important, but hard to prove, contributory factor to many of these infant deaths. The published paper stated that there was no proof of any connexion with mode of feeding. Again, absence of proof is not proof, but this less than fully honest study was widely quoted as proving that there was no difference. I can think of a major Australian study where one of the key researchers expressed similar concerns (off-record) about how the data was presented and interpreted by the senior member of the team...

Statistics can very often be misinterpreted. This is not saying that all scientists whose research is funded by formula companies are venal. Far from it. It is saying that I would feel a great deal happier, and so would many researchers, if important research were fully funded from taxes collected by governments, rather than from 'taxes' imposed by companies upon the purchasers of their products. If companies have so much money that they can sponsor research on a huge scale, why not a prices justification enquiry to ascertain reasonable profit margins, then a government tax on their sales, with the money being available from government for research? A renewable US$1 million grant to the American Academy of Pediatrics buys a lot of goodwill, and doctors are naïve if they think they can become habituated to accepting such funds without subtly altering their mindset to ensure that grants are renewed. 'Financial withdrawal symptoms' can be serious. The double-think obvious in the profession's willingness to use formula profits to subsidise doctors, but to resist quality control of formula on the grounds of unacceptable cost to consumers, shows how far the US profession at least has been unwittingly corrupted by this long association. It was good to see in 1996 the Australian College of Paediatrics, among other groups, working on guidelines for industry sponsorship of research.

But the feature that most disturbed me in 1984 was the emergence of a select cadre of positively pro-infant-formula scientists and spokesmen. Yes, infant formulas are currently necessary, and will be for the foreseeable future. I for one am grateful that they are no longer as bad as they were, and I hope increased oversight and control will make them better than they are now. But present infant formulae are still very experimental. They have begun to capture the mass market since the 1960s; they have modified countless times since then, and scientists are constantly suggesting other modifications. And it needs to be noted that the exclusive use of infant formula for four to six months is *an entirely new experiment, leaving the baby totally dependent on one food source – something that has **never happened before** in the history of formula.* And something which breaches the basic canons of food safety: variety and moderation of sources of food intake.

It may well be that from various perspectives, the older feedings had something to recommend them: evaporated or condensed milk may have been less allergenic,[6] a diet of fresh whole-milk products (supplemented as they always were with fish liver oils and freshly-squeezed juices, and with solids introduced early) may have contained trace elements whose value is yet unrecognised. It was certainly lower in trans-fatty acids than formula made from spray-dried milks! Yet everyone now seems to agree that the older formulas were and are nutritionally inadequate – even the companies which once sold them as 'perfect' infant foods. What guarantee have we that by the year 2020 the companies and doctors may not be distancing themselves just as rapidly from spray-dried, whey-based milks filled with peanut or coconut oil, corn syrup, egg phospholipids, fats derived from genetically-engineered marine algae, and the rest? None at all. The process is well underway!

In our present state of ignorance, how can anyone confidently assert that "modern milk substitutes are so good that there's virtually no difference between them and breast milk", as Sonya Humphreys once wrote in a newspaper article?[7] Yet one dairy technologist/nutritionist clearly argues that formula is at least as good as, if not better than, human milk when he talks of "the rather thin margin upon which most breastfed infants are expected to survive..."[8] As I look at old photos of my now six foot bean-pole adult son at 3 months old and 7.5kg (at 6 months, 9kg) I wonder whether this technologist has ever seen exclusively breastfed babies!

On my visits to scientists working in the general field of maternal and child care (including lactation), I sometimes ask "Are you aware of any doctors or scientists whom you would consider to be hirelings for the formula companies, or simply to have adopted uncritically their line of thought?" It is instructive to see how frequently the same people are mentioned, and my 'black list' is confirmed. These 'company men' will speak out publicly and are rarely challenged. Nobody wants to be thought extreme – those who go public, such as the Jelliffes, in Los Angeles, have been subject to very unpleasant vilification. Just a handful of these well-placed and vocal propagandist professors seem to be able to cow a whole profession. Periodically, mass-circulation medical journals can be relied upon to publish review articles that combine errors of omission and fact to reassure doctors that formula is at least as good as breast milk. It is appalling that there are qualified nutritionists ignorant enough to write such articles, but that they passed uncriticised indicates the condition of medical education and attitudes. I understand, but grieve, every time a professional says to me, "Look, I think you're doing great work, and I support you in any way I can, so ask me for any help I can give. But I can't be publicly seen to support this because it would render me useless among my colleagues. They would dismiss me as another extremist, a fanatic, and stop listening. They don't listen too well now, because they're so sure they're right, but a bit sinks in and they change gradually. They just couldn't handle anyone who doesn't pretend to think like them." So many professionals say this to me that at times I have visions of meetings where everyone vociferously endorses the party line while a majority actually think quite differently but are afraid to be the first to speak and risk censure or ostracism or ridicule. What is the point of pretending we enjoy intellectual freedom when each group has its accepted blinkers which can be changed only when An Authority says so? Freedom of speech must be exercised or it ceases to exist.[9]

Journalists, too, are always very quick to pick up reversals of accepted dogmas. I said in 1984 that I fully expected to see in the next few years a series by defiant bottle-feeders, on the miseries of breastfeeding, and so on. Well, it has happened to some degree. Articles have highlighted the problems and almost accused those of us concerned with this aspect of women's health of being anti-feminist. Part of my reason for writing this book was to try to pre-empt this aspect of the backlash by letting women know why breastfeeding was such a nightmare, and assuring them that it need not be that way. The problem is that if journalists and scientists want to make a name for themselves, challenging apparent orthodoxies is the best way to attract notice – so long as the result is to leave those with money and power feeling comfortable and unthreatened. Well, there are plenty of irrational orthodoxies that could fruitfully be challenged: practices such as weaning breastfed babies because of mild lactose intolerance, or mastitis; or giving glucose to newborns, sensitising babies to cows milk in hospital nurseries, stuffing powerful drugs into infants with reflux...

But to challenge 'medical' practice is risky. Breastfeeding is an easy target, widely accepted as 'best' but nowhere definitely 'proved' in the scientific sense. And breastfeeding lacks a powerful vested-interest group to threaten legal action if the product is slandered or misrepresented; breastfeeding mothers will be annoyed, but they have no real political clout, having chosen thus far not to utilise their potential power. And to sensationalise the problems of, say, pesticides in human milk is much easier than to document the chemical contamination of infant formula – or attempting to halt the pollution at its source. Journalists need have no special scientific training, hence a degree of oversimplification and bias is sometimes unavoidable. These are less excusable in those professionally concerned with infant feeding. The least writers on infant feeding can do is spell out clearly their basic prejudices and assumptions.

My prejudice is clear:

1. *Women's milk of any kind is demonstrably safer for women's children than any artificial substitute, and*
2. *The burden of proof for the safety of those artificial substitutes rests with those who urge or allow their use.*

Those who, like me, urge the continuation of normal physiological infant feeding – i.e. exclusive human milk feeding – do not have to justify their position except in rare cases of obvious abnormality (e.g. the child with inherent defects for whom modification of human milk, or substitution by other feeds, is a necessity). History, logic and physiology all support women's milk as the only normal food for normal infants and, on the face of it, likely to be better than any alternatives for most abnormal infants too.

Other people's prejudices are by no means so clearly stated, or so reasonable, although they are usually very evident from what they write, or what they permit to be published in medical journals without devastating criticism. I find it extraordinary that apparently competent referees can have passed for publication certain articles which concluded that there are no significant health advantages to breastfeeding. Such conclusions do not square with the substantial biochemical and immunological differences between breastmilk and substitutes. Hence I always look first to see how breastfeeding was defined by the authors of such papers.

In almost no instance is breastfeeding exclusive from birth. The mentality that hospital complementary or supplementary feeds are unimportant is firmly entrenched, although it is clearly unjustified to assume that gut flora, motility and infant immuno-competence, all affected by feeding, are insignificant in the aetiology of disease. (Those few studies that do look at exclusively breastfed children always show strong evidence of benefit.)[10]

But worse, all too often 'breastfeeding' is defined as being given any breastmilk at the time of or even before the study. One study[11] considered that a breastfed child was a child receiving "at least 2 feeds" in 24 hours "regardless of other food intake", for at least one of the two months of the study period. Only 15/20 babies had even this small amount to the age of six months, which is (a) a small sample to generalise from; and (b) hardly enough to judge the protective potential of human milk feeding. Breastfed babies were reassigned to the non-breastfed group 'within a month' of further reducing this pitiful amount (presumably any illnesses during four weeks were classified in the 'breastfed' category).

Another study[12] adopted a similar division of infants. 'Breastfed' meant receiving at least two feeds in 24 hours, without mention of other food intake (iron-rich solids negating the protective effects of lactoferrin and gut pH, almost certainly). Those receiving one feed of breast milk, even if it were an identical volume to another child's two feeds, were allocated to the group of those who had "stopped breastfeeding prior to infection" – which would include children totally weaned at four days or four months, or children still receiving one feed from mothers with particularly high/low antibody levels or high prostaglandin levels, or... The third group was those exclus-ively breastfed from birth to six months. Such babies are exceedingly rare in America, where much hospital practice virtually guarantees exposure to formula within the first few days and early supplementation thereafter (with the samples obligingly provided by the hospital as the company's distributor, or mailed direct to the mother using lists sold by hospitals to companies). Despite all this, no 'breastfed' infant developed rotavirus infection in the first three months, and of the seven infants (another huge sample) who developed infection while 'breastfed', only one experienced vomiting as a symptom, compared with 22/25 of those 'who had stopped prior to infection' and 12/18 of the formula-fed infants.

Then there was Adenobojo's study[13] which defined breastfed as "primarily breastfed for three months or longer" and bottle-fed as "breastfed for less than three months". Although this study was done in the early 1970s and can be severely critic-ised, it continues to be quoted[14] in support of the idea that style of feeding has no in-fluence on health in developed countries. This study also quotes the industry argument that there is a one-way flow from breast to bottle-feeding, which is simply not true, as many babies revert from partial to exclusive breastfeeding when they become ill. An-other oft-quoted study of similarly deficient methodology was Dugdale's 1971 study in Malaysia.[15] Common sense would suggest that it is unreasonable to expect huge differences to emerge from comparisons of children given solids at 12½ weeks and thus categorised as 'breastfed', and other children fed human milk to 11½ weeks and then given solids ('bottlefed'); or babies given formula in hospital and breastfed there-after, with babies breastfed exclusively from birth but given solids a week earlier than the first group. None of these or similar studies considers the possible impact of food intolerance in breastfed infants, although in a study by Myers et al.[16] (1984), all three babies "exclusively breastfed" (after 6-9 days: no mention of hospital feeds) began life with rhinitis, which in two lasted for six and ten weeks, while the third had otitis by 12 weeks. To any physician aware of the possible effects of early sensitisation and maternal diet, this would suggest an allergic rather than purely infective disease aetiology, and so early sensitisation in utero or postpartum is a virtual certainty. Interestingly, none of the ten babies formula-fed from birth developed upper respiratory symptoms in the first two weeks, although by weeks 8 and 9, three had upper respiratory symptoms, two had otitis and one had gastroenteritis. Among the seven not exclusively breastfed children three had upper respiratory symptoms, (one with gastroenteritis) and one had otitis: while only one of the three exclusively breastfed children had symptoms (the child with chronic respiratory symptoms). By weeks 12 and 13, four of these 10 formula-fed children were symptom-free, five had respiratory symptoms (three with gastroenteritis as well) and another had gastroenteritis alone. By contrast, no fully or partially breastfed child had gastroenteritis; two out of three exclusively-fed children were asymptomatic, while the third had otitis media. Of the seven partially breastfed children, two were asymptomatic, three had upper respiratory symptoms and two had otitis. Figures like this prove very little, although clearly bottle-fed babies are at increased risk of gastrointestinal disease.

The fact that all ten breastfed children, and nine out of ten bottlefed children experienced upper respiratory symptoms (the tenth being a child who was fed soy formula and who had more gastrointestinal symptoms) seems extraordinary to me. I shall be angry if this study is quoted as showing no ill effects from infant formula feeding, when, as the author said, "it is possible that the results might have been different had we limited our study to breastfed infants whose entire energy intake derived from human milk" **and, I would add,** if the researchers controlled for uterine and neonatal sensitisation. Respiratory symptoms of allergy are indistinguishable from those of viral infection, after all; and the mere presence of a virus does not confirm it as the initial precipitant of rhinitis.

Another study, published in *The Lancet* in May 1982,[17] claimed that "breastfeeding was found to have no significant association with rates of bronchitis or admission to hospital with lower respiratory illness 'when associated influences affecting both health and likelihood of breastfeeding are taken into account'." What astonishes me is the statement: "social changes such as the move from rural to city living and dietary changes other than infant milk feeding may have contributed more to morbidity and mortality differentials"; and control variables such as domestic crowding, parental education, tenure of accommodation, type of neighbourhood and father's occupation "were initially selected *on empirical grounds*" as being likely to contribute to illness. Thus, the universal finding that fewer breastfed children get sick from whatever cause can be explained away.

Why is it more reasonable that one's father's occupation explains a child's illness than that the immense differences between a live biological fluid and a dead processed product should explain the child's illness? Where are the rigidly controlled scientific studies showing that the exclusively breastfed child of a street-sweeper is more often sick than the bottle-fed child of a professor? The assumption that socioeconomic differences can explain away infant illnesses does not explain why, throughout history and across cultures, fewer babies get sick or die when breastfed.[18] An earlier report suggested that regardless of social class, "scarcely any babies with diarrhoea and vomiting or with upper respiratory tract infections... were breastfed."[19] The authors noted that despite appalling squalor for all families, all of the patients admitted were bottlefed. Both living conditions and type of feeding were involved in producing disease.

Here the pro-bottle advocate hastens to concede that breastfeeding is indeed best in places where poverty renders hygiene impracticable and new super formulae unobtainable: breastfeeding is all poor people can afford. But I have yet to see any convincing scientific studies which demonstrate that method of feeding does not matter in any context, or that socioeconomic variables matter more than physiological ones.[20] This seems to me like a convenient assumption to rationalise the status quo, and to allow writer and referee alike to avoid considering the consequences of infant feeding in their lives. This study by Taylor et al. was characterised by retrospective data gathering, poor definition or investigation of mode of feeding, and apparent ignorance about the need to control for allergy/intolerance when assessing infective episodes (as infective episodes need not recur if maternal diet is altered to remove antigens initiating infant symptoms). I would accept that it showed that partial breastfeeding for short periods, as practiced in the United Kingdom in 1975 when almost all babies were fed formula in hospital,[21] may be only slightly better for babies than bottle-feeding – at least where hospital admissions in the first five years of life are concerned. (There was an "almost significant" protective effect against admission in the first year for gastro-enteritis.) But the experience of such messed-about feeding does not entitle anyone to generalise about breastfeeding per se, because its true protective potential has not been explored at all. Exclusive physiological breastfeeding does not include women "breastfeeding for less than a month"! (When did supplementation begin, for a child to be weaned totally by four weeks?) Again, this study is quoted as proving there are no significant health benefits from breastfeeding for children in developed countries, and therefore no need to worry about formula.

Now these are not the worst or the only biased articles passed for publication. Kathleen Auerbach, Mary Renfrew and I collaborated on a later review in the *Journal of Human Lactation*[22] which summarised many more.

The point I want to make is this. *Articles as poor as these would not be published if they showed that there was a marked difference favouring the breastfed child: referees would rightly reject them as unreliable, bad use of data, too small numbers, likely to cause unnecessary alarm about infant formula.* The pro-bottle cadres, some very eminent, would write trenchant criticisms if they were to be published.

Yet when bad articles seem to favour or legitimise bottle-feeding, they are in fact published, and letters challenging them are rarely printed. It is articles such as these which have vitiated medical concern and made it possible for doctors not to take seriously the need to spend time encouraging their pregnant patients to learn about breastfeeding, or to help the lactating woman through the various crises that usually present at some point in time. They make it possible for hospitals to go on with routines that render breastfeeding success unlikely. They make it possible for society to go on being organised around anything except the needs of women and children.

This I believe, is why Finnish work[23] showing conclusively that the introduction of any foods other than breast milk under six months of age has deleterious effects has been studiously ignored, rather than hailed as an important breakthrough. In Finland the logical consequences of that work have been accepted. Hospitals no longer offer formula; maternity leave has been extended from two to seven months; the use of hypoallergenic formula has become widespread for infants unable to be breastfed; human milk banking is thriving. The result: "the incidence of milk-induced gastrointestinal diseases has dropped dramatically and there is every indication that childhood atopic disease will show a similar decline."[24] These studies have found continued benefit to children now in their late teens!

Why do we not insist on more careful studies along the lines of this Finnish work? If we cannot obtain clear-cut control groups, if we cannot do decent epidemiological work, why spend money on expensive bad research when it could be going into preventive health measures? There is no point in 'proving' that partial breastfeeding is only slightly better than partial bottle-feeding – we know enough about nutritional bioavailability and gut flora to have reached that conclusion long ago. What we need to aim for is optimal infant feeding, i.e., human milk exclusively to six months, and continued breastfeeding for the next few years. I believe that this has been accepted by those who are aware of the research: it seems implicit in the comments made by Barness over the introduction of solids debate. It may be true that we can explain away some of the protective effect of breastfeeding by referring to other variables,[25] but it is harder to explain away the fact that even the most negative studies show a constant tendency for breastfeeding children to do better, whether one is looking at respiratory illness, gastrointestinal illness, intellectual development,[26] or much else. If this were an artefact, an odd coincidence, some studies should favour bottle-feeding. In 1998 I am happy to be able to report that we have a few more definitive studies that include a gold standard group of exclusively breastfed babies, and the results are exactly what I predicted in the preceding paragraphs.[27]

Issues of comparative morbidity and mortality are not the only areas where such unconscious bias prevails. A classic example of the medical profession's refusal to accept the obvious is the history of studies proving colic in breastfed babies to be due to maternal diet,[28] and colic in bottle-fed babies due to infant formula, whether cows' milk or soy.[29] I have discussed this at some length in the later editions of my book, *Food for Thought*. More than any other case I think of, this illustrates the reluctance of many professionals to seriously consider a possibility that has far-reaching implications for changes in clinical practice. If breast milk alone can be blamed for sensitisation – fine. But in utero sensitisation due to maternal diet? – we'd rather not know. As for neonatal exposure to formula having long-term effects… just a bit couldn't hurt, surely… people can adapt to most things.

If my attitude there seems cynical, I am merely paraphrasing people who ought to know better. I find it curious how often highly trained scientists ultimately, after a long debate on journal articles, will revert to personal experience as the clincher for their determined rejection of the ideas I propose: "We have two kids and they were normally colicky and active just like the kids you describe, and they aren't food-sensitive." That's what virtually every parent of food-intolerant children said at some stage, myself included. It can be fairly threatening to have to re-think what we thought we knew. We all want to do the best for our children, or want to believe that our mothers did the best for us, and we are all reluctant to believe that we have not. So even scientists will revert to dogma rather than science: I can't out-argue you but I know you're wrong.

As Doris and John Haire argued cogently more than a decade ago, Western medicine has a blind spot[30] when it comes to infant nutrition and its short- and long-term impact. Assessing the differences between breast- and bottle-fed children becomes more difficult rather than less, as populations are further affected not only by artificial feeding in any generation, but also by the massive changes in diet and lifestyle, which make for changes in outcome. The rise in smoking among teenage girls, for example, is likely to have serious consequences not only in pregnancy but also during lactation. The use of steroidal hormones and antibiotics, not merely by humans but also in animals, may have unexpected effects. Human milk composition is fairly resistant to the likely hazards of undernutrition, but there has been no time for adaptation to the hazards of affluence.

Someone will probably argue that there is little point distinguishing between breastfeeding as it is practised today, by women of today, and the possible potential of breastfeeding as a protective force for the newborn and older infant. To my mind, that is like saying that we should have been content with older formula now known to cause harm. If it can be demonstrated that exclusive breastfeeding by a healthy, well-nourished, food-tolerant mother provides better protection than breastfeeding by a malnourished allergic mother, then we can aim to control the allergies and improve the nutrition of mothers. Just as formula manufacturers argue that it is not their present product which does harm, but the conditions under which it is used, so the breastfeeding lobby can argue that mother's milk could sometimes be improved, without conceding anything of their claim to superiority for breast milk. But it remains highly unlikely that any undesirable consequences of breastfeeding could ever be as harmful as the undesirable consequences of artificial feeding!

It would be unfair to blame formula per se for the tragedies that result from leaving feeding bottles in the dirt and heat. (One can blame people who sell formula and bribe healthworkers in places where this is inevitable, but this is no criticism of the actual product.) Similarly, it is unfair to denigrate breast milk because mothers smoke, or eat chocolate biscuits all day, or live on socially acceptable drugs, or have been food-intolerant since they were bottlefed babies. Only the most prejudiced will skip lightly over this point, which could become increasingly important as women from less privileged backgrounds return to breastfeeding.

It remains true that we do all have our prejudices, whether we acknowledge them or not. Only by honest communication of information and ideas can we hope to achieve the best possible results for children. We are all accountable to one another, and none of us can afford to ignore our critics. Those of us who are concerned not about money of prestige or power but about the world's women and children – surely that's most people concerned with maternal and child health? – must recognise the need to work together, and to maintain common sense perspectives. Certainly industry has a role. But we cannot trust any group making sales worth billions annually to provide us with totally objective data: those stakes are too high for inconvenient or threatening truths to survive a process of rationalisation.

Nor can we trust failed breastfeeders, or men whose partners have never successfully breastfed, to tell us about the realities and rewards of breastfeeding. Unsuccessful athletes, or those who have never tried, are not paid to tell us about the realities and rewards of athletics. Breastfeeding is one of the few activities where having failed at it, or refused to try, can make one an expert commentator.

As the saying goes, Self-interest makes fools of us all.

NOTES

CHAPTER 11: THE BUILDING BACKLASH

[1] Phillips, J., *Mothers Matter Too* (Nelsons, 1985) Foreword.

[2] *Food Chemical News*, Jan. 4, 1982, p. 19. This is also a major plank of Dana Raphael's support for infant formula, cf. Raphael, D., "Myths and realities about women and their infant feeding practices", *Baroda J. Nutrition* (1982) 9, 144-153, or *New Generation* (198). A new book, *Only Mothers Know*, reiterates these themes.

[3] Such books deserve a closer look, and if I ever am free to get my next book done, it will happen. Meanwhile, a regular place to find my writing is *ALCA Galaxy* – see Resources.

[4] For this reason I approve of the typical Health Department slow and steady administrative approach, for so long as it maintains real momentum – and it is our job as citizens to see that it does. Despite the cutbacks in government spending this must be a priority. It is encouraging to hear an Australian Health Minister talk in 1997 of breastfeeding as a key preventative health strategy: may he survive the economic rationalists in his government.)

[5] My deliberate refusal to write the right sort of article probably was the real reason for the non-appearance of my WHO Code article, discussed in this chapter. Similarly it was always inevitable that NAACOG, the Nurses Association of the American College of Obstetrics and Gynecology, would not publish the chapter they asked me to write, on the advantages of breastfeeding in developed nations.

[6] It is widely accepted that prolonged heat treatment reduces the sensitising capacities of milks – cf. McLaughlan, P.; Anderson, K. J.; Widdowson, E., Coombs, R. R. A. "Effects of heat on the anaphylactic sensitising capacity of cows' milk, goats' milk and various infant formulae", *Arch. Dis. Child.* (1981) 56, 165-71. It is also widely accepted that some children made very ill by formula in the past were able to tolerate evaporated or condensed milks – hence their almost routine use by some doctors and nurses in the first few days of life, or after gastro-enteritis. The huge rise in food intolerance coincides with the period of change from these extensively-heat-treated milks to spray-dried whey-based ones. I don't know whether that's coincidence. Neither do the scientists.

[7] Humphreys, S., *The Australian*, May 9, 1984.

[8] Packard, V. L., *Human Milk and Infant Formula*. (Academic Press, 1982). This book epitomises the industry approach. It is full of useful information, misleadingly interpreted, and adopts the language of neutrality and 'objectivity'. Its omissions, however, are too consistent to be accidental. I should like to do a page by page critique!

[9] But be warned: speaking the truth, exercising that crucial democratic freedom, has real personal costs. It is a tactic of tyrants, whether petty or great, to persecute (and even prosecute) those who dare to speak a truth they disagree with. When they can draw on organisational or institutional money, such persecution may even be not just wrongheaded, but purely malicious, designed to intimidate and silence, with no real prospect of success, but needing to be dignified with a response because the court process will bankrupt the threatened respondent. Hence the increase in Australia of defamation suits against inconvenient speakers of truth, many settled out of court simply because to continue is so ruinously expensive. As I write a major TV programme is again under threat of lawsuit. When budgets are limited, reporters who target the powerful and provoke such suits may rapidly find themselves unpopular with the management. This tactic works, but is a gross abuse of the legal system which should attract enormous penalties. If lawyers did their duty, first to the court and only second to their client, such abuses could not happen.

[10] e.g. Narayanan, I. et al, "Randomised controlled trial of effect of raw and holder pasteurised human milk and of formula supplements on incidence of neonatal infection", *Lancet* (1984) ii, 1111-3.

[11] Cushing, AH; Anderson L. "Diarrhea in breastfed and non-breastfed infants", *Pediatrics* (70), 6, 921-5.

[12] Weinberg, R. J.; Tipton, G.; Klish, W. J.; Brown, M. R., "Effect of breastfeeding on morbidity in rotavirus gastroenteritis", *Pediatrics* (1984) 74, 2, 250-3.

[13] Adenobojo, F. O., "Artificial versus breastfeeding: relation to infant health in a middleclass American community", *Clin. Pediatr.* 1972, 11, 25-9.

[14] e.g., by Eiger, M. S. et al, "Breastfeeding vs bottlefeeding. A study of morbidity in upper middle-class infants", *Clin. Pediatrics* (1984) 23, 9, 492-5.

[15] Dugdale, A. E., "The effect of the type of feeding on weight gain and illnesses in infants", *Br. J. Nutr.* (1971) 26, 423-432

[16] Myers, M. G. et al, "Respiratory and gastrointestinal illnesses in breast- and formula-fed infants", *A.J.D.C.* (1984) 138, 629-32

[17] Taylor, B. et al, "Breastfeeding, bronchitis and admissions for lower respiratory illness and gastroenteritis for the first five years", *Lancet* (1982) i, 1227-9.

[18] Asher, P. "The incidence and significance of breastfeeding in infants admitted to hospital", *Arch. Dis. Child* (1952) 27, 270-2.

[19] Mann, N. M. et al, "Gastroenteritis in infancy", *Arch. Dis. Child* (1952) 27, 457-67.

[20] Included in these would be maternal nutritional status and immune functioning; composition of breast milk, genetic defects in (say) enzyme functioning, and so on. There is no strict correlation with socio-economic status involved here, although a poor mother is of course more likely to be under-nourished.

[21] Martin, J., *Infant Feeding 1975: attitudes and practice in England and Wales.* (H.M.S.O., 1978), p. 86.

[22] Auerbach KG, Renfrew MJ, Minchin MK, "Infant feeding comparisons: a hazard to infant health?", *J. Hum. Lact.* (1991) 7: 63-71.

[23] Kajosaari, M.; Saarinen, U., "Prophylaxis of atopic disease by six months' total food elimination. Evaluation of 135 exclusively breastfed infants of atopic families", *Acta. Paed. Scand.* (1983) 72, 3, 411-4.

[24] Heiner, D. C., "Modern research relating to food allergy and its implications – Introduction", *Clin. Rev. Allergy* (1984) 2, 1-5

[25] Another study showing significant differences in both respiratory and GI symptoms, where the respiratory symptoms become non-significant after statistical analysis (how sound are those rules for regression?) is Fergusson, D. M. et al, "Infant health and breastfeeding during the first

16 weeks of life", *Aust. Paediatr. J.* (1978) 14, 254-8. Any committed breastfeeding statisticians around? It would make a change to see data analysed with a different set of underlying assumptions!

[26] "Report of the Task Force on the Assessment of the Scientific Evidence Relating to Infant Feeding Practices and Infant Health", supplement to *Pediatrics* (1984) 74, 4.

[27] Eg Saarinen, U.M.; Kajosaari M, "Breastfeeding as prophylaxis against atopic disease: prospective follow-up study until 17 years old", *Lancet* (1995) 346: 1065-9; and, hot off the presses as this edition goes onto them, Wilson, A.C.; Forsyth J.S.; Greene S.A. et al, "Relation of infant diet to childhood health: seven year follow up of cohort of children in Dundee infant feeding", *BMJ* (1998) 316: 21-5.

[28] See Jakobsson, I.; Lindberg, T., "Cows' milk proteins cause infantile colic in breastfed infants: a double blind cross-over study", *Pediatrics* (1983) 71, 268-71.

[29] Lothe, L.; Lindberg, T.; Jakobsson, I., "Cows' milk formula as a cause of infantile colic: a double blind study", *Pediatrics* (1982) 70, 1, 7-20; letters 299-300.

[30] Haire, D.; Haire, J., "The medical value of breastfeeding: do we have a medical blindspot?" Reprinted from *Implementing Family-Centred Maternity Care with a Central Nursery* by ICEA & NMAA, 1974

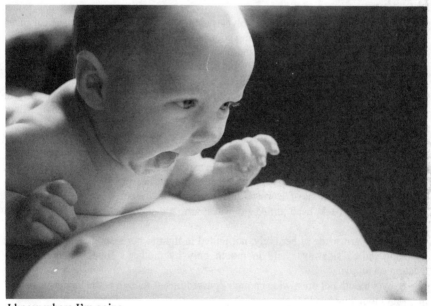

I know where I'm going....

PRACTICAL LEARNING

...persuading mothers to choose to breastfeed and then not being able to give the informed support that can contribute so greatly to success is a sad way which some of us have of failing mothers and their babies.

- C. B. S. Wood and J. A. Walker-Smith
MacKeith's Infant Feeding and Feeding Difficulties
(Churchill Livingstone, 6th edn, 1981), p. 110

Positioning Posers

B reastfeeding management involves practical skills as well as theoretical ones. Future courses for breastfeeding counsellors, professional or lay, must incorporate more hands-on learning and problem-solving. We must first of all learn the correct procedures, not just verbally but visually. The perpetuation in textbooks of inaccurate and misleading photographs is a major source of harm. Our eyes become accustomed to seeing babies wrongly positioned at the breast or mothers behaving in ways that make for difficulties, and we do not spot those problems when counselling: they are 'normal'. (The harmful can be normal.)

So looking at these few pictures should be the beginning of a process of critically re-examining the visual images of breastfeeding and its practice by mothers. Go on from here to look at diagrams and pictures in textbooks, advertisements, brochures and so on. You'll be surprised at what you see, once you learn to look. For example, in Messenger's illustrations of "correct" positioning you will see:

• Baby flat on back, head turned sideways; arm and shoulder between his body and mother's.

• Mother's arm wide of her body, not pulled in tight to her side; therefore the breast is being pulled sideways, held in mouth only by mother's support and/or baby's suction on nipple.

• Baby's mouth not open wide enough - pursed lips as though bottle feeding.

• Hand touching head.

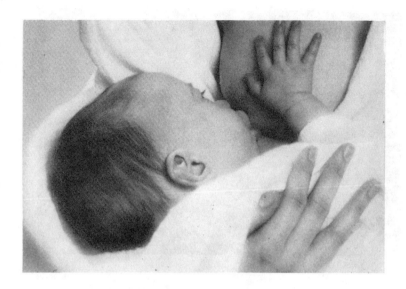

Figure 12.1

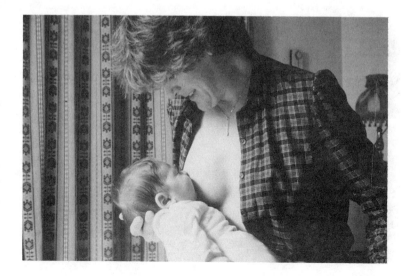

Figure 12.2

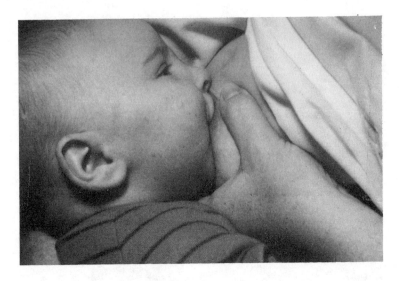

Figure 12.3

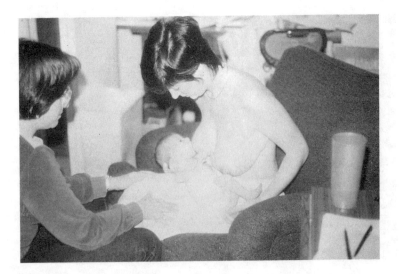

Figure 12.4

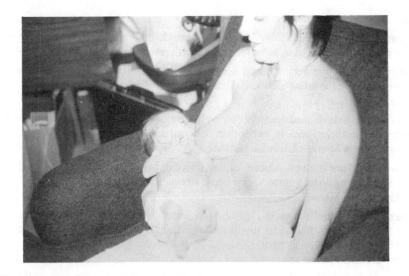

Figure 12.5

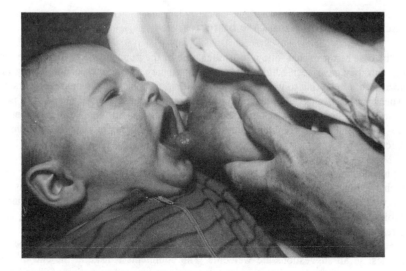

Figure 12.6

The positional errors are as follows:

Figure 12.1: Baby too far from breast, bottle-sucking the nipple (protruding, pursed, 'prissy lips'). This was from some formula advertisement, appropriately enough.

Figure 12.2: Mother very strained across back and shoulders; baby held by head, placing strain on the infant's neck. Baby asleep, rather than feeding.
Photo: © Prue Carr

Figure 12.3: Experienced breastfeeder, well positioned; breast well supported. Baby has bottom lip sucked back in, rather than flattened out and down.
Photo: © Chele Marmet, Lactation Institute

Figure 12.4: Poor latch on. Mother leaning forward, baby insecurely held by head and foot, body falling away from mother's body. Recipe for backache.
Photo: © Chele Marmet

Figure 12.5: Mother shown in Fig. 12.4 has leaned back. Baby pulling on nipple to keep it in the mouth. Recipe for nipple damage. Baby also too far from mother, and at the wrong angle, and on its back.
Photo: © Chele Marmet

Figure 12.6: Experienced breastfeeder, raring to get on. Mouth open beautifully, but nipple off centre. Baby needs to be brought around the mother's body more, or breast lifted and then supported in place until baby is better aligned. Failure to do so will result in pressure on nipple and damage.
Photo: © Chele Marmet

Practical learning from case histories

The case histories that follow illustrate some of the points made earlier in the text. Although they have been edited in places, I hope they retain much of the feeling that comes across in talking to women about breastfeeding. I have taken out much personal or specific criticism of individuals, groups and institutions, because I am not in a position to assess the accuracy or fairness of those criticisms. But believe me, women do have many and bitter complaints about their treatment, far more than this sample suggests.

Most of the case histories report avoidable failures. In future I should like to be able to publish case histories of unusual successes such as the first two histories, from which I learnt new variables to consider when investigating particular problems. An observant reader will notice that oversupply/initial engorgement proved to be just as troublesome for some women as undersupply did for others; that infant crying is as distressing as maternal nipple pain. To provide better solutions to these four problems (or even better, to prevent them occurring) would greatly improve the breastfeeding statistics, so all suggestions are welcome. The comments I make at the end of each case are not meant to be exhaustive, and they presume an understanding of what I have written earlier in the book.

Perhaps one brief comment is in order here, as so many mothers mention NMAA (Nursing Mothers' Association of Australia). It will be obvious that NMAA counsellors did their best for many of these mothers, often going far beyond what could be reasonably expected of people who are themselves busy mothers of two or three young children. That their best was sometimes not good enough is not surprising: why should we expect unpaid volunteers to be able to solve problems that medical professionals cannot? NMAA training can only be as good as the available information and volunteer. It has been far superior to that given to many professionals in the past and present, but it is still imperfect, as NMAA recognises. For every mother here who was not helped by NMAA, I know a dozen who were helped, as their problems were solved by the suggestions that NMAA dispensed. Hence these few failures should be seen in perspective, not as indicting NMAA generally. At the mother-to-mother level, many counsellors do an extraordinary job in helping other women of similar background to succeed at breastfeeding. At the organisational level, a new sense of vision and energy is apparent. For both reasons I am happy to support NMAA – never uncritically, but quite wholeheartedly – and would strongly recommend membership to all my readers, in Australia and overseas. (I have been a member since 1976.)

Case History 1

'My milk has dried up - I need a complementary feed.'

That was how the anxious new mother presented to the hospital. Although they reassured her that to lose one's milk at two weeks is very rare, she wasn't happy till she had a can of formula in hand. They suggested that she come to see me, and her first words were "I'm just not cut out for motherhood, I'm afraid." So we began by talking about how it feels to suddenly have a tiny creature totally dependent on oneself for its every need, and the difficulties all first-time mothers face in adjusting to that role: the occasional feelings of rejection, the anxiety, even panic at times, and all the other normal reactions. When she had calmed down, I asked how baby had been in the preceding two weeks. "Angelic" summed it up: he even slept six hours at night on occasion.

Why had she become anxious enough to seek help? Because all day yesterday and today he had been fretful, difficult to settle, and slept only for an hour or two. What had been different yesterday, or the day before, to account for his change of behaviour? "Nothing." We eliminated diet, drugs including cigarettes, tea and coffee and contraceptives, maternal illness, infant illness. So I asked about nipple problems. Well, actually she had been using a nipple shield until yesterday; could that have had any effect? We discussed types of suckling, the different muscles used in feeding at the breast, and different positions, and when baby woke up we took the time to get him well fixed on the breast – where he sucked vigorously and was full within five minutes on one side. (This was at 6pm after a harrowing day, so the problem definitely wasn't lack of production!) That took quite some time, as the mother, a midwife, clearly hadn't been taught the basics of good positioning for breastfeeding. I pointed out that it was obvious that she had plenty of milk, so perhaps the problem had begun with her let-down reflex, which could be inhibited by pain, fatigue, anxiety, hormones. Had she been upset by anything in particular? (We'd ruled out pain, stitches were all right, nipples were perfect.) She had been anxious because she'd been told that her nipples were small and flat, and she didn't think he could feed without the nipple shield; her sister had just gone home that day, and she had to face the housework and babycare alone for the first time; and she'd been very upset when she had to remove baby's circumcision bandage, and he had been very distressed. Aha! Perhaps his fretfulness had more to do with pain than feeding? We discussed the nipple problem – she had beautiful nipples, protractile, although flat when not in use. I assured her that small nipples were ideal; big ones often became sore until baby's mouth could accommodate them. We talked about fatigue, priorities, and the need to find her own limits of activity and feeding, but that until six weeks or so, her supply wasn't really established and it was in everyone's interests to get that right before the housework! (Fortunately, she had plenty of meals frozen, and wasn't obsessive about tidiness.) I demonstrated the use of a simple baby sling to enable her to get a few chores done if he continued to be fretful.

So we had almost concluded that the problem had arisen because of his pain and her anxiety, when I noticed how well bundled up against the cold he was. So I pointed out that many new mothers actually give baby a heat rash (and described it) because of their concern to keep baby warm; and we discussed how cold could cause an appetite increase because of the need for calories to keep warm (a common cause for increased demand when a baby leaves the heated nursery for his cooler home). "Just as baby needs more fluid if he gets overheated," said I. Eureka! Well, actually, the night before yesterday, she had fallen asleep with him in bed and the electric blanket on, and she woke up to find him saturated in sweat. And from then on he had been constantly wanting to feed and hadn't settled down, until in desperation, just before going into hospital, she had given him boiled water. The fact that he gulped it down thirstily convinced her that her milk had gone.

In the end, we concluded that so many things had been different yesterday that it was no wonder the baby was fretful, but that the whole cycle of negative feedback had probably begun with the baby becoming slightly dehydrated. She was convinced that her nipples were fine, and her supply good, though I warned her that she might have to feed more frequently for the next few days till she'd got over the effects of such a traumatic two days. And knowing that it was normal for the interval between feeds to vary, she no longer felt the need for a 'comp.' bottle. (We discussed its hazards, of course, and how to express and store one's own milk for that sense of security.)

And she decided to press for a new mother's group to be formed through our local Infant Welfare Clinic. As she said, "It would have helped if I'd known that my feelings, and my baby's behaviour, were both normal for us at this stage." She is in fact a nurse herself – does this say something about the curriculum of training?

She reported the outcome to the hospital nurses, who were amazed at the number of significant factors that hadn't come out in their discussion with her. One midwife, who had wanted to breastfeed but had 'failed' after a few weeks, commented that she would probably have gone on feeding had such help been available to her at the time. The midwifery staff are now arranging a seminar on the management of breastfeeding. And there are now two more enthusiastic nurses in the local community.

But what are the chances that a local doctor or nurse would have uncovered so much? It is difficult to switch mentally from all the problems of diabetics, varicose veins, or earaches, and to remember every detail of what might affect breastfeeding. This is where the lactation consultant who takes a detailed history can excel. What may seem like trivia emerging from relaxed conversation may actually be the vital diagnostic clue.

Case History 2

"The baby won't stop crying and wants to feed all the time."

The baby had been born just four weeks premature, at 2975g (16 lb 9 oz) and was three weeks old when I saw him. He had not regained his birth weight. In hospital he had been gavage fed and complemented with formula when he had had difficulty taking the breast. (He was not put to the breast in the first 24 hours; this might have been a longer period of separation had his mother not become very upset.) The mother became painfully engorged and had vast quantities of milk; every nurse told her different things about how to feed him; but all had failed to get him to suck well at the breast, so a nipple shield was provided. This was of the type illustrated in Figure 5.3. The baby was still given top-ups of formula.

Initially I observed the baby feeding from the shield. The mother had forceful and copious let-downs of milk, despite her exhaustion and distress. The baby simply mouthed a little, then lay passively to await the milk. He was content to be there and wait, and fiercely resisted any attempt to detach him, crying vigorously. This was what he did most of the time. The mother believed that he should be feeding only for certain times, but had not tried to enforce this until exhaustion made her try to limit the time at the breast. Despite all this, in the previous week the baby's weight gain had suddenly begun to pick up; he had put on 90gm in two days before I saw him. The mother believed that this had been possible only because of the nipple shield, that without it he would have starved because she had such 'bad nipples'; she had been told her (perfectly average) nipples were inverted and that she would never be able to feed him. The baby had frequent loose stools and a very sore bottom; he was constantly soaked with urine. He was also quite jaundiced, although not lethargic.

Obviously, this was a mother who was quite capable of feeding her baby more than adequately. Equally obviously, the baby had to learn to suckle the breast. At first we let him use the shield to take the edge off his hunger and to soften the mother's breast. Then I stood behind, holding the breast and baby correctly, and tried to get him on. He had no idea what to do, and kept turning his head until he found something hard (my knuckle) and mouthed at that. When, by perseverance and good luck, he finally closed on the areola, he lay there and waited! I had to express milk into his mouth correctly (the 'suckle right or drown' principle in action). He stayed there for some minutes, and came off. After burping and changing, he was ready for more. Again it was difficult to get him on, and he had to be taken away from the breast and comforted when he became too upset, before trying again. The mother felt terrible that it was I who was getting him on, and needed reassurance that once he knew how to suck, and she knew what it felt like to have a baby on correctly, she'd be able to manage alone.

She and the baby had come over at 7 am after an exhausting night, so after this feed I put her to bed and took the baby. He was a bit restless by 10.30, so I put him in a sling. He then slept soundly till 11.45 am, his longest interval ever. For the rest of the day they stayed with me. By the afternoon feed he was lunging at the breast and was clearly getting the hang of it all. The mother was still anxious about managing alone, but her childbirth educator, a midwife (who had got me involved), was able to be with her that evening.

He woke only three-hourly that night, and I saw them the next day. The difference was amazing. His jaundice was almost gone, and his bottom looked much improved. He was generally calmer and very relaxed during feeding. After feeding he made all sorts of contented baby noises for the first time. The mother was delighted. Her nipples had begun to be sore, but there was no sign of positional soreness, so I thought this likely to be initial soreness (described in Chapter 5). The mother still experienced some difficulty getting him correctly positioned, but this was improving rapidly. ("I know where my arms and hands go now.")

Over the following weekend, I telephoned to check that they were doing well. Sunday night he was unsettled, but the mother was confident that feeding was adequate; her nipples were settling down; his bottom had virtually cleared; and he was growing well. (By Monday he had put on 150gm over the previous five days.)

The combination of a very sore bottom and poor weight gain may have been the result of the baby getting too little fat. It is an observation frequently made by those who work with mothers, that the baby's suckling patterns and style seem to influence the composition of the milk they receive. The extraordinary rapidity with which the jaundice cleared once feeding at the breast was established also raises some interesting questions about whether high lactose levels were increasing bowel reabsorption, for instance; or whether fat influenced the clearance in some way. It could have widespread ramifications if this observation were to be confirmed in other women.

The level of incompetence to which women are exposed in hospital is clearly evident in this history. Unable themselves to assist the mother to get the baby on the breast, staff had to explain their failure by telling the mother that her nipples were the problem, thus further reducing her confidence that breastfeeding would be possible. Breastfeeding education for professionals needs to be a practical course, as surgery is. There is clearly a case for in-service workshops for nurses.

And the outcome? Baby went on to be fully breastfed, gaining 300-350gms. per week on average. Mother's main problems related to **over**supply.

Case History 3

Unresolved engorgement, leading to nipple damage and lactation failure

Here in Australia, the problem of the mother with too much milk is emerging as a major one. This case history says a great deal – about the care, energy and emotion many women invest in the process of having children now that we have choices; and about the anxieties we face when things go wrong. I am including with it Margaret's own 'editorial', the letter that came with the account, with which I am in full agreement:

> With your many speaking engagements, it is probably impossible for you to remember individuals. I spoke to you about my problems with breastfeeding because of inverted nipples and the associated guilt feelings I was experiencing. You invited me to recount my experiences as anecdotal material for your next book about breastfeeding. I have done just that, and in many ways it has been 'a load off my chest'.
>
> I feel very strongly that women who try to breastfeed and fail need great support; they need to believe that all women 'fail' some area of childbearing and raising, and that to have done one's best is worthy. Although we all know that breast milk is best, women must learn (before giving birth) that it does not always come naturally.
>
> - M.J.B.

"Guilty... hypocritical... a failure...

"That's how I still feel six months after a healthy, easy, fulfilling pregnancy culminating in a natural straightforward labour, delivering us with a healthy, placid, easy-to-manage son, after eleven years of marriage. So much to be thankful for, surely? Yes, but... I failed to provide breast milk for Martin after the first three months of his life, and now the tears well up again and plop on the paper as I write and remember...

"I did everything 'right' to make my pregnancy and labour problem-free: I gave up my work as a primary school teacher, for the duration of the pregnancy. It was an occupation I found very rewarding, but at times also very stressful, and I wanted to cultivate a relaxed mind and body for the birth. I ate a nutritious and balanced diet and strictly avoided 'junk' items (as I had always done prior to pregnancy). I had no food binges or cravings, and suffered only a little nausea during the first trimester. I had plenty of time to make my own flour, bread, yoghurt, muesli, etc., and to grow my own vegetables and fruit, and thereby remain in an optimal nutritional state. I exercised daily for the entire 41 weeks of the pregnancy – walking, jogging, stationary bike riding, antenatal exercises. I also regularly played tennis, gardened, mowed the lawn, etc. So physically I remained very fit. I believed that this was very important for a woman having her first labour at 33 years of age.

"I prepared my slightly inverted nipples by pulling them out daily and rolling them between my fingers, and by avoiding soap in the shower. My mother and grandmother had both successfully and easily breastfed each of their children for nine months or more, and I assumed I would do the same.

"Well, the 41 weeks passed, with me feeling pleased that everything was going so well. The labour progressed 'naturally', as I had planned for, with much of the first stage spent in a squatting position on the floor. No drugs were taken.

"Martin was a placid little boy, and I was proud that I was so well and mobile after birth. Everything, it appeared, had 'paid off', and smooth sailing lay ahead. How disillusioned I was to become in the days and months ahead!

"Martin suckled at the breast successfully on day one. On day two my milk came in, and my previously flat chest swelled to proportions I did not believe imaginable. My slightly inverted nipples disappeared inwards, buried in this mass of flesh and veins. My breasts became badly engorged, and leaked right through nursing pads, bras, nightdress and sheets to the mattress. The pain was excruciating, much worse than anything suffered during pregnancy and labour. (Why hadn't the books prepared me for this?) And being an antidrug advocate, I was reluctant to accept medication as a means of relieving the pain. I did not want my 'pure' baby to receive drugs through the breast milk when I had made such a concerted effort to avoid such things during his prenatal development and birth. However, the pain made sleep impossible, and on day three I gave in and took half-a-dose of an offered tablet. Immediately I felt guilty, hypocritical, a failure. This course of action was so against what I believed in.

"On day three Martin could not latch on to the breast unaided at all, because the nipples were unprotrusive. Being a placid baby, he would not work hard at pulling the nipple out. Now I was in pain both physically and emotionally, and the tears flowed. (Talk about 'third day blues'!) I had put so much effort into making things go 'right', and now everything was going 'wrong'. Other women who had pregnancy and/or birth problems were breastfeeding well. Why couldn't I do it? Soon there was only one particular nursing sister who could 'get Martin on', and even then it often took six or more attempts (not a great confidence booster).

"The physical pain continued. Bras seemed to add to the constriction, so I left them off but was told this would make matters worse, so I did not know what to do. Martin began to chew on the nipple because he could not get it behind his gums, and the pain was unbearable. The left breast was producing more milk than the right one, and as the left nipple was inverted more than the right one, Martin would soon give up trying to latch on when offered that side. And so a vicious cycle was set up, with the fuller left breast being harder to empty, leading to more engorgement.

"After conflicting advice about whether and how to express some of the milk – under a hot shower, hand express (which I could not then do efficiently, although I became very skilled in later months), have the breast pumped out, or 'put up with it' – the Kaneson pump was used by a member of the nursing staff to just ease the tighter left breast (150ml of milk was withdrawn in this easing, and there was much more milk remaining). Even with the pump, it took repeated attempts to get the nipple out and the milk flowing, and the pain increased and subsided with each pull on the pump.

"For the next two days the only way that Martin could feed was via the nipple shield. My breasts had softened a little, but the nipples were very sore. By day five I was able to squash my nipples up enough to 'force' (terrible word, but apt) them into Martin's mouth, and he did draw the nipples out enough to suck, but not fully, so there was still some chewing action. I religiously applied anhydrous wool fat and was, oh, so hopeful. Martin began to put on weight, and my 'blues' were over, so I thought.

"Not long after getting home, the engorgement and nipple tenderness problems recurred, eventually leading to blocked ducts. Antibiotics prescribed to combat the blocked ducts provoked an allergic reaction in Martin and had to be discontinued. The nipples became cracked and bled. When Martin cried for a feed, I would begin to cry in anticipation of the pain I would experience as he tried to pull the nipple out but instead chewed on it. Martin then contracted oral thrush, and my nipples became painful 24 hours a day, not just during the suckling time. Martin's weight gains became erratic, which seemed to exert an indirect pressure on me to let him suck longer – I had reached a stage where I timed him at the breast and removed him after ten minutes on each side, this being the absolute maximum time I could endure the pain.

"After three weeks of this, with many lumps and bumps now evident in the left breast, and cracked nipples which did not heal in spite of the application of wool fat and daily exposure to sunlight, I purchased a Kaneson pump in order to ease the engorgement and baby-attachment problems simultaneously. By pumping my milk out and giving it back to Martin via a bottle, the ducts were unblocked and Martin received his mum's milk without the trauma of trying to pull out those buried nipples. (I had to go out and buy bottles, teats, steriliser, etc., as I had not purchased any such things during pregnancy, not anticipating I would have need of them.) It was only after commencing expression using the Kaneson pump that I discovered that my left breast was producing four times as much milk as the right one. No wonder it was always engorged and the nipple invisible!

"Over the next few weeks I was forever trying various methods suggested by nursing mothers, doctors, infant welfare sisters, relatives, etc., to get Martin back fully on the breast. It seemed as if I was spending most of my waking hours on attempting to feed Martin, or washing and sterilising pumps and bottles and teats and nipple shields. I became very tired physically and mentally. My weight dropped considerably and I was emotionally always close to tears. Social life was almost non-existent, and visitors were almost unwelcome. My husband was very supportive as I tried such things as feeding via the nipple shield, expressing some milk first to make the nipple more accessible, complete emptying of the breast and then refeeding via the bottle, drawing the nipple out with the pump and then putting Martin on, and so on. Throughout this time of stress I don't know how my let-down reflex continued to work, but it did.

"Eventually I resorted to expressing my milk via the pump six to eight times a day (and night), and then feeding it back to Martin via a bottle at 6 different times a day (and night). This meant that every second hour I was either expressing or feeding; and with each task occupying three-quarters of an hour by the time washing of equipment was undertaken, life became like treading a tightrope. My husband helped by taking over some of the bottle feeds, allowing me to express at the same time as Martin was being fed. This was particularly helpful during the night, but provoked mixed feelings in me because I felt that I should be feeding Martin, as I would have been doing if feeding directly from the breast. I felt like a cow being milked at the kitchen bench.

"As time went by, pressure mounted to stay 'one bottle ahead' of Martin, and eventually I reached the stage where if he took a particularly large feed then there would be nothing left in the fridge for the next time. Although I continued to offer Martin the breast each day in hope that he would eventually be able to resume breastfeeding, he soon would not take it all and would cry for the bottle (another confidence destroyer for me and more anguish, thinking 'he doesn't even want me anymore').

"My longing to breastfeed Martin seemed to become physical as well as emotional. I began to feel ashamed when we had visitors or went out because Martin was drinking from a bottle. I always had to launch into an explanation about how it was my milk he was drinking. I even feel ashamed to go to Nursing Mothers because I wasn't one. The fact that it was my milk Martin was growing on, and my husband's support, enabled me to continue. But I had to introduce formula to Martin before he was one month of age for those times when I could not keep 'a bottle ahead'. Some days he had 100 per cent breast milk; on other days he would have to have one feed of formula. How I dreaded the first meal of formula – I looked for adverse reactions in bowel motions, behaviour, illness, etc., as if to prove to myself that I would be punished for being such a parent by having an unhealthy child. However, there was no discernible change in Martin, which brought some feelings of relief.

"When Martin was 12 weeks old, my husband had to return to his work of primary school teaching. He had taken long-service leave for Martin's birth (and the final weeks of pregnancy), and in addition the six-week school holiday break over Christmas had meant that he had been home since Martin's birth. Alan also had to resume study commitments. I then had to resume responsibility for five out of six of Martin's feeds, and found that I did not have time to express as often as before. Reluctantly, but for my own mental health and physical well-being (and so, indirectly, the well-being of the whole family), we decided to wean Martin fully on to formula. A further deciding influence was the fact that continued use of the pump had led to blood being expressed with my milk, necessitating a change to hand expression in latter weeks. This was gentler but more time-consuming.

"Anguish surfaced immediately as Martin's milk intake gradually dropped from 1000-1200ml daily of breast milk to only about 700ml a day of formula. I worried that he was going to reject the formula and that he would not grow. He became slightly constipated, and his faeces changed in both form and colour. So then we started on fruit juice, advised by infant welfare sister to speed bowel passage; and I felt guilty about what the formula and juice were doing to Martin's intestinal lining. To further complicate matters, my left breast refused to dry up, and it kept producing for weeks after the right one had ceased production (quite an odd unbalanced feeling, really). I again had blocked-duct problems and had to seek medical attention and finally resort to medication. Now that Martin was not relying on breast milk, I did not have the problem of his allergic reaction to antibiotics I was taking.

"Then at four months of age, Martin showed a great desire to begin solid feeding. He indicated this need by reaching for Mum and Dad's food as it was in transit between plate and mouth, by opening and shutting his mouth as we ate, by wanting his bottles at closer and closer time intervals, and by getting grizzly at adult tea time. I had not envisaged embarking on solids before Martin was six months old, and so I wondered if formula feeding was the catalyst – was something lacking in his diet which would have been supplied by breast milk? Would he have been satisfied on breast milk alone for those two extra months? There was no way of knowing. So, after consultation with the infant welfare sister, we started feeding rice cereal and pureed vegetables and fruits. Right from the start he was able to eat from the teaspoon, and he took to all new tastes with relish. He was soon eating a tablespoonful at each meal. Now, at six months, he eats two 'courses' of solids (still limited to fruit, vegetables and rice cereal) at each meal and has sampled more than 20 types of fruit and vegetables, the only rejection being celery.

"With the introduction of solids, bowel regularity and consistency improved and grizzling ceased. Martin continued to be placid and easy to manage, and outwardly healthy. He continued to sleep, through the night, as he has done since eight weeks of age. He rarely cries, and is alert and happy.

"Yet I still feel guilty. Will Martin's intelligence be lower than its potential because he was not fully breastfed? Will he suffer from premature heart disease because I failed? Is he ingesting too much foreign protein, sodium and fat because he is on formula and solids? In many ways I find myself trying to be Superwoman in order to compensate for my breastfeeding failure, sometimes being very rigid about housework and meals and setting unrealistic standards in these areas.

"Well, I can try again next time. I will certainly wear the Woolwich shields as a first step in my nipple preparation. I will be wiser and more skilled with regard to hand expression when my milk first comes in. But even if I do succeed next time, that does not help Martin. Have I harmed him for life? Is it my fault? Did I do my best? Did I give up too soon? Can I ever cease to feel guilty, hypocritical, a failure?"

- M.J.B.

The answer to that last question should be 'yes'. Obviously this mother did absolutely everything possible to ensure success and has no reason to feel guilty. Would that I had been so careful antenatally! What this case illustrates are the problems of the mother with a bountiful milk supply: without skilled help initially, engorgement will lead to nipple problems, which will be exacerbated by any pump, and so on. We need better techniques developed, we need wider availability of physiological breast pumps like the Whittlestone Milker, we need clinical research into management of engorgement. Would small doses of bromocriptine help in cases of oversupply? These women have been ignored by a medical profession which has emphasised the difficulty Western mothers have in feeding even one baby adequately. The other end of the spectrum – those with the capacity to feed the babies – is thought to be a minority who should consider themselves lucky. But if excess milk causes lactation failure, they are just as badly off as the mother with too little.

Educated caring women like this mother face another hurdle. Their concern to do the right thing is admirable and usually results in a thriving baby, just as the health educators suggest it should. "If only other mothers were like that," say those who try to improve child health. When something goes wrong, however, these mothers' concern is seen as excessive, as neurotic and as the cause of their child's problem. "Of course these educated women have problems – they're so hung up on doing everything perfectly that they're so tense that they cause colic/possetting/bed-wetting/night walking." Australian mothers who choose to breastfeed are more health-conscious, and do tend to take their babies to professionals more often for less serious causes, because they take at face value the advice given to do just that by medical authorities, and because they can afford to. Often they do not want any treatment, merely information and reassurance that this apparently minor condition is not some more serious problem. Doctors are happy to encourage this, but also quite often mentally label as 'over protective' or 'anxious' the mothers who take their advice seriously. Some such mothers sense this, and so they seek out 'alternative' practitioners less likely to put psychological labels on them, or rely more on written information.

This case also illustrates another problem: the way in which educated women can use information to torment themselves. Obviously this baby, born of a healthy mother on a good diet, after an easy birth, has done extremely well on the combination of mother's milk, formula, and solids. Equally obvious is the fact that the mother can never know whether he would have been better/worse on any parameter if he had been exclusively breastfed. The only way forward from this is acceptance: "What's done is done; it was the best I could do (and that a superhuman effort); therefore whatever follows, anxiety is counter-productive and guilt is inappropriate."

It's likely that my book will raise spectres for some women, just as my talk did for this mother. For those of you who identify with this mother, take it from me that the last thing I want to do is create anxiety and guilt. Guilt is only appropriate when, with full knowledge and free consent, you deliberately chose something detrimental to your baby for some trivial selfish reason. I do not know a mother who fits that bill – we all do the best we can, within the limits of our knowledge and other constraints. Therefore, we have no reason to feel guilty.

But of course we do. Guilt is born with the baby, because we can never realise all the ideals we have as parents. We always fall short and feel guilty about doing so. But guilt we have to reject as pointless as we adjust to reality. Anxiety we will feel, off and on, as it too is a universal hazard of parenthood, for which there are no easy cures. I'm writing this as a parent. I too did all sorts of things to my first-born, and have an exquisitely hypersensitive food-intolerant son to show for it (but healthy when on his diet). Knowing more meant that my daughters were spared many of his problems, although I too wish that someone else had written my books before I got pregnant, as I learned more with each of my children. So I must regard it as important to spread this message, not to add another burden to already-overburdened mothers – but to try to prevent more women having to face the problems you and I and Margaret have had.

Now that the book has been revised, I can add that with her next baby, Margaret successfully breastfed exclusively to seven months on one breast alone. (The other nipple persisted in cracking even with the best technique, so she dried up that breast.) I actually heard nothing from her until her second baby was 10 months and she needed help to cure deep breast pain due to thrush (fixed with systemic Nystatin in a week, and her doctor was amazed); then again around 17 months when she had had unnecessary surgery for a benign lump (galactocele) and she wanted to know if she would harm the baby or herself by breastfeeding, because the wound was stretching under the pressure of milk in the breast. I said it was the best thing she could do for herself and him; whereupon she said, "Thank God, I did it half an hour ago and it was wonderful relief, but I've started worrying since!" I haven't heard when this baby was weaned: she was determined that this time she would wean when she and the baby felt like it, not be forced into it by any minor problems like breast surgery! Women are wonderful...

Case History 4

Food-intolerance colic leading to maternal despair

"My daughter is almost seven years old. When she was born I decided to give her the best start by breastfeeding. At this stage I'd already reached the point of physical and emotional exhaustion, because of not being able to tolerate food for the final three months of pregnancy and suffering a mismanaged and nightmarish birth. Three days after she was born she started screaming. When I left the hospital she was totally breastfed and she never improved. She improved a little on Merbentyl, but continued to sleep very little and cried most of the time she wasn't being fed. The only relief we seemed to get was when she was carried facing out on my hip, and that was where she stayed for eight months. It was almost impossible for me to eat a decent meal, let alone prepare one, and I was having 0-6 hours of broken sleep per day. How I coped I don't know. I was depressed, lost most of my friends and found criticism from professionals (it must be my fault), indifference and hostility from other mothers, and did not have the energy to search further afield for assistance. My marriage almost collapsed under the pressure [*many do*]. The NMAA literature was so stridently pro-baby, anti-the needs of mothers, that I rejected it as a source of help. [*This is a common criticism, although no longer really fair. Much has changed over time.*]

"My daughter did not improve greatly until I forcibly weaned her at 15 months old. By 18 months she was sleeping through more nights than she wasn't. My feelings about breastfeeding are therefore very confused and rather anti when it comes to myself. This was the most traumatic period of my life – I was living hour to hour and now feel terribly angry about the whole experience and alienated totally from other mothers.

"At present I'm consulting a psychiatrist for a number of reasons, that difficult and unresolved period of my life being one of them. Since my daughter's birth, my health has been difficult. Four years ago I started having chronic 'hayfever' and 18 months ago accidentally discovered a linkage between this and food allergy which continued to worsen. I feel the allergy situation is linked to the battering I took as a mother. Your book, *Food for Thought*, and other literature has made me see that my difficulties could have been due to the baby being 'allergic'. Although her health has been quite good since, it has been deteriorating over the last 12 months and I think she may have to be assessed for allergies.

"What is this confused letter about? I feel that we have suffered badly through ignorance. The absolute desperation I felt then would probably never have occurred if realistic and not ideologically-based arguments were given credence at that time. There is tremendous damage done to mothers like me by so-called expert opinions on childraising, ignorance of 'grass roots' infant welfare sisters, doctors and the NMAA. There is a great need for information for those who are not the 'norm'. It affects the quality of ongoing parenting, and the emotional well-being and health of the family. If I was trained and articulate I'd campaign against the ignorance of the well-intentioned and do something about informing the other women who suffer because they're different. You are the first person who I've heard speak in a flexible, sensible way on this subject. Thank you, and thank you for tolerating the ramblings of a person just starting to put things back together."

My response to the mother's comments: The irony is that I am also the most intransigently pro-breastfeeding person she has ever heard. My approach does not make mothers feel guilty, because they do not doubt that 'breast is best'. What they need is better understanding of management, and of what it feels like to 'fail' despite their best efforts. They need to know that their 'failure' was not of their doing, consciously or unconsciously. When I get letters like this I think, "There but for Mavis Gunther and the medical literature, and my Fitzroy friends, go I…" I remember the disorientation and exhaustion and demoralisation of Philip's early months. This is what undiagnosed food-intolerance can do.

Case History 5

Breast refusal associated with oral contraception

"I successfully breastfed my first daughter for 16 months without any hitches at all, and she weaned herself with no worries. I mentally and physically loved feeding and scorned people who didn't enjoy it, assuming they didn't try! With my second daughter, I learnt the hard way. At three days old she had sucked up huge blisters and appeared cross and fretful, because it seemed the milk just would not flow. I was horrified, but after encouragement from a very patient mothercraft nurse at the hospital I established a good demand-feed pattern and we happily set off home.

"I guess many would say I did successfully breastfeed, as it lasted six months, but then trouble set in. I just couldn't get her to accept the breast, and the harder I tried the more baby Amy fought me. I knew all the nursing mums' advice even before I rang them, but ring I did. And battle we did, for four weeks, with baby losing weight, waking day and night, hitting, biting and flinging herself backward from me as I tried to feed her. I tried drinking more fluids, resting, more feeds (impossible). Then one night at 2 am, with me crying and very upset baby totally rejecting the breast, screaming and cross, we made up 150ml of formula; baby Amy, never having seen a bottle before, gobbled the lot and (I still remember clearly) sat up, smiled, burped and went to bed sleeping soundly until morning. It broke my heart, I cried all over the wretched bottle, and felt totally unloved, unneeded and rejected, I almost hated her for not wanting me. For weeks I even continued trying desperately to offer me first, but it was useless because even if she was starving she'd wait for the bottle and gobble it up quite delightedly. She's one now, and I still feel sad remembering that my first little one was still being breastfed at that age.

"I still blame myself for not being relaxed enough and persistent enough, but I found that with a three-year-old I could not sit down and rest as I know I should have. I also began the mini-pill about this stage and blame that, too. But I am now convinced that some babies just don't like breastfeeding, and I have certainly learnt to be more tolerant of mums who say to me they couldn't feed.

"From eight weeks to the fifth month I had been ill with an infection of the cervix, and yet it didn't affect the feeding, nor did the endless and varied antibiotics that I took for those few months. It was just that instantly Amy didn't want me. Now doubtful as to whether we will have another baby, I often feel sad that I may never feed again. If we do have another child I imagine I will be terrified it would happen all over again."

What is there to say? Clearly breastfeeding matters to mothers, and clearly professionals are not very sensitive to that possibility. Maternal illness did not affect the baby, and the fact that the first six months were so trouble-free (despite initial positioning problems, leading to blisters) strongly suggests that the cause of breast refusal of sudden onset had little to do with maternal tension or tiredness. This sort of instant dislike is not uncommon; in my experience it often relates to changes in diet or the use of chemicals on or around the nipple (spray underarm deodorants, for example) or oral contraception. Some mothers who notice this fussiness in feeding within a few days of their beginning the Pill have gone back to other methods of contraception, and the baby has stopped fussing as suddenly as she started. We are all different hormonally. Some of us can swallow steroid hormones without any problems; others seem unable to do so. Doctors prescribing oral contraceptives to lactating women should warn mothers of this possibility. However small the minority affected, lactation failure is not an acceptable outcome.

Case History 6

Poor supply associated with initial engorgement, nipple pain and bad management

"During my pregnancy, the doctor told me to roll my nipples out and rub wool fat on them, because they were flat. I worked diligently morning and night rolling them out and trying to toughen them. I lacked confidence about my ability to breastfeed because my mother had had trouble and I kept thinking about that.

"My son was born, and all I wanted to do was feed him. I fed him on one side on the delivery table. I was pleased until the next day, when the trouble began. To make matters worse, I had a fantastic milk supply. I have extremely sensitive skin, which I didn't realise was as bad until my son began sucking. Each sister at the hospital told me to do different things, and I became so confused. I got information from the NMAA (which I'd joined when I was pregnant), and they were helpful. Anyway, I tried creams, ray lamps and everything else suggested to no avail. When I left hospital my milk supply decreased rapidly because of the tension I was experiencing.

"I cried for the first month because I felt such a failure as a mother and a person. It used to upset me incredibly when I had to give my son a bottle. I hated going out, because people would see me giving him a bottle and they would give me strange looks, or so I imagined! I was also upset when people would ask me if I was feeding him. When I would have to reply in the negative, people seemed to make a judgment of me, and my sense of failure seemed to increase. Even now, after 15 months, I am still sensitive about the subject. I can talk about it now, whereas before I would avoid the subject.

"When I become pregnant again, I am hoping to breastfeed and I will attempt to toughen my nipples up more intensively during the pregnancy."

This illustrates the usual engorgement/nipple trauma syndrome. The decrease in milk supply after leaving hospital probably had as much to do with restricted suckling and poor positioning as to inhibition of the ejection reflex due to pain. 'Tension' is not an accurate description. But this letter is included because of the mother's confusion about conflicting advice, and the distress over bottlefeeding. How do we converse about feeding? What should we say after a mother announces that baby is on the bottle? To leave it up in the air, in some embarrassment, leaves the mother to suppose that we are judging her, when we may not be. I usually hazard one further question: "Did you decide to bottlefeed her from the beginning or did you find breastfeeding difficult?" This usually leads to a long conversation about why she 'failed', from which we both learn something.

Case History 7

Probable nipple confusion due to early conditioning; oversupply/food-intolerance colic.

"Even now, as I am two-thirds through my second pregnancy, I still envy happily nursing pairs. To this day I am worried that all may not go well with my second feeding experience, as my first was so disappointing and heartbreaking.

"Andrew was born three weeks early and suffering from hyaline-membrane disease. I was not allowed to feed him myself until day five, but he was fed expressed milk from a bottle from day three. We left hospital on day nine, and Andrew was fully breastfed on demand. Even at that stage he was showing signs of being 'windy' and difficult. I had not bonded as I had hoped to, and I was dismayed when at two weeks it was clear that Andrew was becoming very colicky indeed. At about this time he began refusing at various times and for varying lengths of time. I had no idea what was causing him to refuse the breast, and the lengths between feeds (about six hours) frightened me because he was so young and had previously fed about three-hourly. He was having Merbentyl from a bottle and always sucked greedily from the teat with no sign of refusal.

"At about four weeks Andrew refused for about 19 hours, and I had no choice but to express and feed him my milk from a bottle which he accepted readily. My NMAA counsellor was a tower of strength during this distressing time and encouraged me when I flagged. I was becoming increasingly worried as feed time approached, always wondering if he would fight and kick or feed eagerly. I generally had no problems with the night feeds at this stage, and he usually returned to the breast during the night, often after not having fed from me all day. During this period the colic continued, sometimes three attacks a day during which he would not feed at all, bottle or breast. My main feelings at that time were of terrible rejection and worthlessness. I was disgusted by my abundant milk supply and the fact that Andrew would happily drink my milk from a bottle but not touch me. All through the refusal he continued to stack on the weight, and at times I felt I could never do anything right for my baby.

"When Andrew reached six weeks he refused for 31 hours during which time I practically lived with my NMAA counsellor. He happily drank my expressed milk but screamed and pushed away if I tried to offer the breast. We tried squirting milk into his mouth first, honey on the nipples, ice on the nipples, feeding him while he was asleep and feeding him with a nipple shield. I was coming to resent my son very much, and my poor counsellor had run out of ideas too. At his six-week clinic check, my local Child Health Nurse suggested that I substitute one feed a day with Prosobee as this sometimes reduced colic. Game to try anything, I replaced the afternoon feed with Prosobee and Andrew (typically) drank the new food readily.

"I was nearing breaking point and was so tired I dreaded each new day. It would take me nearly half an hour to express enough for a feed and then a half an hour to feed him by bottle (with tries at the breast in between times), so I did the natural thing and replaced yet another feed with Prosobee. Immediately my supply dropped, but the refusal and colic continued so all his feeds except the two night feeds came from a bottle. I was desperately ashamed of my 'weakness' in resorting to the bottle more than the breast, but I was so tired and despondent that I knew I was fighting a losing battle. By the time he was eight weeks old I even stopped expressing, as I was so resentful and depressed. I would cry as I fed him by bottle but I still offered him the breast first and on very rare occasions he would suck for a brief time. My counsellor still encouraged me and tried to make me understand that I had not failed Andrew, in fact he had failed me.

"I gave Andrew his last breastfeed at nine weeks three days, and to my absolute disgust he never had another attack of colic! I finally put him on to S26 and he never gained weight as well as he did on breastmilk. He happily bottle-fed until he was 14½ months, but I felt rejected for many of those months and ashamed to feed him a bottle in public.

"I'd like to point out that I had a good quick let-down reflex and an abundant supply and that Andrew had no physical reason for refusing the breast. I have dissected the problem a hundred times and still have no solution, but I console myself that he is now a very happy and well adjusted toddler, and with the new baby coming I hope to feed for a long time, although I will take it as it comes.

"I have the greatest compassion for those who I meet through NMAA and elsewhere who are forced to stop feeding for some reason or another, but I have never met a case quite like mine. I was so sad and confused at that time, and I had to put up with a lot of hurtful remarks from relatives and friends who insisted that I was trying to 'force'-feed Andrew. I still resent the fact that our relationship was so short, and I pray that I won't make the same mistake twice."

This is the sort of case where seeing the baby breastfeed is essential to diagnosis. Possible explanations lie in the early exposure to formula (up to day three) and conditioning of suckling patterns. A baby who was difficult by day nine also suggests intrauterine sensitisation and colic in response to maternal dietary antigen; it is more usual for neonatal exposure to formula to result in colic 10-20 days after birth. Episodic breast refusal fits the food-intolerance hypothesis, as does the willingness to feed at night but not during the day. (Why, I don't know, but several mothers of food-intolerance children have commented on this as a notable feature.) Why should Andrew accept milk from a bottle? It could be that the strong chemical/rubber taste disguised the taste of the allergen in the milk sufficiently for him to accept it – babies can be proper little gourmets! Or it might be that Andrew had trouble coping with the abundant supply, rapid ejection reflex, or just the way he was being held to breastfeed, or had never learned to suckle the breast comfortably after his early bottle conditioning. Here one would need to observe the feed carefully.

I suspect that this was a combination of both problems. The disappearance of colic when breastfeeding ceased strongly suggests that something in maternal diet was a contributing factor. Did this mother smoke? Drink lots of tea and coffee? Have a history of food addiction/aversion? Binge in pregnancy? Take vitamin supplements, brewers yeast, etc? To suggest the most reasonable course of action for the future, I would need to have much more information.

Note again the pain the mother felt, both when difficulties were in progress and when bottlefeeding. An experience like this makes many mothers give up more quickly next time because they no longer believe that they are capable of successful breastfeeding.

Is it fair for a counsellor to suggest that the mother did not fail the child, he failed her? Will this help the mother who perceives her child as responding negatively to her, as refusing, rejecting, 'difficult'? I have seen families shattered by the realisation that they have unfairly categorised one child as difficult, when they now see clearly that the causes were totally outside the child's personality. So please, do not encourage mothers to see their babe in arms as having failed them. Rather, the professionals have failed them all.

Case History 8

Probable low supply

"I am 29, a teacher and mother of Kate who is now eight months. I tend to be the sort of person who expects the worst (secretly knowing that it probably won't happen) so that I can be pleasantly surprised when it doesn't. I 'expected' to cop all the problems of pregnancy... and breezed through it with only a little back-ache. I 'expected' a long painful labour... instead Kate was born less than five hours after my first contraction. Funnily enough, I had never given a thought to the possibility that I might fail at breastfeeding. All my friends and relations fed their babies (apparently effortlessly), and in fact I was inwardly very critical of people I saw bottle-feeding. I read Virginia Phillips' book *Successful Breastfeeding*, and how also Dr Llewellyn Jones' *Breast-feeding: How to Succeed*, and I knew that all you had to do was relax, feed frequently, use anhydrous lanolin on the nipples, and any problem could be simply overcome! I also knew that the hospital here is a little old-fashioned, and babies are 'comped' while the mother's milk comes in. I decided that I would not argue with the nurses, but I would feed my baby whenever I wanted to and just hope for no problems!

"In fact I didn't really have any problems in hospital – slightly engorged breast for a short time. Kate was keen to suck and in fact would suckle as long as I let her. She usually would not settle well after a feed, and I would pick her up and suckle her again. The nurses said 'She's only using you as a dummy' or 'She won't suck long on an empty breast' so I did get a little confused and was glad to get home.

"I was surprised how little Kate would sleep. Feed her, put her down, hang out the nappies, come inside, crying baby! I kept waiting for her to settle into a pattern of three- or four-hourly feeds, but she never did. This is where contact with other mothers or NMAA would have been useful, as the books didn't stress the fact that some babies need very frequent feeds. I was never sure if I should feed her. Her worst time was the evenings when I'd go to bed, and my husband would spend a couple of hours walking Kate around. Looking back, I'm sure she was hungry. In fact I wrote in my diary when she was only 11 days old, 'She seems to be satisfied with 10 minutes each side if she has a swallow with each suck. When it's three or four sucks to a swallow, she wants to keep going all the time.'

"When Kate was six weeks old, it suddenly dawned on me that she was hungry most of the time. Up until then I had felt quite competent and confident – lots of people commented that I didn't seem like a 'new Mum'! I started expressing in the morning to try to build up my supply, and in the evening I would feed her and then give her my expressed milk, which she'd gulp down in record time and want more! I once gave her some glucodin and she slept for a record six hours! Because all my efforts to build up my supply didn't seem to work as the books promised, I got more and more worried – the thought of perhaps having to bottle-feed gave me a knot in the stomach, so although I tried to relax, I was obviously very uptight. I never had that real 'let-down' feeling, but that didn't seem to be the problem – there obviously just wasn't enough milk there. In the morning there was quite a lot, my breasts would sometimes leak, and I could express an ounce or two after a feed. But as the day went on, even if I did virtually nothing, my supply dwindled. However, Kate has always gone three or four hours at night; I think she was so tired after feeding and being awake most of the day, that she would sleep from sheer exhaustion.

"The infant welfare sister was very supportive and was surprised that all my efforts were not really succeeding. She was also surprised that I got a dose of mastitis when I was attending a conference, leaving expressed milk for the baby. In fact, because Kate was putting on a little weight and had quite a few wet nappies, the only way I knew she was hungry was from her unsettledness, the five or six sucks before she had enough milk to swallow, and the way she would gulp down the expressed milk.

"I came home from a (Thursday) visit to the Health Centre determined to give it another week before giving in to comping Kate. I fed her almost non-stop for three hours and the rest of the day seemed quite good (although she was awake from 6 pm till 11.30 pm as usual). The next day I fed her almost constantly from 10 am till 12.30 am (i.e. over 14 hours), but on the Saturday morning my breasts were not even tight.

"In Dr Llewellyn Jones' book there was a drug mentioned, called metaclopromide, which was known to release prolactin. I asked my doctor about it when I was at seven weeks for my check-up. He had not heard of this use – his book indicated it was used to stop vomiting, hiccoughs, etc. The infant welfare sister was much more interested and rang the Queen Vic. Breastfeeding Advisory Clinic. She found that they were using it there under the name Maxolon, to help mothers of prem. babies keep up their supply. So on the Saturday morning, I went to my doctor and told him this, and he gave me a script. On the Saturday/Sunday there was no improvement and on Sunday night, exhausted, I gave Kate a bottle of half-strength formula. She totally demoralised me by drinking 150 ml, sleeping for two hours, and drinking another 150 ml. I continued to take the Maxolon and gave comps only in the evening – Kate put on 250 g in five days! I started to feel very 'woozy' from the Maxolon and, as my husband was at home on holiday, did virtually nothing but sleep and feed Kate all day. Everyone said I looked like a zombie and I really felt as if I wasn't all there. When I would lie down, I wouldn't really sleep, and could feel myself dribbling. I stopped taking the Maxolon and immediately felt better.

"Suddenly, Kate started going three or four hour between feeds, and I didn't have to 'comp' her for two days. By this time it was Christmas, and I was really happy to be fully breastfeeding again. We had a quiet Christmas and at home. On Boxing Day, my supply again ran out in the evening and at 1 am I let John give her 120mls of formula. I was really upset, and this was the time I needed someone to talk to. The infant welfare sister was away, and I tried contacting NMAA members, but no one answered their phones.

"From then on, the comps gradually got earlier and earlier, and Kate became less keen on suckling at the breast. She had always been happy to suck as long as I let her, but as she got older, it became more of a battle. I battled on till five months, until she was only feeding from me first thing in the morning – and finally she rejected that feed too. It was almost a relief to not have to try any more.

"At about four months I tried to use NMAA Supply-Line and found that helped a little to build up my supply. But at that stage it was a battle to get Kate to feed. I feel that if I'd used it first, instead of comping, it would perhaps have been helpful.

"I use to believe that people who said that they 'couldn't' breastfeed had not really tried. Perhaps I tried too hard. In a way, having bottlefed, and realising that it isn't as bad as I thought it would be, I will at least not panic if future babies have the same problems. In other words I will be more relaxed and hopefully more successful.

"The sense of failure I feel over this has been very strong. I would feel myself close to tears whenever I spoke about it and for months it was my only topic of conversation. It's only since Kate was fully weaned that it no longer upsets me, although writing this brings it all back! I used to silently condemn bottle-feeding mothers, and therefore I feel people will condemn me. In fact I was never embarrassed about breastfeeding in public – I am about bottle-feeding. I feel that people will think I am one of those who didn't really try. Most people can't understand why I feel such a sense of failure. I think that part of it is that I am used to being able to do the things I really want to. It is very frustrating when your body lets you down. In some ways I would feel better if I could put my finger on what I did 'wrong', then I could do the 'right' thing next time. Surprisingly, I feel confident about 'next time'."

This seems to me like a case of low supply of hormonal origin: the genuine 'poor milker' like me. The pattern of evening insufficiency is common; I and many other mothers have since managed this by organising to express milk in the mornings while feeding (see p. 111) and store it for supplementing in the evening. While the rate at which baby gulped down her bottle is related to the teat hole, the suck/swallow ratio at the breast makes it clear that baby is not getting enough. Of course, this may be due to something other than hormonal pattern; if the baby were not correctly positioned she might be unable to milk the breast efficiently. If the mother has sufficiently elastic breast tissue and protractile nipples, it might be possible to be badly positioned without nipple damage ensuing, although this is unlikely. Mothers need to know, however, that some babies will guzzle down any amount from any bottle, even if they regurgitate it all later, so simply taking milk proves little about what they need. It is a little unclear whether this baby was frequently fed in the early days of 'ten minutes each side'... this may have been a case where early ad libitum feeding may have improved the outcome. But I am not sure that the Supplyline could be expected to achieve more than frequent early feeding (Philip, after all, suckled constantly without apparently increasing the volume produced, through his vigorous suckling on an 'empty' breast certainly seemed to extract plenty of fat, if his weight was any guide!) This baby may have needed more self-regulated suckling. The evening wakefulness and unsettledness may also have had other causes; mothers also need to know that babies' sleep patterns are very varied.

The reaction to Maxolon is interesting. Have other readers has experience of this drug, and with what results? Does anyone know of controlled clinical trials assessing dosages, indications, contra-indications, and so on, in breastfeeding?

Note again, too, how much this biological process matters to the mother.

Case History 9

Possible transient milk intolerance; nipple pain; traumatic birth

"My daughter was born after 15 hours of labour; during labour I used gas, pethidine and finally a epidural. Her birth was induced, she was a forceps delivery and had the cord around her neck. I mention this because I feel that the birth was partly responsible for the trouble we had feeding.

"She spent her first 24 hours of life in a humidicrib. I had tried unsuccessfully to feed her on the delivery table, but to be honest, I was more interested in sleep than suckling my daughter. Whilst in the humidicrib, the nursing staff were bottle-feeding her, and I distinctly remember one sister being more than a little annoyed that the baby would not take the quantity required, much less in a reasonable time. During the four days I stayed in the hospital, the nursing staff tried help me feed, although I felt we were doing fine. One of the sisters was quite rough when helping, and she and I became rather miffy with each other because I refused her help on several occasions.

"The hospital was rigid about four-hourly feeding. I used to sneak in feeds and, if caught, received very black looks; however the staff were not quite game to say much. I felt very sorry for the girl in the next room, who after having feeding difficulties with her first child, started from scratch artificially feeding her second baby (born the same day as mine). I remember her getting upset when the staff would not let her make up a bottle because her son wanted a feed an hour earlier than allowed, and eventually she had to wheel him back to the nursery because his crying was upsetting her too much.

"When we finally got home (I was pleased to be out of hospital) the feeding became more of a chore than I could have imagined. On reflection, I remember worry about dirty nappies that needed washing, dinners that needed preparation, and all the general household duties that I felt needed doing. I can remember that many times when I was feeding I was tense thinking about what should have been done but wasn't. In a nutshell, I believed my breastfeeding failed because I could not relax. The baby was like a little magnet when it came to picking up tension, which in turn caused 'colic' and so the circle kept going round. I think we kept trying for about three weeks. After that time I just gave up and put her on formula.

"With regard to pain during breastfeeding, I remember when she first took the nipple it hurt like hell, just like a wild animal latching on. I remember when I had put her on the bottle I felt relief, on the one hand, and a feeling of inadequacy on the other. The relief, because she was satisfied and because I could measure what she was eating and knew she wasn't starving. The feeling of inadequacy resulted from the idea that I was going to breeze the whole breastfeeding business. None of the literature I read even hinted at the hassles one could have. Pride was also a big factor in my feelings.

"Just before I decided to give up breastfeeding, my husband and I took the baby to our paediatrician to see if there was any reason for consistent crying. He rightly suggested that I should go home and do nothing but feed her when she wanted it. He also was adamant there is was no such thing as 'wind' and that burping was unnecessary. This latter I would dispute. Well I went home and tried to do nothing but feeding the baby. However, nappies don't wash themselves, and my husband was not inclined to be helpful, so feeding was abandoned. Also the baby had lost more weight than was considered healthy, and this reinforced my decision to artificially feed her.

"In summing up the reasons I failed to feed, I would say that she was a lazy feeder, I was too tired and tense to relax when feeding her, my husband could have helped with housework (no grandmothers within 1000km), and overworked nursing staff could have been gentler and more encouraging than they were. If we have another baby, I feel I will be wiser regarding feeding, probably more competent (I felt lacking in the mothering department), and if I fail again, I have promised myself no guilt or feelings of inferiority.

"Regarding current feeding, she eats everything. Until yesterday the only thing she had a dislike for were fresh strawberries, but she has since changed her mind and now absolutely nothing in the house is sacred. Included in her list of edible food, is avocado, fried onions, garlic bread, fish… you name it, she'll eat it. Since taking on more solid foods, her whole personality has become very contented, whereas the first three months she was constantly waking in the middle of the night, would not sleep for long during the day, and was, to say the least, a real little grizzle. I could not complain about her behaviour now. She is very alert, sleeps very soundly during the night and is generally a very content little girl.

"One thing you may be interested in is that fresh pawpaw after milk feeds seem to settle the stomach of even the most vomit-prone child and keeps the milk down. My baby was a persistent vomiter, and an old lady told me to give her pawpaw. It works!"

Again, iatrogenic failure which the mother ascribes to the wrong causes. This mother had fissured nipples, in itself a cause of inhibited supply and a sure sign of inadequate attachment: yet she has been persuaded that tension was the problem! The pawpaw bit is interesting: perhaps the enzymes helped digest the protein?

Case History 10

Probable food-intolerance-induced failure to thrive

"I am writing in response to your request in the NMAA newsletter re feeling a failure of breastfeeding, as I have experienced this emotion after each attempt at breastfeeding. Just briefly I'll relate my history.

"I had read books and literature before the birth of our first child, e.g., *Successful Breastfeeding* by Virginia Phillips, and in one book I remember reading that 98 per cent of women can successfully breastfeed given optimal knowledge, encouragement and advice. So with this in mind I fought against clinic sisters and doctors who told me otherwise: that not all women can breastfeed and I just happened to be unlucky, even though I gave all my energy and effort and was bitterly disappointed when I had to stop because the baby was not thriving. Then followed about 12 months of minor depression which was rooted in the thought that I had failed as a mother. I can remember thinking: 'this baby doesn't need me now... anyone can give her a bottle... only her mother can breastfeed her now.' While I was suffering from depression I couldn't look at or talk to easily with other women who were breastfeeding, and if I was in a position where I had to give the baby a bottle in front of others I felt they were judging me as a poor mother. So I used every opportunity to talk about my reason for bottle-feeding, and I would try to impress on people I really thought breastfeeding was the best though I couldn't do it.

"Our second daughter was born when Lisa was two and a half years old, and I joined NMAA at this stage. Our experience with Lisa had resulted in a lot of tenseness in the family, and combined with my inexperience as a first-time mother we attribute a lot of Lisa's early behavioural problems (poor sleeping, nightmares, extreme temper tantrums) to our 'bad' start. Marie was born, and right from the start she slept heavily. Often I'd have to wake her at the four-hourly intervals for feeds. I'll admit I was reluctant to break this pattern to rely on more frequent breastfeeds in hope it would boost my supply – my experience with Lisa was still too raw. So Marie was 'comp'-fed on a regular four-hourly right from hospital, and needless to say breastfeeding soon suffered; she was weaned by three and a half weeks. (Then followed a quite bad allergy reaction to cow's milk, so she was put on soy milk, then goats' milk. Now at three years of age, Marie is still having problems with failure to thrive – she's tall but underweight. She has already had blood, urine and faeces tests which showed no disease. And a breath hydrogen test for lactose intolerance was negative, even though she had quite positive reactions: watery puffy eyes, sneezing and a running nose for a week afterwards, loose frequent motions for 48 hours after, sleepy and irritable for a week after. I believe this isn't very reliable so my next step is to go to a good naturopath for advice.)

"Prior to the birth of our third child I read lots of literature, spoke to lots of people and was again convinced that optimal knowledge and encouragement, I could 'do it', i.e. breastfeed. Well, I battled on for three weeks breastfeeding Peter exclusively, in consequence exhausting myself as he literally latched on for what seemed like 24 hours a day. He had lost 250 g of his birth weight and took three and a half weeks to regain it: no weight gain in the first week, 85 g by 10 days, no weight gain in the next week, and 165 g in the third week. This see-saw pattern was of great concern to me, as I was keen to see a definite improvement in the success or otherwise by following all the advice and recommendations I had been given. But with the other children and my very long-suffering husband to consider, I (or we) made the decision to complement-feed him to ease the pressure on the constant attention being given to Peter. This put us in a dilemma, because with cows' milk allergy present in the family I was against giving any form of cows' milk formula; but as I had had skin allergy tests done on myself, which showed an allergy to soybean, I also decided against giving a soybean formula. This left goats' milk, which we decided on. The decision was still a very difficult one to make, after all the high hopes. I gave the complement by the Supply-Line to avoid the easy teat of a bottle, but this took ages so I wasn't gaining any extra time for the rest of the family. Therefore, more and more I relied on giving a bottle which was quicker.

"About the time he was 10 or 12 weeks old it became apparent that a lot of his crying and feeding problems (he would cry unless being carried over the shoulder and would frequently baulk at both breast and bottle) were caused by a medical problem, and sure enough we found out that he had gastric reflux with probably oesophagitis (although an endoscopy wasn't performed). Once we started treating him with Gaviscon and Mylanta and started him on cornflour blancmange and rice cereal, he improved very quickly and gained weight rapidly. During the fourth month I battled on with breastfeeding hoping as he took more solids he would want less bottle complements, but alas that didn't happen and by five months I gave up breastfeeding.

"Now I'm pregnant with our fourth child (unplanned, but welcome all the same), and I'm in a real quandary as to what to do for this one. I'm definitely strongly committed to breastfeeding being best – especially with allergies in the family – but honestly, what do I do for the best? My experience with Peter has convinced me that I've done everything possible and I still haven't succeeded. When I look back at photos of Peter in those first few weeks I realise how skinny and drawn he looked, and yet at the time I didn't want to admit that he wasn't getting enough.

"Please advise me; do you know anyone in Brisbane who researches breastfeeding, someone I could talk to at length and who could give me some explanations for my low supply. Is it hormonal, or am I so uptight in my emotions about breastfeeding that I can't relax? [*No! She'd know if she was.*]

"Also how reliable are the skin prick allergy tests? I had them done when I was seven weeks pregnant with Peter and showed 17 reactions including strong reactions to cows' milk, beef, pork, coffee and soybeans. I've tested myself by elimination diets and cows' milk, beef, pork and coffee do make me feel sick, but I didn't like the taste of soybeans so I didn't persevere with testing."

This mother needs specialist help from a lactation consultant who knows about allergy and intolerance. She might be one of the small minority who for physical reasons cannot lactate adequately. But until feeding techniques have been reviewed in careful detail, and then food intolerance investigated in both mother and baby, that conclusion is premature. Nor should it be made without some investigation of maternal hormonal levels, breast structure, and so on.

Many such mothers, neglected by conventional medicine, resort to alternative medicine and are then condemned as neurotic and obsessive. The negative breath hydrogen test on her daughter may (or may not) have ruled out lactose/milk sugar malabsorption, but its positive accompanying symptoms strongly suggest cows' milk intolerance, as no commercial lactose is so pure as to be without traces of milk protein to which sensitive children can react. Had the test been positive, a diagnosis of lactose/sugar intolerance would have been accepted. But doctors do not believe protein intolerance is common, so these symptoms will be ignored. The prospects for her fourth baby are not encouraging. Should breastfeeding be impossible the baby should be fed a low-allergy formula, preferably Neocate, an elemental formula. However, in Australia babies must usually prove they need this by becoming very sick after being made intolerant, first to cow milk and soy milk, and then cow-milk based hydrolysate formulas. Such fun for everyone…

Case History 11

Simple hospital-induced lactation failure – and success

"Jason and Natalie were born in a fairly large hospital when I was 23 and 25 years old, respectively. Adam was born in a small but good country hospital. When Jason was born the hospital was very rigid and did not really encourage breastfeeding. Mothers were permitted to cuddle (not feed) about six hours after the birth, and allowed(!) to feed after 24 hours because the baby must have only glucose water first. Then the baby was brought at four-hourly intervals accompanied by a bottle of formula, usually hoarse from crying, and full of wind. Being rather shy and having no knowledge of breastfeeding or advice – except 'wash the nipple, cream the nipples and feed for two minutes only at first' needless to say I was discharged from hospital with very little milk, no let-down, a bundle of nerves and a screaming baby. Jason was only two weeks old when I gave up trying to breastfeed and gave him formula completely.

"When Natalie was born two years later, I was optimistic about breastfeeding and thought things were going fine. I still had to beg to see my baby after about five hours and was not to feed her till next day, but no bottle arrived with her, which I thought was great. They even brought her to me during the night. I loved it until, on day four, my hopes were shattered when the aide who brought the babies (we were not encouraged to visit the nursery except to show baby to visitors) demanded to know what I was feeding Natalie as the poor kid was starving. No one had said jaundiced babies are sleepy babies, and I thought she'd been contented. I also discovered they were tube-feeding her as well. I was down but not out, so I went home armed with formula for 'complements only'. I was told not to feed under three hours, breastfeed for only 10 minutes each side, and then complement. This I did faithfully (with her bringing up most of the comp), for four weeks, until the demands of a two-year old and a clinic sister who said that 110g weight gain in one week was not enough, made me decide to give up the breastfeeding.

"I was devastated and was tempted to try again after 24 hours of being engorged, but didn't think it would be the right thing to do. No one said, 'don't give up the breast, give up the bottle'. I felt very depressed and a failure. Even five years later I felt cheated and would shed a tear. I should add that because of financial problems I went back to work part-time when Natalie was three months old, so bottle-feeding was more convenient for baby-sitters. My supply was never abundant, so expressing milk would have been out of the question. I felt I wasn't a good and proper mother as all my friends had been able to breastfeed (although I realise they were fortunate in having a good supply early and may not have been really committed because they all put their babies on the bottle by three to five months).

"When we moved to a small country town two and a half years ago I was able to give up work. After a while we decided to have another baby, and this time I was determined and my husband also was adamant I would breastfeed. As soon as I became pregnant I joined our local NMAA, which was the smartest move I ever made. With the help and encouragement from NMAA leaflets, counsellors and suggested books, I can now joyfully say I've succeeded. Adam was born in early January. The hospital sisters were pro-breastfeeding so when he was an hour old I cuddled and suckled him. He roomed-in during the day, and the only top-ups he was given were with expressed breast milk and only after my permission had been sought. It hasn't been easy. I still didn't have an overabundant supply and I also had an alert non-sleepy baby, which meant I seemed to be always feeding him, but I persevered and it was worth it. No bottles to prepare, no solids until five and a half months, no cranky baby waiting for a bottle to warm. I feel fulfilled now, and while I love all my children equally, I feel closest to Adam because of the experience of breastfeeding from the first hour after birth."

Case History 12

Nipple and breast problems; poor medical advice leading to abrupt weaning
"My baby (first child) was born five weeks ago. During our stay in hospital the sisters were very supportive in trying to establish the feeding. I seemed to have no pain whilst in hospital and was convinced that all would go smoothly.

"When I got home my left nipple became badly cracked, and I eventually developed an infected breast. The doctor prescribed antibiotics and asked if I thought I could hand-express for the next five days. I couldn't even touch the breast itself because it was so sore, let alone having to pull on it to express milk. I there and then made up my mind to put Michelle on the bottle, and the doctor prescribed tablets to dry up my milk.

"I was a bit upset when I got home from the doctor, but I certainly didn't feel a failure. However, when certain friends found out I had changed to the bottle, they made me feel guilty. These women had successfully breastfed their children and made it known to me that I had given up too easily. I was told that my baby would suffer from the changeover to the bottle and that breast milk was much better for the baby. I was very angry with these people for telling me these things and more. They made me feel that I was depriving Michelle of the best thing I could offer her. She has not suffered from the change, and even though I can't look down and see her suckling on my breast, I can still look into her eyes and convey the love I have for her. Her weight has gone from 3685g at birth to 4535g at five weeks, so I can see she is not doing too badly at all.

"To sum up my experience, I would like to say that in failing to breastfeed I have not suffered in any way with the relationship with my baby. However, I have suffered in the friendship field with a couple of my closest friends. I plan to breastfeed my second child if I can, and try not to take too much notice of other people's views on the subject."

The outcome for the baby of this abrupt weaning due to poor management is not yet known. The mother was fortunate to escape breast abscess. However, the loss of intimacy with some of her closest friends may prove to be a serious break in the network of support that all mothers need, especially with their first baby. While the friends are quite correct (although some babies cope well with the change to formula), to blame the mother for following the doctor's advice is unreasonable. They would do better to accept the mother's decision and help her cope, while writing or talking to the doctor to tell him how poor such practice is.

Case History 13

Food intolerance colic; iatrogenic lactation failure

"My daughter Kiri was born five and a half weeks premature, and it was a very long and tiring labour (25 hours). Despite this she was in good condition and the only problem was that she hadn't developed a sucking reflex. Due to the incidence of allergy in my family, I was particularly anxious to breastfeed and was surprised to be asked (while still in the labour ward) what formula I wished her to be fed. When I requested the use of pooled breast milk, because of the family history, I was told that it was kept for babies much more premature than mine.

"Unfortunately all my worst fears were realised. At about four weeks, just before I left the Mothercraft Hospital, Kiri was still only partially breastfed and was being comped with Nan, and she began to develop extreme colic. After my return home this became worse. A typical pattern day would be that I would feed her, she would be fine for half an hour and then start screaming for two hours, and then fall into exhausted slumber for an hour or more before the whole cycle started again. Despite this I managed to get her fully breastfed at eight weeks. However, she then stopped gaining weight, and because of my exhaustion my milk supply would not increase. Even though now fully breastfed, she screamed with colic as before.

"By about 12 weeks I had to reintroduce comps, and the clinic sister at Karitane suggested that the mixed feeds (of breast milk and Nan) might be upsetting her. I decided to wean her. After two weeks on milk formula, I changed her to Prosobee. This gave a substantial improvement in the colic problem for a while; however, within a month she began to throw up all the time. Despite this she continued to grow very well, and I continued feeding her Prosobee. At about five months she was admitted to hospital with diarrhoea, and at six months she started suffering from middle-ear infections (an ongoing problem). When she was 12 months, I took her to the allergist who diagnosed an IgA deficiency (which would have been ameliorated by breastfeeding). She also has multiple food allergies.

"In this respect I feel I have failed to provide her with extra protection she needed because of her genetic makeup. I put these developments down to several things: feeding of milk formula in hospital; her premature birth; poor advice from the clinic sister, who did not seem to understand (and should have) the likely problems of my ceasing breastfeeding and the cause of my baby's 'colic'. I am particularly angry with the hospital for not feeding her with pooled breast milk as requested, especially as I later discovered that they were being closed down; and their stocks of frozen milk would have been sufficient for Kiri's needs.

"Although not available at the time, a Lact-Aid would have been very useful to me, as continuous expressing was aggravating my tenosynovitis. Since I am a single parent I do not intend having any more children. I would otherwise have loved a chance to get it right. I can only regret not using NMAA before my baby was born."

Toni Adams

I only regret that *Food for Thought* was not published in time to spare this mother such problems. Kiri's food allergies should have been evident to any health worker from this history, long before 12 months. Curing this colic would have meant modifying maternal diet, as outlined in *Food for Thought*. In the process, some degree of maternal food intolerance would no doubt have become obvious. In many such cases on record, members of the family in three generations have come to realise that their 'allergy' problems, whether asthma, hayfever, joint pain or skin rash, all have a food component that can be readily modified.

Case History 14

Cardiac defect leading to poor feeding; immediate worsening when formula feeding inappropriately prescribed

"I successfully breastfed our first son for 21 months and was looking forward to feeding our next baby. When our second son, Graham, was born I automatically breastfed him and continued until he was three and a half months.

"Our problems began at three weeks, when he started to have a low weight gain (about 55 g per week) for no apparent reason. I fed him every three or four hours and was sure he was taking enough; he would go to sleep for two or three hours at a time. I thought we had a perfect baby. But at six weeks a heart murmur was diagnosed, and still he wasn't putting on enough weight because although he seemed to be happy with what he was getting he tired easily. At 11 weeks further tests were done; it was discovered he had two holes in his heart. We weren't sure how big they were.

"I was in a mothercraft hospital for eight days. I expressed my breast milk as they used a squeeze bottle to feed him (in other words, forcefeed). He was put on a sedative before a feed, so that he would feed a lot better. [*where is the logic here, when sedation makes for poorer feeding?*] I knew he was sick, I also knew and kept telling them that he didn't belong there, I knew that his heart was a lot worse than it was made out to be. My efforts to convince people were getting nowhere, and eventually after eight days I was allowed to go home. In the meantime he had several fevers and a cold or two. Six days later, after a tiring time and a refusal to feed, we saw a top cardiologist who said that an operation was needed but not just yet. We went back into the mothercraft hospital under pressure from my doctor, and Graham was put on a formula because he was losing weight. By then I was really cross as I knew that my son belonged in a proper hospital, he was sick and in distress, his condition was deteriorating every day. After the second bad night he was transferred to the local hospital; by the end of the week he was transferred to a Sydney hospital by air ambulance.

"In Sydney, we were informed that the baby needed open heart surgery or would die within the year. He was being fed Isomil by tube, which was the best they could feed him so that he wouldn't tire as much, and in July he was operated on. He did not have the strength to suck on my breast, so has been bottle-fed [*which takes more effort!*] and has a dummy helping him to suck; also we found that when he was getting breast milk he had a rash on his face and the food used to go straight through him. [*Possible intolerance to foods in maternal diet; this in turn may have been part of the reason for poor weight gain.*] Since the operation our son has been thriving on Isomil. I no longer care what food he gets as long as he can tolerate it. [*40% of cows'-milk-intolerant children become soy-intolerant too.*]

"I didn't fail to breastfeed Graham, but it ceased too soon: through his heart condition he was unable to suck hard which is required to suckle the breast. [*nonsense: cf. p. 100*] I know that the bonding won't be the same but I plan to use baby massage on him and carry him in a possum pouch, so that I won't miss out on the closeness. I am looking forward to having him home and bringing him up as a normal little boy.

"My experience in Sydney opened my eyes as to the number of babies who couldn't be fed because of hospitalisation quite soon after birth. In some cases the mother continued to express, but for the majority of babies long-term hospitalisation meant it was awkward for mothers to keep expressing. A lot of mothers gave up, and I realise how hard it was for them not to feed their children."

Did a change to cows' milk and then soy milk benefit this sick child? Would elimination of maternal dietary antigens and continuance of breastfeeding have provided him with better nutrition and immunological protection? Is drinking from a bottle and sucking a dummy less tiring than breast feeding? Is it true that 'bonding won't be the same'? Will sedatives help a baby suckle more vigorously? No prizes for guessing that I think four out of five answers are probably 'no', though this requires individual assessment.

As for the general question, everyone accepts that a few babies cannot be breastfed because of illness. The number involved is fewer nowadays than ever before. However, it is reasonable to ask whether it is not those babies who most need human milk available to them, whatever the problems of collecting and storing and using banked human milk. Yes, there would be problems. But there are problems with synthetic substitutes too. Mothers would feel less distress about giving up breastfeeding if the alternative also offered substantial immunological benefits and was easily bioavailable.

Case History 15

Low supply despite good knowledge and motivation

"I'm very interested in your research into breastfeeding as I've been unsuccessful twice now and would love to succeed if there's a next time. I must admit that finding out why it doesn't work for me and overcoming the problems would influence my decision about having more babies. The depression and utter frustration I felt when I 'failed' remain – a year after giving up the battle to partially breastfeed my second child.

"Before my first child was born I read widely about feeding and took it for granted that, like my sister and my friends, I would fully breastfeed my baby and continue to do so until the child initiated the weaning process. That was my theory! However, the reality proved different. Firstly, after an uncomplicated labour, the newborn baby did not want to suck and thrashed about trying to escape the delivery room staff's efforts to 'latch her on'. Secondly, she had a blood incompatibility problem which meant she was taken away to the Special Care Nursery for a couple of days, and I had to use a breast pump to try to encourage milk to come. She was never interested in sucking from me and I did not produce much milk, so the paediatrician who was treating her insisted that she be given formula as well.

"Once home (and still determined to breastfeed) I contacted NMAA and was told to feed more frequently, to spend days in bed with her, 'increasing supply'. I tried that and found it one of the worst experiences of my life! Imagine a baby who did not enjoy nipple sucking and who never found her efforts rewarding enough to fill her hungry tummy sufficiently to put her to sleep, trapped with a determined mother. She thrashed and screamed with hunger and I cried with frustration. At the six-week check-up, the family GP (who, unlike some doctors, believes breastfeeding to be a good thing) announced she was not progressing under this regime and really needed food.

"Back to the Nursing Mothers' counsellor, who had two suggestions. My being 'uptight' was preventing 'let-down', so a $10-a-sniffer prescription of oxytocin was recommended. (I went through three of these.) And the baby should be given the formula through a Lact-Aid device which drips formula from a capillary tube on to the mothers' nipple so the baby must still suck her to get the goodies. This was rented to me by NMAA, with many anecdotes about the successful users and much positive propaganda about how my own milk would gradually take over from the present "necessary evil" of S26 formula. My baby put up with her mother's idiosyncratic feeding beliefs until she was able to rip the capillary tube out of the plastic bag of formula which I had to wear around my neck. We were both saturated in smelly milk formula, and she was still very hungry and angry that the milk supply had ceased. A part of this regime was that to increase supply I was supposed to be 'frequency feeding' every one or two hours, but the mixing of the formula and the sterilising of the complicated capillary tube device took at least half an hour, and feeding at the imitation breast took another half an hour, so there was just time for nappy changing and nappy washing before it all began again.

"Eventually, the two or three night feeds became bottle-feeds, and by five months the baby made the decision that nipples, capillary tubes and all that were not for her! So she settled into being a much more contented bottle-fed baby, and I gradually learned to cope with the adverse reactions of family, friends, and even mothers at adjoining cafe tables who expressed their surprise that such a young baby was not receiving the proper care and attention symbolised by breastfeeding. Those who knew the real story told me that it was all because of her 'bad start' in the Special Care Nursery and my subsequent inability to be calm and relaxed about the whole process. I was told that breastfeeding was successful if you 'fed with your head' (i.e. if you believed in it).

"Before my second baby was due, I felt hopeful I could improve on my previous efforts and re-read all those things about supply and letdown reflex and thinking positively. Another uncomplicated pregnancy, a trouble-free delivery and a baby with no blood problems made me very hopeful during my time in hospital. My family doctor, knowing I wanted to breastfeed (and was afraid of failure) organised for us to leave hospital without the usual weigh-ins to check that the baby was getting enough milk and let us go home to do as much 'frequency feeding' as we felt necessary. So we did and felt much more successful and believed we were doing well.

"Unfortunately, at the six-week check-up, it was obvious that the baby was dehydrated and certainly not gaining weight, so the GP suggested we augment faith with formula. Determined (again!), to succeed, I continued to breastfeed and supplemented the baby's food with half-strength formula after each feed if she was still hungry. This went on until the baby was about 10 months old, and she gradually lost all interest in the breast. This second attempt was slightly less painful and marginally more successful (though two-thirds of her food supply came from the bottle) than the first, but I always hoped my supply would increase and always listened with envy to other mothers' accounts of 'leaking in public' and their problems of weaning their dependent offspring.

It's a year now since I gave up the struggle to keep my second daughter interested in breastfeeding and it really doesn't seem nearly as vital an issue as it was then. However, I know how irrationally eager to succeed I shall be if ever I have a third child. My most enduring feeling about these two experiences is the utter frustration of being able to convince people that I really wanted to breastfeed (because I believe it to be the best thing for both baby and mother) and yet being unable to manufacture that essential commodity, breast milk."

This case history, like the others, indicates the need for more careful clinical diagnosis and management of real physiological problems, and the destructive effects of pseudo-scientific 'psychological' explanations.

Future writing will include other case histories. If you have some, or wish to recount your own case, please send me a typed account, and indicate whether you are happy to be acknowledged in the event of publication.

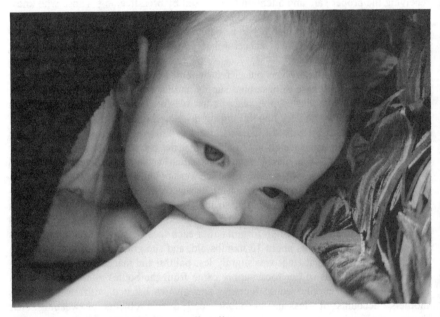

Sleepy older baby at flexible breast: all smiles
Same stretch by young baby on tight breast → nipple fissure

13. CONCLUSIONS

For Kuhn the history of science is a story of
(i) the emergence and establishment of a new way of looking at phenomena;
(ii) the detailed working out of the consequences of the new approach (this is the phase of 'normal science');
(iii) the gradual emergence and accumulation of anomalies with which the now-received view cannot cope;
(iv) the breakdown of the accepted view and the emergence of a radically new view, discontinuous with the older one, which is eventually accepted and endorsed by the scientific community (this is the phase of 'scientific revolution'!).
This process is repeated over and over again in the history of science.

- Max Charlesworth, *Science, Non-science and Pseudo-science*
(Deakin University Press, 1982), pp. 34-5

When I have finished public lectures on the hazards of artificial feeding, one of the usual responses is "How on earth did we reach this stage where intelligent, caring, thoughtful people accept at face value the idea that the bottle is 'nearly as good nowadays'?" That is a very large question, which deserves a book rather than a chapter. But I hope that the narrative in Chapter 10 will help to make some sense of what is an extraordinary state of affairs: that people blindly accept and truly believe that science and commerce have been able to create an adequate equivalent of one of the human body's most complex and under-researched fluids. The equally ridiculous idea that women have a true choice of these apparently almost equal alternatives is very recent. Even the very new idea that scientists could do better than evolutionary processes in making a food for babies has some adherents!

This new way of looking at infant feeding (stage i of Charlesworth's schema) began in the late nineteenth century. Before that many substitutes were used, but no one believed them to be equivalent. Not until perhaps the 1960s was the idea of the equivalence of modern formulae and breast milk popularly accepted – although different groups in different countries were 'converted' at different rates. The 1960s and 1970s were the period of Charlesworth's stage ii, 'normal science', when (thanks largely to industry marketing and healthworker naïveté) it was taken for granted that infant formula was equivalent to breast milk. Many scientists have now moved into stage iii, as they see anomalies and problems which imply that perhaps this uncritical belief in the safety of artificial formulae is due for some drastic revision.

But the real quantum leap comes in moving from stage iii to stage iv, from quali-fied belief to disbelief. The religious analogy is quite apt, for we can never prove our views to be definitely true, beyond all question. The organising framework we use in thinking about infant feeding reflects our life experience, whether we recognise that openly, as I do in this book, or have become so habituated to living in one framework that we cannot recognise its pervasive influence, or merely consider it the 'right' perspective. This latter is, of course a real danger for all of us, but most especially for scientists in a society that reveres them, and has found few ways of rendering them accountable to the larger community. That this is a debasement of all that science is meant to be[1] will not prevent it happening: I remember reading (and failed to note) an article reporting that first year medical students have a capacity for critical evaluation that is lost as their training progresses.

But this generation is not responsible for the failures of previous generations. Why have we continued to ignore the obvious potential for harm involved in feeding human infants non-human milks? One reason is that it was, and is, in no one's immediate interests to publicise the possibility, in the absence of clear-cut studies demonstrating gross immediate harm. Once a substantial number of women have bottle-fed, to raise such issues is to invite controversy. In the small world of orthodox medicine, the suggestion that one is 'extreme' has such professionally damaging overtones that few doctors or nurses will risk being so labelled. And no other groups have had access to the information needed to disturb their accepted beliefs. It took me a long time to realise that all these problems and deficiencies should make me question the one most basic belief, that artificial feeding was 'close to' breast milk. I was as well-indoctrinated as any other modern mother or midwife or doctor.

Another reason probably lies in our agricultural origins. Farmers breed animals for a variety of short-term traits: the ability to produce plenty of milk in dairy herds, the ability to put on the desired type of flesh efficiently in beef herds, the right quality and quantity of wool in sheep, and so on. Resistance to disease is a consideration only where the disease causes unacceptably high losses of productivity and/or no cheap veterinary solution exists. Development of the animal's mental capacities is neither possible nor desirable in breeding programmes – a 'stupid' cow which puts on plenty of condition is preferable to a 'smart' one which might be better able to survive in hostile environs. We have been breeding animals for external measurable qualities such as growth.

The mind-set earlier this century (and still in poor communities), when life was simpler, was that big equals better. When babies overall began to grow bigger and fatter on very strong concentrations of milk, we assumed that this meant that cows' milk was safe for babies, perhaps even better than human milk. The 'runts' who failed to thrive, or died, were not surprising to those used to animal models. Maternal rejection is not uncommon in animals, particularly those raised in artificial environments, and it was an easy progression to see infants who failed to thrive as responding to their human mother's overt or more subtle rejection. (Sometimes so subtle that no evidence for it could ever be unearthed, but why spoil a good theory with facts?) This is still a dominant theory for explaining failure to thrive in children.[2]

What such studies fail to appreciate is the devastating effect on the mother (and therefore on the relationship between mother and infant, and both parents) of a child which fails to thrive despite her best efforts, while her friends' children have no such problems. The change in maternal attitudes that results when food intolerance is controlled (rarely thoroughly investigated by those who believe 'mothering' is the key) has to be seen to be believed. And, as discussed earlier in this book, such studies also conveniently overlook the historical and cross-cultural evidence that children raised in conditions of appalling deprivation thrive while breastfed.

Because animals are bred for slaughter, mental traits are irrelevant, and the long-term degenerative diseases caused by their early feeding need never be investigated. Feeding human infants is much more complicated precisely because we do not wish to diminish or destroy the child's innate intellectual potential,[3] and we do not wish to see the child suffer from degenerative diseases any younger than is truly inevitable. Yet hand in hand with the rise in formula-feeding of American infants has been a steady decline in national IQ and a steady rise in the incidence and earlier onset of serious degenerative diseases. We are still not asking whether changes of formulation are linked to rising rates of allergy, or whether it takes a few generations to reach maximum harm potential for artificial feeding (as it does in animals). How much of the disease normal in developed countries is due to infant feeding, we don't know. That at least some of it is due to infant feeding seems a reasonable probability, given the way in which human milk is so specifically designed not only for the needs of the neonate, but also as a biological programming agent, designed to activate and influence the development of the child's own immunological and metabolic systems, and to do so for life.

A further Pandora's box of problems is also opened by the possibility of inter-generational effects of infant feeding. Damage done to the female in one generation may have an impact on her children, gestated in her body, with an immune system developing from 12 weeks after conception. It is quite clear that whatever factor causes an infant to have high serum total IgE levels at birth is responsible for much allergic disease. Clearly, in food-intolerant families children are at risk of sensitisation in utero and at risk of ill-effects while being breast fed. Such effects could become cumulative unless the causes are recognised and controlled. Combined with the ability of medical science to keep alive yet more damaged children, who in their turn reproduce, this could lead to a geometrically progressive increase in allergic and auto-immune disease with each succeeding generation. Such mechanisms could also explain why it was that babies seemed to have suffered fewer obvious ill-effects from far less satisfactory feedings in earlier generations: they came of healthier stock in societies where the weak died in infancy, they were carried in a body relatively healthier because breastfed for longer, and they were not as exposed to so many toxic chemicals. This may be speculative, but is not unreasonable.

One of the most important reasons why it has taken us so long to realise that breastfeeding is much, much better than formula-feeding lies in the character of Western medicine. The close nexus between medicine and industry outlined in chapter 10 was natural, given both the society of its time (its assumptions about the truth, women, progress, and much more) and the structure of medicine itself. As I outlined in an earlier book examining the development of nurse registration in the state of Victoria, the earliest nurses were little more than glorified parlour-maids,[4] and there was fierce medical opposition to every increase in their knowledge and responsibility. This ensured that until very recently, nursing was not a fully autonomous profession; that the perceptions of women were not recognised as valid where they were manifest; but that mostly women in medicine had no perceptions outside the accepted medical modes. To stand up for likely merits of woman's milk as against the carefully measured male substitute, at a time when male-dominated research was not even looking at the human product, required confidence and knowledge unattainable to most nurses of the time.

There were such doctors and nurses, men and women alike. The profession generally regarded them with tolerance as long as they were not 'extreme' – that is, as long as they agreed that modern formulae were safe, that many women under modern conditions would 'fail' at breastfeeding, or would not want to, and that none of that was the doctor's business or responsibility. Less tolerance was extended if they tried to insist that breastfeeding mattered enough to be taken too seriously. In every case, their work in this area was ignored,[5] as being of little or no importance.

Western medicine developed as an interventionist, controlling, paternalistic profession/science/industry.[6] The organised profession (as distinct from many individual doctors) often opposed any basic preventative medicine not controlled by doctors, such as maternal and child health care clinics.[7] It assumed that people seeing doctors frequently for minor problems would be healthier than those taking responsibility for their own health and seeing doctors only in serious illness – a proposition that is at least debatable nowadays. It therefore opposed many public health education measures: it was a doctor's task to tell patients what they needed to know, and to decide what they needed to know as well. (The example of labels on infant foods given in ch. 10 is symptomatic.)

While this medical model persisted, important feed-back from the patient was largely impossible to assimilate into the system. The system's failures were, and often still are, rationalised away under convenient psychological labels. The system's successes were bruited abroad through a sycophantic uncritical media, and served to increase people's dependence on god-like medical figures. That such medicine did have triumphs, I would be the last to deny. But that this was and is at considerable cost is now emerging from the profession's own literature. Infant feeding was one such area, but there were many others.

It is partly the successes of Western medicine – its analytic skills – and partly its failures, and the humanity induced by the recognition of iatrogenic problems, which now enables us to consider more impartially the consequences of earlier experiments with infant feeding. Human nature being as it is, this is not easy for people who have thought this subject uncontroversial for decades, and who have publicly committed themselves to the idea that infant feeding doesn't matter much. As I sat waiting to do paediatric Grand Rounds at one major maternity hospital, two doctors were overheard to say: "Going to Grand Rounds this morning?" "Nah, it's only breastfeeding." Typical of too many.

I think that infant feeding does matter. It probably matters more than we can currently know, given the limits of nutritional understanding at present. But we do know that for many children the parents' 'choice' of breast or bottle is a life-and-death matter. Not only poor children in every society, but pre-term, hypersensitive or particularly vulnerable children of the rich, may die or be profoundly brain-damaged as a direct consequence of bottle-feeding. For others, it matters less; unrealised intellectual and physical growth potential, chronic or intermittent illness, and/or shorter life span may be the only consequences. Perhaps for some others there are no consequences, though I have yet to meet any such children myself. For all these children, there may be profound psychological consequences due to the disturbance of normal parental attachment by those conditions we (unlike many other societies) have accepted as normal – colic, crying, night wakefulness, growing pains, etc. – but which have quite clearly been due to minor food intolerance in many Australian families. Those parents who are driven to desperation by their baby's 'difficult temperament' may or may not become baby-batterers. But their relationships are affected, in ways which custom often builds into life-long consequences.

All these effects are 'normal', in the sense of being so common as to be unremarkable. They are not normal, if by that one means something programmed into the physical development of all human beings. If they were, then infant crying and colic would be universal, and eczema, asthma and the rest would occur in similar proportions in underdeveloped countries. Professionals must learn to enquire in great detail about infant nutrition as part of their normal routine. We have to overcome our 'medical blindspot' despite the possible embarrassment our findings may prove to be.

For I believe that it is profound conservatism that prevents many professionals from examining the significance of early infant nutrition. If it should prove to be – as much evidence suggests - an important contributory factor in diseases ranging from liver and kidney malfunctions to autism, schizophrenia, auto-immune diseases like diabetes, and cot death, consider the upheaval this could generate. A great many parents would be very upset, and some with good reason would be angry over the information or management they received at the hands of professionals they paid and trusted. Many commercial interests would lose a great deal of money. (Only those who reinvested in the business of human milk formulae and availability, for a much smaller market, would stay in business.) Professionals would have to learn new skills, adopt new routines, and involve themselves in a new way of thinking about breastfeeding problems. Society at large would have to be reorganised to enable women to participate fully without weaning their babies. And so on. Inertia and the desire for a peaceful life conspire to maintain an undesirable status quo, where the majority of babies receive less than optimal nutrition.

This inertia/laziness factor is sometimes tacitly recognised. In asking about what instructions were given on feeding during gastroenteritis and fasting before anaesthesia, I have often been told that this doctor/hospital does not discriminate between human milk and other forms of milk because 'it's easier and less confusing' theoretically for mothers. Poor dim creatures that we are, there are not many of us incapable of recognising the difference between breastfeeding and bottle-feeding, and I would suggest that it is not terribly difficult to write instructions on what to do in either case, and why. However, a clear-cut discrimination on these grounds would start mothers thinking and probably asking questions awkward for staff to handle, such as "If I had been breastfeeding would my baby have become sick this time?", "Would it help my baby to get better if I could get her some breast milk?", "Do you have human milk available for sick babies?", and so on.

We must insist upon this sort of clear-cut distinction between human milk and its artificial substitutes, and not permit breastfed babies to suffer because of some desire to average it all out and keep everyone happy. This moral cowardice masquerading as pragmatism is best exemplified by the current recommendations for the introduction of solid foods. The American Academy of Pediatrics Committee on Nutrition made a recommendation in 1980 that babies be introduced to solid foods between four and six months of age, after previously exclusive breast milk or formula-feeding. As a later letter pointed out,[8] their reasoning was: disappearance of the extrusive reflex at four to five months; ability to indicate satiety by five to six months; development of appreciable IgA levels by seven months. A more appropriate recommendation (but unpopular) would thus have been to introduce other foods no earlier than six to seven months. This squares with Kajosaari and Saarinen's work on allergy,[9] where exclusive human milk feeding to six months rendered negligible the rates of food allergy at 12 months. For infants given solids between three and 6 months, the incidence was 37 per cent. For infants given solids after six months, it was 7 per cent. The children had strong family history of allergy, yet only 14 per cent (compared with 35 per cent) had eczema at 12 months. Indeed, these children still show benefit at the age of seventeen.[10] Clearly six months' exclusive human milk feeding must be the minimum goal.

But why exactly did the AAP Committee in 1980 recommend between four and six months? A letter from the Committee Chairman made this clear: because of the possible risks of prolonged exclusive artificial feeding. He said, "Trying to convert from previous practices of feeding solids at 1 month of age to the present recommendations must be done step-wise. A compromise was felt to be necessary. For breastfed infants there seems no advantage and some disadvantage[11] to early supplements. When one uses an artificial formula, no matter how good, one must beware of possible missing ingredients. Weighing advantages and disadvantages, the Committee on Nutrition felt that 4 to 6 months of age was reasonable with present evidence."[12]

But how many parents choose to bottle-feed knowing there is a risk of possible missing ingredients? And why penalise breastfed infants because of "possible missing ingredients" in formula? Why not have two distinct sets of recommendations for the breast- and bottle-fed infant?

• Exclusive human milk feeding for so long as growth and health remains good – in Dr Barness's own case, this was 12 months, and that is not exceptional. Only a generation ago many mothers took it for granted that 9 months was the age for giving other foods, and many thriving Australian babies are exclusively breastfed for similar periods.

- Exclusive use of a new, yet-to-be developed low-allergy formula[13] for infants unable to be given human milk, with the addition of other foods after three or four months to try to guard against possible unsuspected deficiencies in the formula, industrial accidents, and the like   Why not a two-part policy, for such different groups of babies as the breastfed and the artificially-fed? This is clearly the logical solution, but it would cause mothers to ask questions about the 'equivalence' of formula. It would enrage the manufacturers who contribute so generously to the Academy. It would upset the status quo. Paediatricians really ought to "eschew endorsement for the sake of palatability [sic] of popular trends, and to present unpopular recommendations if they can be justified and if they offer the opportunity to lead a misdirected community toward more desirable health care patterns", as one so aptly put it.[8] They ought to, but they often do not.[14] This is a marker of how corrupted medicine has been by its long association with commerce. In 1998 it is clear that the world health bodies agree that breastfed babies can be breastfed to 6 months, but there is still no clear voice saying, "But beware of missing ingredients in formula and widen the bottle-fed baby's diet by four months at latest..."

To restore public confidence in the profession will require more than assurances of financial integrity, which is not the issue. (Though I find contemptible many of the practices Rawlins discusses.) The issue is whether many paediatricians are now capable of thinking outside the mindset created by company marketing messages, of perceiving the truth that breast and bottle are not equivalent, and of formulating crystal-clear messages based upon the differences between the products. To talk about promoting breastfeeding while continuing to write identical recommendations for introduction of solids, feeding during gastroenteritis, fasting before anaesthesia, or any other contingency, for breastfed or artificially fed infants has to be either stupidity or hypocrisy. Mothers are not stupid. They get the message quite clearly, as they are meant to: 'Yes, breastfeeding would be nice, but it makes no real difference.' Many people, doctors included, truly believe that. But only those with enormous vested interests could maintain such a belief after a careful reading of the research literature pertaining to the composition and activity of human milk, and the peculiar vulnerability of the neonate. Vested interests, of course, are not always monetary in nature. All of us find it difficult to admit having made mistakes. Only now we are beginning to realise how much we didn't and don't know.

Ironically, it is this new realisation that constitutes our last major obstacle to rapid progress. Those earlier doctors and businessmen were confident that they had discovered perfect, or perfectly adequate, infant foods – and in the absence of any regulations, they made and sold them. Nowadays, however, even when we are aware that these products may be deficient, our knowledge of the complexities of bioavailability means that we cannot advocate rapid change, even when we have good grounds for thinking it might be an improvement. We could end up doing even more damage, as the Syntex company did with Neo-Mull-Soy, for the best of motives. Having accepted the status quo, we are stuck with defending it, assuring parents that it is adequate, relieving their anxieties on learning of material such as is found in Chapter 1. And in doing that we perpetuate the status quo. **Our society's acceptance**

of bottlefeeding as normal and nutritionally equivalent to breastfeeding is the major obstacle to change.

Of course, the adoption of universal exclusive breastfeeding and the supply of human milk formulae in the first months of life is no panacea for the world's ills. There are countless other risk factors, chiefly poverty and its attendant ills: lack of clean water and of sanitation; overwork and under-education; oppression and exploitation, particularly of women; the chemical nightmares created by indiscriminate use of socially accepted drugs and compounds, and the horrifying possibilities being opened by recombinant gene technology and mass animal husbandry. Affluence, too, creates its own risks: chemical pollution and global environmental degradation; and nuclear disaster, whether from 'peaceful' atoms, weapons testing, outright war, or simple accidents. I am not asking anyone, therefore, to abandon their concern about other areas of risk to human life and health. I am asking them to lend what support they can to the promotion of breastfeeding and a right ordering of priorities in infant nutrition. For infant feeding has been shown to be one of the few risk factors that can be relatively readily and cheaply altered.[15] This is a tribute to women's concern for their children's well-being.

I should like to suggest that we and the government set long-term goals:

• to provide pre-pregnancy and pre-natal help to women in order to reduce the possibility of in utero and breast milk sensitisation.

• to promote exclusive breastfeeding for six months, as almost all women are capable of successful lactation;

• to organise and then promote the widespread availability and modification of human milk for all infants unable to breastfeed, in the first three to four months of life; ultimately and ideally for the first six months;

• to accept the responsibility of paying for all infant formula (cows' milk or other) powder and water needed by those mothers who cannot breastfeed and who cannot afford infant formula (this would be strictly means-tested) after those first few months of human milk;

• to promote the development of better 'normal' infant formula for all children requiring it; and to subsidise the excess cost of specialty formulas (above the cost of normal formula) only for families able to afford normal formula.

• to set strict controls on artificial feeding equipment and its marketing, and to police those controls.

Would this result in a massive cost increase in an age of cost-cutting? At present, yes. If planned and worked towards intelligently, no. If the government were paying for infant formula, its devotion to improving hospital practices, community attitudes and support, maternity/lactation benefits, and so on, would improve remarkably. If those changes took place, there should be plenty of donors, perhaps even wet-nurses, available to supply human milk for babies unable to be breastfed in the first few months. This should greatly reduce the need for specialty formulas of all kinds (as well as bills for hospitalisation of sick infants) and by six months most babies could begin changing over to a normal mixed diet. What would drop dramatically would be the consumption of infant formulae of all kinds and, very probably, infant morbidity and mortality in the first six months, hospitalisation costs, and so on. "We would be giving a good example and saving ourselves money as well as avoiding a variety of illnesses in our children," as Wood and Walker-Smith have said.[16] Of course, if the government could be motivated by ethical or scientific stimuli (rather than financial ones) to actively promote exclusive breastfeeding, it need not accept the responsibility for paying for infant formula. However, I believe this would be a good idea for a number of reasons:

• If a national government were paying, it would end the current anomalies where a low-income supporting mother in an urban slum uses evaporated milk because she can't afford formula and her child vomits carton milk, whereas a wealthy society mother gets virtually free Pregestimil or Neocate because her child is intolerant of cows' milk. Need should govern support from taxpayers' funds, not access to specialist medial services. The poor child's need of good nutrition is almost certainly greater than his wealthy counterpart – and infant formulae are too expensive.[17] But the chances are slim indeed that poor families will have babies diagnosed as allergic.

• If the government were paying, it would have a compelling motive for reducing the inflated costs of formula, standardising the product and ending wasteful advertising, competition, and distribution of largesse to doctors, all paid for by formula users. (This is a major reason why such a proposal would be bitterly opposed by industry.) Infant formula should not be advertised to the public at all; if it is necessary, it will be used, and doctors can be kept up to date on new products through professional, not commercial, channels. And of course, a standardised product, or products, with regular testing built in to the system, would reduce the risk of the deficiencies which have plagued infant formula thus far.

• If the government were paying, it would have good reason to resist pressure from vested interests of all kinds. The WHO Code of Marketing of Breastmilk Substitutes would suddenly be seen as an inadequate minimum, rather than as an inappropriate ideal. Food marketing might be subject to some stringent objective scrutiny, and manufacturers and advertisers taught to educate consumers, not merely motivate or manipulate them, and so on.

This will offend the sacred cow of free enterprise and be seen as infringing the consumer's equally sacred right to variety. But babies only get one chance at life. They are more important than profits. Their first six months may well be critical to their later health. Whatever needs to be done, **(a)** to promote exclusive breastfeeding and **(b)** to create and make available the best possible alternatives for the non-breastfed child, must be done.

I am concerned about the fact that underprivileged children get carton cows' milk rather than formula, just as I am that any baby gets formula when she could have been breastfed. Conversations with doctors reveal that only cost constraints prevent them from prescribing less allergenic products more often, or investigating prospects for human milk banking: this in a society where in vitro fertilisation, liver transplants and coronary bypass operations are paid for from public revenue.

Impossible? No. Idealistic? Of course. But without ideals to work towards we will continue to move in the wrong direction: towards ever more complicated, ever more expensive, ever more unaffordable high technology infant formulae which the wealthy can afford while the poor make do, as they always have, with cheap and inadequate substitutes – or else spend huge proportions of their inadequate income on feeding one family member. This early malnutrition thus ensures that they remain poor, a fact which the rich are very ready to overlook because it serves their interests.

But change is possible. As Brindlecombe said, "To change behaviour is always difficult, but trends in infant feeding show that it can be done, and in a relatively short time too. A national campaign in which the media play a big part, and in which a less desirable commodity is made difficult to obtain is likely to produce results."[15] The motivation of such change is universal and deeply felt, for all parents want the best for their children and are willing to sacrifice to that end. Just as advertisers do, health educators should capitalise on this desire to do the best possible for the child.

No one regrets that an infant formula industry exists. Substitutes for human milk are currently necessary, and I for one am grateful that they are no longer as bad as they once were, even if they are not half as good as doctors and parents assume them to be. But to quote Professor Leif Hambraeus, "Unfortunately, the progress in food technology, in addition to developing substitutes for breastmilk for feeding infants of mothers who, for various reasons, do not breastfeed, has included an intensive commercial promotion of the proprietary formulae. This has led to a rapid decline in breastfeeding... It should therefore be emphasised that the introduction and marketing of breastmilk substitutes and the explosive expansion of artificial feeding of infants is an extraordinary example of a large *in vivo* experiment performed without any research protocol including a control series."[18]

Artificial feeding of infants is, in fact, the largest uncontrolled in vivo experiment in human history. Its effects are so widespread as now to seem normal.

Breast is best. Almost all babies need human milk exclusively for a minimum of six months, and with other foods for some time thereafter. This is my basic belief. I also believe that social change is inevitable; and that everyone concerned about infant nutrition can help bring about that change, at personal, local and even national levels.

When I consider the scope of the changes needed, I can understand those who lapse into apathy because they believe nothing significant can be done. But all of us can do something about this: complimenting a mother brave enough to feed her baby as she needs it, whether in public or not; writing letters to comment on some aspect of infant feeding practice; observing how infant formula, bottles and teats, and other baby foods are manufactured, marketed and used in the community.

All of us must do something about it, for it is true that "if you are not part of the solution, you are part of the problem". So let us see a revolt of women – and those near to them – against the hydra-headed tyranny of artificial feeding and its offshoots – poor breastfeeding management, uncritical diagnosis of 'psychological' ills, and a lack of financial support for postpartum women who want to work as mothers without losing their home or all possibility of any subsequent career. Let women have some real choice about infant feeding, in fact. For babies, only the breast will do.

Appendix

Areas where change is possible: a brief list

Consumer education

- Beginning with very young children, and certainly through the schools, contact with local breastfeeding mothers and education about the benefits of breastfeeding, hazards of substitutes. Education creates motivation both to begin and to persevere through difficulties.
- The creation/strengthening of mother-to-mother peer support networks liaising with professionals educated about lactation.
- The creation and strengthening of consumer networks monitoring industry practice.

Professional education

- Education about breastfeeding management.
- Improved hospital practices.
- Improved clinic advice and facilities as needed; vastly improved medical management of breastfeeding problems.

Availability of human milk

- Human milk banking.
- Human milk modification (even commercial processing?)[19]
- Wet-nursing, or cross-nursing.

Changes in the workplace

- Improved maternity leave (a minimum of six months unpaid leave after a period of three months paid leave).
- Workplace provision for breastfed babies, as prescribed under the ILO Convention of 1919.[20]

Changes in social practice

- Paid lactation leave.
- Special support for the mother at home with under-5s.
- Volunteer counsellors to receive unemployment benefits.
- Changes in media images, cultural attitudes and stereotypes.[21]

Changes in industry practices

- Implementation of WHO Code as a minimum.
- Careful independent monitoring.
- Checks built into manufacturing processes, with routine sampling.
- Encouragement (not suppression) of whistle-blowing on defective product.

NOTES
CHAPTER 13: CONCLUSIONS

[1] cf. Chalmers, I., "Scientific inquiry and authoritarianism in perinatal care education", *Birth* (1983) 10, 3, 151-66; letters (1984) 11, 1, 43-7.

[2] Casey, P. H.; Bradley, R.; Worthan, B., "Social and home environments of infants with non-organic failure to thrive", *Pediatrics* (1984) 73, 348-53.

[3] This highly controversial topic will be discussed in volume 2 of this series. But parents should know that there are indeed indications that breastfed children have an advantage intellectually. cf. "Report of the Task Force on the assessment of the scientific evidence relating to infant feeding practices and infant health", *Pediatrics* (1984) 74, 4, suppl. p. 634-7.

[4] Minchin, M., *Revolutions and Rosewater: the evolution of the Victorian nurse registration 1923-1973.* (Available from the Victorian Nursing Council, 555 Collins Street, Melbourne 3000), p. 97-100

[5] cf. Illingworth on self-demand feeding: *Lancet* (1952) i, 683; Gunther on nipple pain: *Lancet* (1945) ii, 590; Newton on nipple damage: *J. Ped.* (1952) 41, 411; Waller on engorgement: *Arch. Dis. Child* (1946) 21, 1 – and so on.

[6] Willis, E., *Medical dominance* (George Allen & Unwin, 1983); Starr, P., *The Social Transformation of American Medicine* (Basic Books Inc., N.Y. 1982).

[7] Starr, op. cit., p. 260-1. In 1921 Congress passed the Shepherd Towner Act establishing pre-natal and child health centers. In 1927 the American Medical Association persuaded Congress to discontinue the program, as doctors moved into these areas. Although such clinics were established and survived in Australia and the U.K. their potential as primary health care centers has long been circumscribed by their sensitivity to the wishes of the medical profession, on whose tolerance they have thus far depended. Their future evolution will be of interest.

[8] Ganelin, S, "The feeding of solids debate", *Pediatrics* (1981) 61, 165.

[9] Kajosaari, M.; Saarinen, V., "Prophylaxis of atopic disease by six months' total solid food elimination. Evaluation of 135 exclusively breastfed infants of atopic families", *Acta Paed. Scand.* 1983, 72, 3, 411-4

[10] Saarinen, U.M.; Kajosaari M, "Breastfeeding as prophylaxis against atopic disease: prospective follow-up study until 17 years old", *Lancet* (1995) 346: 1065-9.

[11] Quandt, S. A., "The effect of beikost in the diet of breast-fed infants", *J. Am. Diet. Assoc.* 1984, 84, 1, 47-51. This article showed that early introduction of solids 'may lead to a significantly lower weight gain than continuation of the exclusive milk diet.' And of course, as discussed elsewhere in this book.

[12] Barness, L. reply to Ganelin, *Pediatrics*, 1981, 67, 166.

[13] Heppell, L. M. J.; Cant, A. J.; Kilshaw, P. J., "Reduction in the antigenicity of whey proteins by heat treatment: a possible strategy for producing a hypo-allergenic infant milk formula", *Br. J. Nutr.* (1984) 51, 29-36.

[14] Rawlins, M. D., "Doctors and the drugmakers", *Lancet* (1984), ii, 276-8.

[15] Brindlecombe, F., *Public Health* (1977) 91, p. 117.

[16] Wood, C. B. S., Walker-Smith, J., *MacKeith's Infant Feeding and Feeding Difficulties* (Churchill Livingstone, 1981), p. 107.

[17] In Australia, a week's supply for a 5-6 kg baby would presently cost at least $9-11 at least. The supporting mother's benefit is $115 per week. Rental costs – when accommodation can be found – range from $100-150 per week for very ordinary places. (An additional $15/week rental supplement is available for rents above $40.) What mothers receive can also be reduced by the fact that action to secure maintenance from the father is a pre-condition for receiving the benefit at all. Australian men are noted for not paying such maintenance awarded against them – it will

take time to prove this to authorities. It is therefore not surprising that less expensive substitutes for human milk continue to be used despite the joint medical/industry campaigns to persuade parents to use formula.

[18] Hambraeus, L., "Proprietary milk versus human milk in infant feeding", *Ped. Clin. N. Am.* (1977) 24, 1, 17-36.

[19] Rao, A. R., "Human breast milk as commercial infant food", *J. Trop. Pediatr. & Envir. Child Health* (1977) 24, 1, 17-36.

[20] This Convention specified 12 weeks paid maternity leave, free medial/midwife attendance; nursing breaks of half an hour twice daily. In 1952, this was extended to "a total period of at least 1½ hours during the working day, and adjustments in the frequency and length of the nursing periods should be permitted on production of a medical certificate." As well, "Provision should be made for the establishment of facilities for nursing or day care... at the expense of the community or by compulsory social insurance." In neither case was pregnancy or breastfeeding a legitimate cause for dismissal, without evidence of serious fault by the woman, and "During her legal absence from work before and after confinement, the seniority rights of the woman should be preserved as well as her right to reinstatement in her former work or in equivalent work paid at the same rate."

I.L.O. – Convention 3 – Convention concerning the employment of women before and after childbirth. Washington, 29 November 1919. – Recommendation 95 – Recommendation concerning maternity protection. Geneva, 28 June 1952.

[21] To depict a bottle-fed baby on television is 'advertising', whether it occurs in a show or as a commercial. It reinforces the normalcy of bottlefeeding, which is all that has to be done now that the market has been created. (The role of advertising and the media generally in legitimating antisocial behaviour is sometimes – as with cigarette smoking – extremely important and usually overlooked. Advertisements don't just sell products, they create and make 'normal' certain behaviour patterns, whether chewing gum with one's mouth open, drinking beverages approved for one's subgroup, smoking in public, or bottlefeeding babies.)

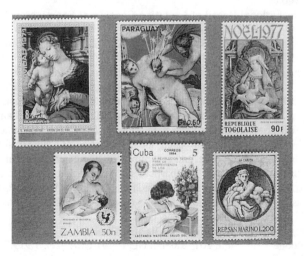

Breastfeeding stamps around the world: card by IBFAN Germany

*B*REASTFEEDING RESOURCES

Addresses are as up to date as possible in 1998, but changes are frequent. There are also many useful resources that I have not listed. This is mainly because WABA (the World Alliance for Breastfeeding Action) is now funded by UNICEF and other donors to act as a world-wide central clearing house for information about breastfeeding. Hence I am merely selecting some resources, in a list biased towards the providers of practical help, though it does include some central advocacy resources. WABA should have many more listings, and the new edition of Bestfeeding (Renfrew, Fisher & Arms) will carry a larger list. I would appreciate feedback on the usefulness of contacts or materials you receive from those listed, to guide future inclusions.

International Resources

• **WHO (World Health Organisation)**
Nutrition Unit (James Akré or Randa Saadeh) or CHD (Felicity Savage), 1211 Geneva 27, Switzerland. Tel: 41.22.7913316 Fax: 41.22.791 4156; e-mail: akrej@who.ch; saadehr@who.ch; savagef@who.ch. WHO has a web page with addresses. Try http://www.who.ch
• **IBLCE (International Board of Lactation Consultant Examiners)**
PO Box 2348, Falls Church, VA. 22042 USA. Fax: 1.703 560 7332. E-mail <iblce@erols.com>. Australian contact: Ros Escott, IBLCE Regional office, PO Box 13, South Hobart, TAS 7004; tel: 61.3.6223 8445; fax: 6223 8665. E-mail <escoa@mpx.com.au> (IBLCE). Regional offices for Europe and New Zealand also exist. IBLCE is the organisation which examines and then certifies Lactation Consultants as basically competent to practise. Its examination, held internationally since 1985, serves as a focus for the profession that is developing in the US and elsewhere. While in British-origin countries there may seem little need for a separate profession, many midwives and physicians are using the examination as a way of focussing their efforts to update their knowledge, and as a minimum competency standard for those of them who wish to specialise in this particular part of the health professional's role. Although expensive by non-American standards, the exam is well worth the effort involved. Passing it is a pre-requisite for voting membership of most democratic professional LC organisations.
• **ILCA (International Lactation Consultants' Association)**
4101 Lake Boone Trail, Suite 201, Raleigh NC 27607 USA. Tel: 1.919.787 5181; fax: 787 4916. E-mail: <ilca@erols.com>; website: <http://www.ilca.com>. ILCA is an

international professional association for lactation consultants. Its annual Membership Roster and its *Journal of Human Lactation* are useful resources.

• **ALCA (Australian Lactation Consultants' Association)**

PO Box 192, Mawson ACT 2607; tel/fax: 61.2.6290 1920. E-mail <alcagalaxy@ interact.net.au>. The only Australian national professional association which requires IBLCE certification as its entry criterion. But people in many countries subscribe to *ALCA Galaxy* for current information on all aspects of infant feeding and the International Code.

• **NMAA (Nursing Mothers' Association of Australia) and the NMAA Lactation Resource Centre**

PO Box 4000, Glen Iris VIC 3146. Tel: 61.3.9885 0855; fax: 61.3.9885 0866; web <http://home.vicnet.net.au/~nmaa/lrc.html>; e-mail <nursingm@vicnet.net.au>. Another very useful global information centre; LRC membership and subscription to *Breastfeeding Review* is recommended.

• **LLLI (La Leche League International)** PO Box 4079, Schaumburg, IL. 60668-4079 USA. The first and still the largest breastfeeding mothers' support group. Contacts and leaders in many countries. Has a Center for Breastfeeding Information. Tel: 849 519 7730; fax: 847 519 0035; e-mail <OrderDepartment@llli.org> for catalogues. Website: http://www.lalecheleague.org/

• **UNICEF**

UNICEF publishes *BFHI News*, only some issues of which can be found on the website at <http://www.unicef.org>. Editor's e-mail address: <pubdoc@unicef.org>. Fax: 1.212.824 6465

• **WABA (World Alliance for Breastfeeding Action)**

PO Box 1200, 10850 Penang, Malaysia. Tel: 60.4.658 4816; fax: 657 2655; e-mail <secr@waba.po.my>; website: <http://www.elogica.com.br/waba>. Intended to act as an umbrella group for and to assist global networking by all breastfeeding advocates; anyone can join in by signing an endorser form. A WABA Directory was to have been part of WABA's role as initially envisaged, though none has yet been published. However, individuals can ask for contacts in any region. WABA has produced much printed material of varying cost and usefulness in particular regions; its main public focus seems to be the promotion of World Breastfeeding Week each year, and monitoring via the GLOPAR project. WABALink appears sporadically, and distribution is unpredictable, so you need to keep renewing your endorsement and asking for mailings, if Australian experience is any guide. The website is generally well-maintained, and has lots of interesting items.

• **<http://www.cdinet.com/womensrights>**

Women's rights to maternity protection: an important and useful report, by the Clearinghouse on Infant Feeding and Maternal Nutrition, APHA. Can be downloaded, and contains many relevant street and website addresses, although several are now wrong.

Other useful national groups

AUSTRALIA [if dialling from overseas drop 0 from area code; country prefix 61]
• ACOIF, the Australian Coalition for Optimal Infant Feeding, the Australian Alliance for breastfeeding action, can be contacted by writing to Sue Byrne, c/o NMAA, PO Box 4000, Glen Iris, Vic 3146.
• ACE (Associates in Childbirth Education) and ACE Graphics, PO Box 366, Camperdown NSW 2050. Tel: (02) 9660 5177; fax: (02) 9660 5147; e-mail <andrear@mpx. com.au> The Australian source for subscriptions to MIDIRS (see UK entry).
• ACMI (Australian College of Midwives Inc.), 3 Bowen Cres., Melbourne. Vic 3000. Tel: (03) 9804 5071.
• ALC (Australasian Lactation Courses), PO Box 336, Unley SA 5061. Tel: (08) 8271 8740; e-mail: <mcintyrea@onaustralia.com.au>.Correspondence course for health professionals. (NB: a private business unconnected to ALCA, despite initial similarity)
• ALCA (Australian Lactation Consultants' Association) – see above.
• ALCA Victorian Branch, 1st floor, Queen Vic Women's Centre, 210 Lonsdale St., Melbourne 3000. Tel/fax: (03) 9650 5391.
• ALMA Publications and Seminars, 14 Acland St., St. Kilda, Vic. 3182;tel/fax: (03) 9537 2640. e-mail <minchin@netlink.com.au>.
• LIFE Inc. (Lactation and Infant Feeding Education), 27 Argyle St., Chadstone Vic 3148. A group of experienced Australian breastfeeding advocates who provide education in Australia and overseas on request. E-mail: <midwyf@ozemail.com.au>.
• Allergy and Environmental Sensitivity Support and Research Association, PO Box 298, Ringwood, Vic. 3134. Tel: (03) 9888 1382. Library; publishes a useful newsletter called *Sensitivity Matters*.
• Supplier of innovative wooden foot pump that interacts with the Medela pump set and is a cheap low-tech alternative: Stewart Lyons (03) 9702 8562

AUSTRIA [country prefix 43; always check area codes]
• Verband der Still- und Laktationsberaterinnen Österreichs IBCLC (VSLOE) (Austrian Association of Lactation Consultants IBCLC), c/o Anne-Marie Kern, Lindenstrasse 20, A-2362 Biedermannsdorf. Tel/fax: 22 36 72 336; e-mail <e.kern@online.edvg.co.at>.
• Verband Europaeischer Laktationsberaterinnen IBCLC (European Association of Lactation Consultants IBCLC), c/o Ilse Bichler,Steinfeldgasse 11, A-2511 Pffaffstaetten. Organises conferences every two years (simultaneous translation); comprehensive training programmes in German and French. Tel/fax: 22 52 46 511; email <101507. 2311@compuserve.com>

BRAZIL [country prefix 55; always check area codes]
• Grupo Origem, Av Beira Mar, 3661 Loja 18, Casa Caiada-Olinda, PE Tel/fax: 81 432 1599; e-mail: <origem@elogica.com.br>.

CANADA [country prefix 1; always check area codes]
• CLCA/ACCL Canadian Lactation Consultants Association, c/o Maureen Fjeld, 2125-29 Avenue SW, Calgary, ALTA. T2T 1N6. Tel: 403 244 4791; e-mail

<fjeldm@cadvision.com>
• Compleat Mother, RR#3, Clifford, ONT. Canada N0G1M0. Tel: 519.327 8785. Irreverent and funny, a refreshing alternative mothering style.
• INFACT Canada, 10 Trinity Square, Toronto M5G 1B1. Tel: 416.595 9819; Fax: 591 9355.Excellent website, newsletter and resources relating to the Code and breastfeeding.

FRANCE
• French Association of Lactation Consultants, c/o Lea Cohen, 116 rue du Général Leclerc, F-78420 Carrieres sur Seine. Tel: 01 3968 1081
• IFAM, c/o Giselle Laviolle, 65 Allée du Lac Inférieur, 78110 Le Vesinet.
• La Leche League France, BP 18, L'Etang la Ville, France 78620.
• Info-Allaitement, c/o Dominique Couturier, Bayers 16460, Aunac.
• Solidarilait, Centre Puercultrice, 26 Bvd. Brune, F-75014 Paris.

GERMANY [country prefix 49; always check area codes]
• Arbeitsgemeinschaft Freier Stillgruppen, Gertraudgasse 4R, 97070 Wurzburg. Tel: 09 31 57 34 93; fax: 09 31 57 34 94; e-mail <AFS-Stillgruppen@t-online.de>. Website: http://www.stillen.org/
• Bund Deutscher Laktationsberaterinnen (German Association of Lactation Consultants) Elke Sporleder, D-30457 Hannover, Delpweg 14. Tel: 511 46 71 64; fax: 511 46 59 06 website: http://www.stillen.de

GREECE
• Greek Association of Lactation Consultants, Anna Patsourou, Anaximandrou 93 GR-54250 Thessaloniki. Tel: 031 656 703

INDIA [country prefix 91; always check area codes]
• BPNI (Breastfeeding Promotion Network of India) PO Box 10551, BP 33, Pitampura, Delhi, 110034 India. Tel: 91 11 2 11 435; fax: 91 11 713 4787

IRELAND [country prefix 353; always check area codes]
• Association of Lactation Consultants in Ireland (ALCI), c/o Nicola Clarke, 26 Violet Hill Park, Glasnevin, Dublin 11; or Eileen O'Sullivan, 223 Forest Hills, Rathcoole, Dublin. Tel: 1 458 9532

ISRAEL
• Israel Lactation Consultants (Evi Adams), P.O.Box 14099, Ashdod. E-mail: <evadams@ibm.net>.

LUXEMBOURG [country prefix 352; always check area codes]
• Initiativ Liewensufank a.s.b.l., BP 1075, L-1010, Luxembourg. Tel: 36 05 98; fax: 36 61 34; email: maryse.lehners@ci.educ.lu

MALAYSIA [country prefix 60; always check area codes]
• Parenting Concepts Sdn Bhd., 2776B, 1st floor, Jalan Cangkat Permata, Taman Permata, 53300 Kuala Lumpur. Tel: 3 405 3872/3; fax: 3 406 8914. e-mail: <tasmim@tm.net.my>.
• PPPIM (Breastfeeding Advisory Association of Malaysia), 25A, Jalan Kampong Pandan 53100 Kuala Lumpur.

NETHERLANDS [country prefix 31; always check area codes]
• Vereniging Borstvoeding Natuurlijk, Postbus 119, 3960 BC Wijk bij Duurstede. Tel:

0343 576626; website <http://utopia.knoware.nl/users/vbn>.
• Nederlandse Verenigung van Lactatiekundigen (NVL), Postbus 5243, NL-2701 GE Zoetermeer. Tel: 79 32 13 693.

NEW ZEALAND [country prefix 64; always check area codes]
• NZ Lactation Consultants' Association, Po Box 29-279, Christchurch, NZ. Publishes *Issues*, an excellent journal. Editor's tel: (03) 473 8677; fax: (03) 473 8097.
• LLL New Zealand, Box 13383, Johnsonville, Wellington 4. Te: 04 478 1315; email: lllnz@clear.net.nz; website: nttp://www.lalecheleague.org/LLLNZ/

NORWAY [country prefix 47; always check area codes]
• Ammehjelpen, and AHIG, c/o Ammehjelpens sekretariat, 2423 Østby, Norway. Berit Marie Øyeshaug (secretary/administrator). Tel: 6245 5251; fax: 6245 5105.
• Ammefagrådet (Breastfeeding resource group) c/o Grø Nylander, Kvinneklinikken, Rikshospitalet, N-0027 Oslo. Tel: 2286 9215; fax: 2286 9235.

SOUTH AFRICA [country prefix 27; always check area codes]
• SALCA (Southern African Lactation Consultants Association), PO Box 1227, Roosevelt Park, 2129. E-mail <lynn@mod.co.za>.
• NABA (National Alliance for Breastfeeding Action, South Africa), PO Box 222, Auckland Park, 2006. Breastfeeding Liaison Groups in the nine provinces fall under this umbrella.
• LLL-SA, PO Box 10153, Aston Manor, 1630. Tel: (021) 968 537
• BFA-SA, PO Box 4055, Old Oak Village, 7537. Tel: (021 646 8363

SWEDEN [country prefix 46; always check area codes]
• Amningshjalpen, Box 54, 274 03 Rydsgard. Tel: 0411 44 333.
Website: http://www.amningshjalpen.se
• Svenska Amningsinstitutet, Kronhusgatan 2 E, 1tr, Goteborg, S-41113

SWITZERLAND [country prefix 41; always check area codes]
• see WHO above.
• Berufsverband Schweizericher Stillberaterinnen (BSS), (Swiss Association of Lactation Consultants), Postfach 686, Berne 25, CH 3000. Fax: 41 31 333 3187. Tel: 671 0173 Fax: 671 0171 e-mail: BSS.Geschaeftsstelle@gmx.net
• Geneva Infant Feeding Association (GIFA), PO Box 157, 1211 Geneva 19. 41.22 7989164. Fax: 41.22.7984443. Publishes *Breastfeeding Briefs*. E-mail: <philipec@iprolink.ch>.

UNITED KINGDOM [country prefix 44; always check area codes]
• Healthlink Worldwide (formerly AHRTAG) 29-35 Farringdon Rd., London EC1M3JB; tel: 0171 242 0606; fax: 0171 242 0041. Website <http://www.poptel.org.uk/ahrtag>. Publishes useful inexpensive newsletters.
• Association of Breastfeeding Mothers, *PO Box 207, Bridgewater TA6 7YT. Tel: 0171 813 1481; Fax: 0117 966 1788. Email: abm@clara.net; Website: http://home.clara.net/abm/
• Baby Milk Action, 23 St. Andrew's Street, Cambridge, CB2 3AX, UK; tel: 01223 464420; fax: 01223 464417; e-mail <babymilkacti@gn.apc.org>.
• Breastfeeding Promotion Group, The National Childbirth Trust, Alexandra House, Oldham Terrace, Acton, London W3 6NH; tel: 0181 992 8637. Publishes *New*

Generation.
• Breastfeeding Network, PO Box 11126, Paisley PA2 8YB, Scotland. Newly-formed by ex-NCT counsellors. Tel: 0870 900 8787 E-mail: <broadfoot@btinternet.com>.
• International Confederation of Midwives, 10 Barley Mow Passage, Chiswick, London W4 4PH. Tel/fax: 0181 995 1332
• Lactation Consultants of Great Britain (LCGB), 111 Pilgrim's Way, Kemsing, Seven Oaks, Kent TN15 6TE. Tel: 585 493873.
• MIDIRS, 9 Elmdale Rd., Clifton, Bristol BS8 1SL; tel: 0117 925 1791; fax: 0117 925 1792. Email: midirs@dial.pipex.com; website: http://www.midirs.org/ Superb database and information pack: the best in the world for those who cannot afford numerous journal subscriptions. Available in Australia from ACE (above).
• Royal College of Midwives, 15 Mansfield St, London WIM OBE; tel: 0171.872 5100; fax: 0171.312 3536.
• TALC, PO Box 49, St. Albans, Herts ALI 4AX. First-rate, CHEAP slides, books, etc. Tel: 0 1727 853869; fax: 01727 846 852.
• Tropical Child Health Unit, Institute of Child Health, 30 Guilford St., London, WC1 N 1EH. (TALC materials can be viewed and bought here, excellent library, MCH courses and resources.)

USA [country prefix 1; always check area codes]
• Breastfeeding Support Consultants (BSC), 228 Park Lane, Chalfont PA 18914; tel: 215 822 1281; fax: 215 997 7879; e-mail <bsccenter@aol.com>; website <http://members.aol.com/bsccenter>.
• Bright Future Lactation Resource Centre, 6540 Cedarview Court, Dayton, Ohio 45459; tel: 937 438 9458; fax 937 438 3229; e-mail <lindaj@bflrc.com>; website <http://www.bflrc.com>. Free catalog of posters and teaching aids, videos, games, buttons, etc.
• Lactation Institute and Breastfeeding Clinic, 16161 Ventura Blvd, Suite 215, Encino, CA 91436. Tel: 213 995 1913. Directors Chele Marmet and Ellen Shell pioneered the concept of Lactation Consultancy; they offer a variety of mainly US-oriented courses.
• LLLI (La Leche League International) PO Box 4079, Schaumburg, IL. 60668-4079 USA. The first and still the largest breastfeeding mothers' support group. Contacts and leaders in many countries. Has a Center for Breastfeeding Information. Tel: 849 519 7730; fax: 847 519 0035; e-mail <OrderDepartment@llli.org> for catalogues.
• NABA (North American Alliance for Breastfeeding Action), 254 Conant Rd., Weston, MA 02193. Tel: 617 893 3553; fax: 617 893 8608; e-mail: <marshalact@aol.com>.
• UNICEF: UNICEF H8F, 3 UN Plaza, New York NY 10017. Try <http://www.unicef.org>.
• Wellstart San Diego Lactation Program, 4062 First Ave., San Diego CA 92103; tel: 619 295 5192. USAID-funded, international, culture- and development-conscious programmes for health professional teams. E-mail: <inquiry@wellstart.org>. website: http://www.wellstart.org/
• Women's International Public Health Network, 7100 Oak Forest Lane, Bethesda MD 20817; tel: 301 469 9210; fax: 301 469 8423.

ZIMBABWE [country prefix 263; always check area codes]
• Southern African Lactation Consultants Association, 10 Camberwell Close, Borrowdale Harare. Tel: 04-883500; fax: 498870 Email: mhc@harare.oafrica.com

INTERNET RESOURCES
Again, there are a zillion of these now available, and no one can read everything that's out there. Nor is it all of consistently excellent quality, so read critically! Once you locate a site, links are routine, so I will just list a few useful or less well-known ones.
• **LACTNET** An e-mail list for lactation consultants, other medical professionals, and lay breastfeeding counsellors. Lactnet archives and joining instructions are now available on the WWW: <http://library.ummed.edu/lsv/archives/lactnet.html>. Basically you need to send an e-mail to LISTSERV@library.ummed.edu, saying "subscribe Lactnet", and all else follows.
• **LACTNEWS** A website with listings of conferences, new resources, and other lactation-related advertising. Find it at <http://www.moontower.com/bwc/lactnews.htm>.
http://www.vicnet.net.au/vicnet/nmaa/nmaahome.htm
Nursing Mothers Association' of Australia home page.
http://www.latrobe.edu.au/www/microbio/milk.html
Information about breastmilk's protective properties by a top microbiologist.
http://www.lalecheleague.org
La Leche League International home page, where you can connect to general breast-feeding information, news about LLLI, and most of the LLL catalog to peruse. You can also find webpages for many LLL groups in different countries.
http://www.mcs.com/~auerbach/lactation.html
For help in finding a lactation consultant and information on what LCs do
http://together.net/~kbruce/kbbhome.html
Kathleen Bruce's page with information about lactation consultants and LC services
http://www/infactcanada.ca
INFACT Canada's new homepage.
http://www.catalog.com/fwcfc/growthchart.html
Growth charts for breastfeeding babies
http://www.prairienet.org/community/health/laleche/fullworth.html
For information on support for women harassed while breastfeeding
http://www.gn.apc.org/babymilk
Baby Milk Action is dedicated to ending the promotion of artificial milk.
http://trance.helix.net/~lois/bfem.html
WABA materials on the importance of breastfeeding for feminism.
parent-l-owner@uts.edu.au
PARENT-L is an Internet e-mail list which discusses all ages of nurslings, as well as general parenting topics (with a special fondness for attachment parenting). A Dutch version is at **bv-list-owner@knoware.nl**
http://www.prairienet.org/community/health/laleche/dettwyler.html
Anthropologist Kathy Dettwyler has been a frequent contributor to PARENT-L.
http://www.clark.net/pub/activist/bfpage/bfpage.html

Good breastfeeding advocacy page with a variety of links, including the Newman *Scientific American* article – <bfpage/ scientific_american.html>.

http://www.prairienet.org/community/health/laleche/BonWeb.html
Quick reference to breastfeeding resources on the Internet.

http://webzone1.co.uk/www/cathus/janelink.htm
Jane's Breastfeeding and Childbirth resources website is excellent

http://www.parentsplace.com/readroom/bf.html
ParentsPlace maintains a list of breastfeeding articles, many of which were written especially for them by experts in lactation.

http://www.geocities.com/HotSprings/Spa/3156
Eclectic breastfeeding information by an American living in Sweden, Ted Greiner.

http://web.superb.net/apastras/index.html
Action pour l'allaitement website.

http://www.fmed.uba.ar/mspba/lacred.htm
Lacmat, a Portuguese and Spanish speaking site.

http://www.ecobaby.com/default.htm
EcoBaby. Equipment for breastfeeding: pumps, apparel, breast pads and more.

http://www.Amazon.com
Great cyber-bookstore, useful if you have cannot get a book from a group where the profits will support breastfeeding.

See also websites noted under country addresses, for the groups listed there.
And remember that journals like the *New Scientist, British Medical Journal, Pediatrics,* and many more can be found and read via the web. Medline can be searched via Medscape or BMJ.

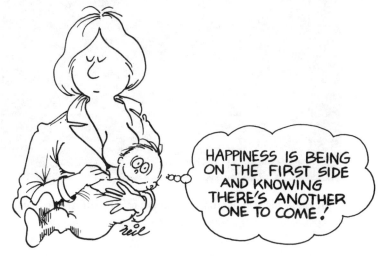

Courtesy of Neil Matterson, from *Is he biting again?* (Marion Books, 1984)

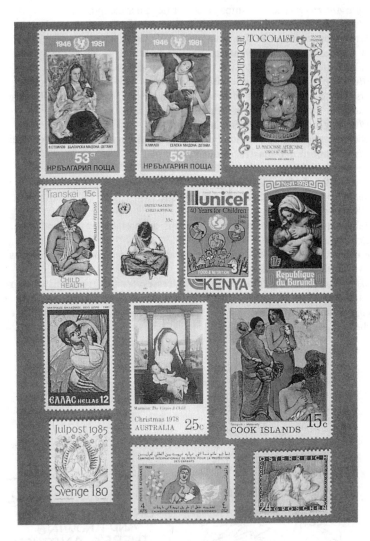

Breastfeeding stamps around the world: card by IBFAN Germany

MIDWIVES AND MOTHERS

Breastfeeding does matter; it matters to the individual child, the mother, the family, and society. This is now clearly recognised, both by professionals and parents. This book is timely because it picks up where many of us have left off; at the point of acknowledging that breast is best, but not feeling too sure what to do about all those 'buts'. This book starts from that point, shows us why breastfeeding matters profoundly, and challenges us all to eradicate the 'buts'.

This book is also timely because it celebrates what is possibly the most powerful force in our fight for successful breastfeeding; the partnership between parents and professionals. Maureen Minchin had succeeded in the almost impossible task of presenting her arguments in an informed yet sensitive and understandable way. Her knowledge of the science of lactation is extensive and her understanding of the art of breastfeeding is deep. She has presented a vast amount of material with an insight and honesty that scientists and health professionals will benefit from reading, and she writes in a way that parents will find enjoyable and informative. As a midwife who has watched and been involved in the development of the ideas in this book, I have experienced closely that collaboration between parent and professional that is essential in developing our knowledge of breastfeeding. For too long, scientists, doctors, midwives and nurses have known some of the science of breastfeeding, while mothers have known many of the problems and feelings associated with breastfeeding. Good management and successful breastfeeding requires both of these perspectives to be brought together.

This book is timely because parents are asking for more involvement in their own health care, while health professionals are recognising that parents are indeed the primary health care givers for their children, and as such should be actively involved in their health care. The hierarchical medical model of 'doing to' people is thankfully being superseded by the democratic model of 'doing with' people, involving health promotion and education. With this latter approach, health professionals see their roles as giving accurate information and helping parents to care for themselves; a partnership of care which empowers women to take control of their own lives and health.

The opportunity to work with Maureen Minchin on this book has proved to me that the partnership between parent and professional is essential, and deeply rewarding. Midwives are the professionals who are most involved with mothers' success in breastfeeding, and I have seen how the combined insights of a mother and a midwife have led us both to a clearer understanding of the field. We both believe that all babies have the right to be fed with human milk, and that to achieve this, fundamental changes must take place in the attitudes and knowledge of professionals, of parents and of society. Our sharing of ideas and close collaboration has brought us both a little closer towards seeing how these changes are possible.

I am pleased to contribute to this revised edition of 'Breastfeeding Matters' and to welcome it as a book which has been, and continues to be, of importance to parents, health professionals, and scientists who ask and answer questions. This book brings both perspectives together with an insight and honesty that will help all of us to improve our practice and to increase the success of breastfeeding.

HUMAN MILK FOR BABIES

The benefits of human milk for babies are now beyond dispute, although many questions remain to be answered. Maureen Minchin demonstrates this in chapter 1, which is a comprehensive synthesis of research on human milk. Despite the ability of some scientists to doubt the existing evidence, we now know that not only is breast feeding best, but it is essential. Perhaps, though, the scepticism of the doubting scientists is useful, since it provokes more questions to be answered; it is never to good to become complacent about complex issues. And it is true that much of the early evidence in the 'breast v. bottle' debate was questionable; that emotion often overwhelmed scientific validity; and that studies were published which could be criticised. However, recent studies confirm many of the arguments previously attributed to emotion, though much remains to be answered. In some ways we are only beginning to know the right questions to ask. The startling thing is that little of this heated debate was generated when artificial milk feeding was first introduced and widely available. Little outcry greeted what was in fact the most radical change in nutrition of the human race. Perhaps, indeed, wisdom comes with hindsight. We have realised the mistake we made then, and are turning back to the best food for human babies; human milk.

CHANGING PRACTICES IN BREASTFEEDING

My interest in breastfeeding was first generated by observing mothers, babies and midwives in the mid 1970s, as a student midwife in Britain. At that time, hospital practices were rigid, babies were 'taken out' of the nursery to the mothers at 'feeding time', complementary feeds were routine, and all babies were given formula feeds overnight so that their mothers could sleep undisturbed. All formula intakes were carefully calculated according to a standard equation, and babies had to be given the required amount. I became concerned watching well-meaning nurses and midwives give a breastfed baby a bottle of formula, persuade her to swallow more than she wished and then sit her up while she vomited. This may have been 'scientific', (i.e. measured) but it was surely not helpful. Far from sleeping comfortably, mothers would often lie awake listening to the babies crying (because two midwives could only feed two babies at a time), and become painfully engorged as they spent the night with no baby to suckle. Even without having read the literature which had been available since the 1950s and 60s on breastfeeding regimes in hospitals [i] I could see clearly that present practice was not effective.

It has been encouraging to watch and participate in the revolution in hospital practices since that time. Flexible feeding, banning of the complementary feeds, and freedom of contact between mother and baby are all practices that have been initiated in many hospitals, supported by the WHO/UNICEF Baby Friendly Hospital Initiative.

PROBLEMS, ADVICE AND SUPPORT

But I have some questions. In spite of mothers choosing to breastfeed, they don't often continue for as long as they plan to, or for as long as the baby needs . Throughout the western world, we find that of the mothers who start to breastfeed, about one third to one half of them have stopped by the time the baby is three months old.[ii] This trend, disturbingly, is being echoed in non-industrialised countries, with appalling consequences for child and maternal health.

Why do mothers stop breastfeeding? Studies suggest that the main reasons are a feeling of 'insufficient milk', and problems with breasts and nipples.[iii] Both of these problem areas, discussed in Chapters 4 and 5, can be helped by knowledgeable support and advice, available at the right time for every mother. I carried out a survey of over 100 mothers in Scotland in 1981-82.[iv] Part of the extensive interview was designed to elicit information on feeding problems and reasons for stopping or continuing breastfeeding. Almost all of the mothers, whom I interviewed at 12-16 weeks postpartum, had encountered problems of some kind. The difference between stopping and continuing lay not in the problems encountered, but in the support received by the mother; the quality of that support, and the time at which she received it. If help was available at the right time, and if it was knowledgeable and accurate, mothers would continue and overcome the problems. Sadly, many mothers did not receive this support at the right time, and bottle feeding became the solution.

I found very few mothers who had chosen to stop breastfeeding; the decision to stop was a difficult one, often accompanied by grief and guilt. One reason often given by professionals for the high discontinuation rate is that mothers do not really want to breastfeed. This is not borne out in any literature I have ever read, or in my own extensive discussions with breastfeeding mothers.

KNOWLEDGE GAINED FROM MOTHERS

I have learned a great deal from talking with breastfeeding mothers over the years. I have learned to listen to them, and to take their insights and feelings seriously. Often they say things that are not yet given academic credibility in the scientific literature, but that are part of the store of knowledge built up by experienced breastfeeding mothers and sensitive and experienced breastfeeding counsellors. I have learned not to be possessive about my professional role; other mothers can often provide the insight and support that a breastfeeding mother needs, and we need to find the right way of tapping into this vast store of experience and accumulated knowledge. Of course being a mother and a health care practitioner are not mutually exclusive categories. It is now possible to combine a career with motherhood, and many midwives and doctors are parents themselves. Hopefully that will increase their insight and improve their practice. I spoke to a doctor who was breastfeeding her first child. Describing her new views on breastfeeding, she said, 'there is nothing in the world that makes me feel so important, or so content. . .' The experience of feeding my own children was just the same.

I have also learned that academic knowledge combined with good clinical skills are valuable and necessary to be a successful practitioner in the field of breastfeeding; up-to-date knowledge and good, applied skills will help in solving the difficult or intractable problems. There is a need to disseminate this knowledge, and to up-date it continuously, for the benefit of mothers and those working with them. The concept of a breastfeeding clinic, as exists in the USA and proposed here (chapter 2) is important in providing a focus for collection and dissemination of this information. There is a profound ignorance among many practitioners of the importance of breastfeeding, and of the techniques and problems involved. This must be changed - and soon - to prevent the continued widespread failure of breastfeeding.

Changes are required in other, more fundamental aspects. Breastfeeding is part of a woman's life - an important part, but not the only activity she has to do. It must not become another burden that women must fit into a life already over-loaded with the physical and emotional demands of child rearing, career, relationships, marriage and housework. It must become part of life in a way that will demand changes in provision of child care, maternity leave, support from fathers, perceptions of breastfeeding in public places and access to facilities to express and store breast milk safely. These factors will not change easily, but they will change if breastfeeding is recognised to be a fundamentally important factor in child health, and if that recognition is backed by appropriate action (see Chapter 13).

MIDWIVES AND MOTHERS

This commentary is called "Midwives and Mothers", because these are the people most intimately involved in successful breastfeeding. This is not to say that fathers, doctors and others are not involved in the process, but the relationship between mothers and midwives (and nurses in North America, where midwives are scarce and often not legal) is crucial.

Midwives are involved in the care of mother and baby from the beginning. They are there at the birth of the child, and are responsible for that important first feed (see Chapter 3). Thereafter they will be the principal practitioners and teachers in the sometimes difficult business of establishing breastfeeding. Their contact with mother and child gives them an understanding and knowledge quite different from that of doctors who will see the mother occasionally during the post partum period. Midwives are responsible for planning and carrying out hospital routines, and for giving the mother the information she may need to continue breastfeeding successfully at home.

Nursing and midwifery have been moving away from a model of controlling behaviour of patients, towards working together with people in their care for some years now. We are now coming to see that mothers and midwives are partners in the process of breastfeeding. A midwife will be able to teach the rights and wrongs, and to suggest solutions to problems, but the mother is the one who must learn, and who must carry out any proposed solutions. Responsibility for this is joint; both midwife and mother must acknowledge that they have a contribution to make to successful breastfeeding. They must also have a commitment to it, which arises out of their knowledge that breast is best, and which motivates both of them to overcome difficulties.

Many women establish their babies at their breast with no real difficulty at all. But it can be hard work to help some mothers breastfeed their infants. It may take hours of back-breaking work, and it seems easier to say. . .'just give her a bottle. . .' Not saying that means that the midwife wants the mother to give her baby the best food, and that she accepts her responsibility in that process.

It is often not an easy task for midwives to encourage breastfeeding. Hospital routines and attitudes of other staff may still interfere with successful breastfeeding. What is needed here is the support of midwives for mothers and mothers for midwives, to demand change in an ineffective system.

IN THE LONGER TERM. . .

When mothers return home, the midwife and community nurse continue to play an important part. Our western culture is the only culture in the world that does not care for its new mothers by giving them the attention and teaching of an experienced older woman. We expect women today, who may often have little or no previous experience of child rearing, to learn to adjust to all the demands of mothering, including learning to breastfeed, with only the help of a partner and immediate friends and family. The new mother may find that no one around her has any knowledge of breastfeeding; where does go for help? She may go to a voluntary group, such as NMAA, National Childbirth Trust, or La Leche League, or she may go to her midwife; or to no one. It is hard, as a new and tired young mother, to go anywhere; it is good if help comes to you. We must look seriously at the provision of home care for mothers; (Holland provides 'maternity aids' who come in and help with basic household chores for 10 days after the mother returns home[v] [15.]); and in particular, we must look carefully at care for mothers whom we know are likely to have extra problems. We know that mothers of sick or premature babies, mothers who are young, or unmarried, or less well-educated, may need more support. Do we bias our care towards these mothers to give them that extra support?

How this care is given will vary from situation to situation. Some mothers will only need the support that other mothers can give them, while others will need the additional assistance of a trained midwife. Often a combination of these will be the answer. The important thing is that appropriate advice and help is available when breastfeeding, the more women will be available to share their experiences in the future.

I would like to thank Maureen Minchin for writing this book, and for updating and producing this latest revised edition. I believe it has had and will have a profound impact on the value placed on breastfeeding. I would also like to thank her for giving us both the opportunity to learn and develop our knowledge and convictions as midwife and mother. Our relationship has been very special and immensely rewarding, combining learning with caring, honesty and a good dose of humour. We believe that women have the right to make their own choices and control their own lives. Their ability to do this depends on accurate information being available to them, and caring support being given by health professionals. This book provides much of that important information.

We can learn so much from each other, if we only listen. It can be a painful process breaking down the barriers that we have learned to build up in our training as professionals, and to truly listen to and work with parents. But these barriers, as Anne Oakley demonstrates in her work,[vi] are impediments to true understanding of each other and our true worth. Midwives are immensely valuable in the success of breastfeeding; they hold a key role. But they are only valuable if they listen to mothers and use knowledge to guide their practice.

I look forward to the time when breastfeeding will be widespread and accepted; to the time when mothers will be supported by a network of experienced women who have all successfully breastfed. That time will come more quickly when parents and professionals work together in a supportive and knowledgeable way.

Professor Mary J. Renfrew (formerly Houston)
Director, Mother and Infant Research Unit,
University of Leeds, UK

[1] Illingworth, R.S. & Stone, D.G., 1952. Demand feeding in a maternity unit. Lancet 1, 683; Gunther, M., 1955. Instinct and the nursing couple. *Lancet* 1, 575-578.

[2] Foster K, Lader A, Cheeseborough S. *Infant Feeding 1995.* Office for National Statistics. (HMSO 1997)

[3] Renfrew MJ, Woolridge MW, Ross McGill H. *Enabling women to breastfeed. Interventions which support or inhibit breastfeeding. A structured review of the evidence.* (HMSO, in press)

[4] Houston, M. J., Howie, P. W., McNeilly, A. S., 1983. The difficulties of breastfeeding and the care offered to breastfeeding mothers at home. *Nursing Mirror* 156(6), i-viii.

[5] Kloosterman GJ. 1978. The Dutch system of home births. In Kitzinger S, Davis JA (eds) *The Place of Birth* (Oxford Medical Publications) 85-92

[6] Oakley, A., 1981. Interviewing women; a contradiction in terms. In: Roberts, H. (ed). *Doing feminist research,* 30-61. Routledge & Kegan Paul, London.

S UPPING WITH THE DEVIL??

A personal addendum made necessary by international gossip by the unaccountable.

The vexed question of healthworker interaction with industry will be the subject of a complete chapter in a later book, but here I want to record two examples of what I personally have found possible. My readers can assess whether my judgment on these issues has affected my writing. I am not suggesting that only my chosen course of action is right: I believe in trusting my conscience and the judgment of my colleagues, while accepting that we will all make mistakes, and so extend that courtesy to others. The important principle is to be open and accountable. I am writing of these issues here because I have been the subject of vicious gossip by the less scrupulous.[1] I don't really care what such individuals think, but I am very concerned that good information or worthwhile arguments might not reach good people because their source has been slandered as tainted. We should all remember that McCarthyism was effective as well as evil, and with hindsight good people regret having been taken in. And we should insist on individuals' right to reply to any allegation we hear about them, and which they often have not heard. Natural justice demands this, and we are failing ourselves and acting without integrity if we listen only to one side of any story and rush to judgment, or pass on gossip.

Firstly, after giving a presentation at a major teaching hospital interstate, I was asked by the staff to make an educational video on positioning the baby as part of a series for the hospital to use for its other staff and sell. I agreed. The Educational Resource Centre which was making the series later informed me (at the suggestion of the company) that they were using a grant from Nestlé to subsidise the series. Obviously this would be a useful video, and money for making such things was virtually non-existent. So I inquired as to the degree of freedom the Resource Centre had in its choice of topic, content and speakers. This was total. I inquired as to the control of sales, and where profits from sales would go: this was to the hospital, who retained full rights over the film once made. (Nestlé simply could get so many copies free for distribution to professionals, and thereafter had to pay for copies if wanted.) This ensured that the film could not be made difficult to obtain, as seems to have happened to *Helping Mothers Breastfeed*, another excellent film Dr. Felicity Savage[2] and Chloe Fisher made, with an independent producer, but for Nestlé Switzerland's ownership and distribution. So I agreed to participate, provided that it was agreed in writing that I had total control of content, complete right to change and edit and to refuse permission to proceed if things were going wrong; that Nestlé had no such rights; that I was paid **nothing** beyond the cost of travel and accommodation in the time needed to make the film. (This clause is necessary to avoid financial dependency: if I can earn money doing other things, but earn nothing from working with industry, there is no danger of gradually finding that I am dependent on industry!) The film was made. Along the way it acquired a very strong introductory piece about the hazards of formulas and bottle feeding per se, before the material on positioning. It was made in 1986, when no-one but myself talked publicly of formulas "lacking the fatty acids needed for proper brain growth after birth." I gather it was heavily copied in Manila at the IBFAN Forum in 1989, and (minus identifying logo) has created discussion in many places in the world, as well as generating independent income for the hospital's resource programme.[3]

So was it worth doing? I think so. Did it help Nestlé Australia look like good guys? Probably, with a few people: those who did know and respect me would not have seen it as anything more than sound advertising by Nestlé, while for those who did not know me as the author of *Breastfeeding Matters*, the association with me would have meant nothing to Nestlé, and it might even have made my words believable! As one Director of Nursing said, "You know, I never would have believed what you said about infant formula if it hadn't had the Nestlé logo on the video: we show it to all our pregnant mothers and our breastfeeding rates have gone up." Do I repent of doing it? Not at all, because the Nestlé logo on the video meant more babies got breastfed.

When the Nestlé Boycott was revived again in 1987[4] many long-term breastfeeding activists in Australia and overseas had concerns. I was consulted about this by a key member of IBCoCo, said that I could not support it in Australia, and suggested instead a co-ordinated global year-long appraisal to identify the worst offender in each market, then a co-ordinated international boycott targeting the worst in each market: which would have allowed us in Australia to target a company other than Code-compliant-in-Australia Nestlé, and still be part of the global movement. That year of evaluation could have caused a great deal of change world-wide as no company would have wanted to be targeted. The reasons given to me for rejecting this were less then convincing, although the time is not right to publish these openly.

I'm still feeling quite comfortable about my decisions both to make that Nestlé video and refuse to support the revived Boycott in Australia despite the hassles this has caused me since, again better not recorded in this book. Integrity is not in the eye of the beholder but in one's actions and one's motives. I suspect that careful historians may find that the principal, presumably unintended, effect of the 1987 US revival of the Nestlé Boycott was to assist the US companies fight Nestlé's then-current attempt at US market penetration. If this is so, it indirectly led to direct advertising to the public, as Nestlé were locked out of the lucrative institutional contracts by good people trying to save babies.[5]

The second example of personal industry liaison was also a useful experience. I was asked to write an article on the WHO Code for *Nursery News*, a free handout produced independently, but paid for by Nestlé and given to maternal and child health nurses and others. I agreed to do so on condition that

- what I wrote was not edited without my consent;
- I was not paid for this;

• Nestlé had no right to change what was written;

(All these conditions go down in writing and are signed by the person I am dealing with, or we do not proceed.) In the end, the article was not printed: too long, they said. However, the company later asked permission to run the article in *Australian Doctor Weekly*, another of their free publications funded by general advertising, which goes to every doctor in the country. As a result I had quite a number of requests for *Protecting Infant Health*, the IOCU Guide to the Code for healthworkers. So it was worth the time it took, and my integrity was not in question.

Yet I have had some unpleasant flak about being prepared to associate with Nestlé (or any other formula company) even so indirectly as this, as well as flak about being prepared to question or criticise in-house (as I have done) whatever I see as counter-productive, unjust, wasteful or undemocratic actions by some breastfeeding advocates. I have been libelled on Lactivist and elsewhere by fellow IBFANers as having sold out to the companies. Some of these consider the above Nestlé 'link' explains what they say is a change of strategy or policy by me. Some have responded, not with answers to my questions or criticisms of my actions, but with denunciations of my character and speculation as to my psychological state. When reason is replaced by vituperation I feel certain that there is something to hide, and my questioning was truly justified. An independent critic's task is to be independent and a critic, not the propagandist for any group. Good guys with good intentions, myself included, can make dreadful mistakes and need to be held to account. The expert who says African women never have breastfeeding problems is harmful to the cause of breastfeeding and women's health, no matter what his intentions may be; he needs to be told so. Publicly if he talks publicly. The group that spends $350,000 of UN money for worldwide breastfeeding promotion in a year needs to explain to all of us in predominantly women's breastfeeding groups starved for funds, especially in developing countries, why $70,000 of it ever went to an American university and so much seems to go to men, and so little to grassroots women's groups, relatively speaking. Who has been paid what and why? Who determines the priorities? What democratic processes put those people in power and how may others attempt to join them? Such questions need to be asked and answers need to be documented. Accountability is not a virtue only infant formula companies should practise.

Clearly anyone who thinks I've changed in essentials never read the first edition of *Breastfeeding Matters* carefully, and noted my even-handed criticism of any behaviour that I consider damaging to the cause of breastfeeding. *Breastfeeding Matters* criticised healthworkers at least as much as it criticised industry, as the Royal College of Midwives was mature enough to recognise. I am aware of the potential dangers of industry liaison, but also of benefits flowing from it. The genuine willingness of Australian industry to consider our proposals and negotiate has been a crucial aspect in the development of all these initiatives in Australia, and seems notably absent in some other countries. That willingness to negotiate only comes in a climate of respect, in which people are not categorised as White Hats and Black Hats automatically just because they claim to be breastfeeding advocates or are working for industry. Of course I have also worked with industry via my role as Consumer Alternate on APMAIF 1992-1995, and in many other situations. While industry remains co-operative this is essential. But I think my ongoing, entirely self-funded voluntary work and its results should persuade all but the most irrational that I have not sold out to in-dustry. If I'm wrong about that, too bad. What others think of me personally cannot be allowed to influence what I do, or I am of no value as an independent critic. Of course I invite reasoned argument and debate, and remain willing to be convinced on any point that I am now or have been wrong. I just don't care much for those whose response to differences of opinion on strategy is to call it heresy and excommunicate fellow believers. If I and other volunteers like me are not members of IBFAN (as one long-term IBFAN paid staffer circulated in writing) because we refuse to follow overseas suggestions where to do so would harm local breastfeeding, then IBFAN is not "a worldwide coalition of citizen groups working for better child health by promoting breastfeeding and eliminating irresponsible marketing of commercial infant foods, bottles and teats".

There may be renewed suggestions that I have misused the title of IBFANer, which I am proud to claim for myself and anyone of the vast numbers of Australians who have worked so long and hard for breastfeeding in this country. IBFAN is a wonderful loose network, full of marvellous individuals, but not an organisation. This is a strength in that no one can target the whole easily; and so reprisals against individuals are less likely. It is a weakness in that the largely self-perpetuating governing group, a small centralised IBFAN Coordinating Council (IBCoCo), can make pronouncements for which it cannot be held accountable by membership. Even within IBCoCo there is an even smaller rapid response group which may not consult all IBCoCo members before speaking or acting. Too often only these people can speak for IBFAN; too often the rest of us are claimed as IBFAN when numbers and credibility are needed, but disregarded as "not really IBFAN" if we ask questions about money and power in IBFAN, or seek to make change. Most ordinary IBFANers have very little power or opportunity to join these inner circles, are unlikely to be invited if they are critical of existing policies (such as "the Code must be made law"), and indeed may be abruptly cast out of IBCoCo (and the area they represent ceases to be represented) if they try to maintain such a position. All organisations, even loose networks run by small groups, can experience problems of accountability, while still being worthwhile organisations. My criticism of some actions by some IBFANers, and some policies, is not the same thing as criticising IBFAN per se. Only those individuals who think they are the organisation are likely to confuse the two.

But it is support for IBFAN's principles is what makes one an IBFANer.
IBFAN stands for
- the right of infants everywhere to have the highest level of health;
- the right of families, and in particular women and children, to have enough nutritious food;
- the right of women to make informed choices about infant feeding;
- the right of women to full support for successful breastfeeding and for sound infant

feeding practices;
- the right of all people to health services which meet basic human needs;
- the right of health workers and consumers to health care systems which are free from commercial pressures;
- the right of people to organise in international solidarity in order to secure changes which protect and promote people's basic health.

I offer my thanks and love to my fellow IBFANers everywhere who are working to improve maternal and child health, to oppose and expose unscrupulous industry tactics and to create more democracy and accountability in IBFAN as in the rest of the world. And I invite your critical response. IBFAN needs you, and it needs you to be involved and to insist on being taken seriously, at every level. The world needs an even stronger IBFAN. (Perhaps we should add to that IBFAN list of rights, the right of all IBFANers to knowledge about and involvement in decision-making and strategy development in IBFAN, and to knowledge about IBFAN finances!)

---

[1] I have no objection to any honest mistake, as made by a naive BMAC worker who reported the gossip on Lactivist and so gave me a chance to clear my name, and who apologised for his mistake very promptly. But I believe we are all remiss if we allow gossip about individuals to be published covertly without the subject of the gossip being told of it and being given an equal opportunity to respond. And I would urge readers not to trust any person who is willing to pass on such gossip as fact in private mailings or circulars.

[2] Felicity Savage too has done and continues to do wonderful work for breastfeeding. Now employed by the CHD Unit at WHO Geneva, she has created an excellent training programme, and her simple book for healthworkers in developing countries, Helping Mothers to Breastfeed, is a classic which has been translated into many languages. Her earlier "collaboration with Nestlé" over the video referred to earlier has in no way affected her zeal for breastfeeding, any more than mine has. And certainly no one who knows Chloe Fisher considers this video compromised her care for mothers!!!

[3] Called *Latching-On, the key to Successful Breastfeeding*, it is available from the Education Resource Centre, Adelaide Women's and Children's Hospital, Fullarton Rd., North Adelaide, S.A. 5006, Australia.

[4] By an American group in 1996 publicly outcast from IBFAN for a liaison with a US company, how justly I cannot assess as yet. Did this liaison exist earlier and influence the decision to set the Nestlé Boycott going at a time so convenient for US companies? Or was it a recent development, as the result of working in a confrontational style and eventually realising that the solution of complex problems must involve industry? Historians of this issue in the United States will have some interesting trails to follow.

[5] Should this principled unwillingness of myself, ALCA, and NMAA to endorse the Boycott 1987-1991 have led to subsequent destructive overseas interference in Australian affairs, so that in the end a professional association was split and breastfeeding advocacy divided in this country? I think not. Yet it ultimately did.

Revising *Breastfeeding Matters* has been a convoluted process. It was very much a book of its time, addressing the people and the issues of the time, on the basis of the evidence then available. On the other hand, its fundamental themes – the magic of women's milk, the risks of all substitutes, and the need for serious societal action to enable women to breastfeed – have not become less true or important, nor will in the foreseeable future. In many ways it would be easier to write a whole new book than revise this one, and indeed the material for two new books is already on my computer. I confess I was tempted to simply reprint the 1989 version and get on with the new material, but deliberately wasting paper on spreading even one outdated fact is unethical. In the end I have tried to strike a balance: amending only that which needs major revision, such as the history and politics chapter, all the clinical/management material wherever there was something new to add, and anything which in 1998 I would now approach differently. Chapter 1, the summary of the hazards of infant formula and benefits of breastfeeding, I have by contrast left largely untouched. There is certainly more proof of formula's inescapable risks, and since 1985 it has continued to be imperfect and subject to change and recalls, yet chapter 1's conclusions are the same as they were in 1985. I have left it untouched because it is in many ways more powerful to say, "We knew this in 1984. This is not new. Why has so little changed?"

My personal academic-activist tension referred to in 1984 also remains. Having been splendidly vindicated by ongoing research, professional recognition, and increasing peer support in the thirteen years since I wrote the first edition, I am now confident of the soundness of my philosophical basis, and have not lapsed into complacency about ongoing study of the field. However, being under considerable pressures, I cannot take the time to be as precise in my referencing of this update as I would be for a truly academic exercise. (I did that last time against the advice of the publishers, but because I knew it was important for credibility when breaking such new ground.) Readers thus will find that I have not included detailed references for every section of the new material I am adding. Such evidence does exist. What makes this omission possible is the new ready access to reference material by anyone with a computer and modem, or able to ask NMAA or MIDIRS to do a search for them. What makes the omission necessary is the fact that detailed referencing takes far longer than any other aspect of writing, and I have not had time for my own work, already rescheduled too often as a result of other people's requests for (usually unpaid) help.

In many ways that is symbolic. Since 1984 I have written the equivalent of several books, but largely in support of various professional bodies which have developed their interest in breastfeeding over that time. Submissions to government on a variety of topics have been the equivalent of a chapter each time. Involvement in ACOIF (the Australian Coalition for Optimal Infant Feeding), as a member of the Professional Advisory Board and Director of ILCA (the International Lactation Consultants Association), as an ad hoc consultant to groups as diverse as UNICEF, WHO, Wellstart and IBLCE; work on BFHI and the International Code in Australia and overseas: all of these and much more explain my lack of published tomes. As an elected ALCA Council member 1989-1995 I was involved in the national development of the Lactation Consultant profession in Australia, and thirteen issues of *ALCA News* from 1990 took vast amounts of time. (But stand as a valuable chronicle of events in Australia and elsewhere: I strongly recommend the purchase of back issues August 1990 to the present by anyone wishing to chronicle this period.) Having helped establish and support many of the professional lactation consultant organisations and other breastfeeding advocacy groups now in place around the world, I have naturally spent a lot of time working behind the scenes not only as worker and adviser, but as commentator and constructive critic. Before I wrote *Breastfeeding Matters*, I saw much to be critical about. I still do. And I think honest critics play a crucial role in any social enterprise.

There is, however, a high price to pay for being an honest critic. Not everyone knows how to distinguish between the writer and what is written, and some indulge in unworthy and hurtful personal vendettas rather than rational or valid textual criticism or argument. A critic expects to be criticised, but it is a shock to find oneself personally defamed, when serious and legitimate questions about their actions prove uncomfortable for those with power or money who do not wish to be held accountable. It is even more of a shock when the persons doing such things claim to be fighting for the same cause. I believe strongly that the cause of justice is never advanced by unjust actions. I also believe that we must oppose injustice whenever it presents itself in our lives, even when that is not the easiest course of action. Freedom of speech would not exist long if every time a writer spoke the truth and was threatened with a lawsuit the writer cravenly retreated from the truth. Those with access to money may try to bully into silence those of us without it; but when we have the support of our friends and colleagues they will not succeed. And despite the personal costs we will survive and be stronger for the experience.

Historians are educated to be critical observers. The world-wide infant feeding situation demands intelligent and ongoing comment if sustained progress is to be possible. I hope that the next decade will see many more first rank academics (whether historians or sociologists or anthropologists or economists or midwives or whatever) using the skills of their discipline to investigate infant feeding realities; and actively joining with all those who have a genuine desire to achieve optimal infant feeding outcomes for infants everywhere. We who want to help babies cannot afford to perpetuate dilettante versions of history, simplistic diagnoses of the problems, and doctrinaire solutions based on very little understanding of the realities of women's experience of infant feeding or of the societies in which they live. Within the broad range of groups that are part of the infant feeding movement, we need to be flexible and mature enough to debate strategies and develop pragmatic solutions, step by step towards the ideal. The conservation movement, seen as so radical in the 1970s, has now evolved to include a mainstream pragmatic element which has achieved a great deal by what powerful minorities still see as "working with the enemy", i.e., those sections of government and industry which have evolved enough from their once-extreme 1970s position to act a little more responsibly. The conservation movement retains its radical elements, but these no longer dominate the substantive debate as they once did (even if they can still be sure of achieving headlines by their tactics). While helpful in raising public awareness of a problem, such radical elements may sometimes vilify moderates and pragmatists as traitors to the cause. Yet in fact it is often persistent moderate groups which create the longest lasting changes in attitude and action. Extremism is alienating in all walks of life: the person who rants hatred about any person or group is not attractive to the onlooker, and often generates sympathy votes!

Sadly, such elements do emerge in discussion of infant feeding, and many people feel uncomfortable when they do. I believe that such elements on 'our side' are feeding the backlash which is so absurdly labelling child health advocates as "LactoNazis", "breastfeeding fascists", and so on. Books such as *Bottle Feeding without Guilt* (Robins) seem to me to be the logical outcome of certain types of breastfeeding promotion. Breastfeeding advocates need to do more than condemn the factual inadequacies of such books: they need to understand why they are written, and join forces with all women wanting the best for their children.

Of course, such 'extremism', however counter-productive, is entirely understandable, and perhaps even justified by the extreme prejudice, ignorance and callous cynicism which still characterises the actions of some participants in the world of infant feeding. Industry behaviour, for example, however improved over its earlier excesses, at least where we can record it, remains a huge problem, thanks to the gullibility of their target audience, which is increasingly doctors and the general public rather than midwives (who have educated themselves more than any other group). But that is another story, for another book. Industry apologists should draw no comfort from this book, as while it makes it clear that industry was and is not the sole factor creating the situation we now face, there is little evidence that they are doing much to stem the harms they have done world-wide, and more and more evidence that their pursuit of profit will continue to be over the bodies of children, whatever their avowed intent.

I thank all those readers, among them respondents from multinational industry and its vociferous opponents, and especially those parents who failed to breastfeed, who have given me such direct and overwhelmingly positive feedback. I thank my family, now increased by a grandchild, for supporting this work and being willing to accept cheerfully that my personal crusade has caused us all to struggle within a very limited income. I thank my many dear friends and colleagues, who have supported me through a period of unprecedented difficulty related directly to my chosen role as an independent critic of all that is destructive of women's ability to nurture their babies at the breast. I particularly thank those who have taken time to advise on the new material in this edition: you know who you are, and also why you have chosen not to be named.

I also thank those many writers whose life bears witness to the fact that telling the truth without fear or favour is a guarantee of persecution by the powerful, who have money or prestige or patronage to lose by exposure. Nothing is more controversial than the truth, plainly told. That is what my writing will always be about. As a historian I am aware that truth is hard to discern, and am willing to listen to others' truths plainly told. But sloppy research, suppression of evidence, distortion of facts, self-aggrandising claims that fail to acknowledge the work of others, inexcusable tactics such as unsubstantiated generalisations about individuals and vilification by association: these tactics have no place in advocacy and in fact harm any cause. If we who advocate breastfeeding do not hold ourselves to the highest standards of truthfulness, professionalism, and democratic accountability we are not credible demanding such standards of others, including industry. We will all fail to some degree, as none of us is infallible and the perfect book cannot be written, nor the perfect association created. But there is a difference between failing despite trying, and simply not bothering to do the hard work needed to make a reasonable effort, but instead waffling on from a basis of dilettante interest and personal prejudice, or setting up personal fiefdoms in which the chosen elite control everything from pennies to policies, while the masses are disempowered or disenfranchised. I have tried in the past, and in the future will continue to try, to work to reasonably high standards of both scholarship and accountability, and I do not apologise for being critical of actions or writings which seem to me to fall short of those standards. If my readers ever feel that I fall short of these self-imposed standards, I hope you will write and tell me so.

Infant feeding matters... so, breastfeeding matters!

Maureen Minchin, January 1998

If you have enjoyed my books to date (*Revolutions and Rosewater: a history of the Victorian Nurse registration authority 1923-1973*; *Food for Thought: a parent's guide to food intolerance*; and *Breastfeeding Matters: what we need to know about infant feeding*) and would like to be on the mailing list for more, please send me your name and address.

The absence of biographical details on end covers is deliberate.
I believe that writing should be judged on its merits.
The worth of a book has nothing to do
with the weight of titles and length of cv that
an author lists (and mine is too long anyway!)
If you have read this book
you know a great deal about its author,
and can test the book's worth for yourself

Potentially lethal? But perfectly legal, because we have no bottle/teat standards...

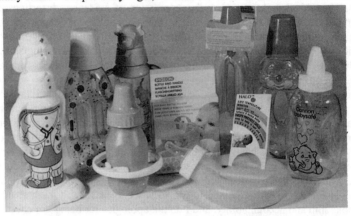

Nor do we monitor water quality too closely, especially in rural areas...

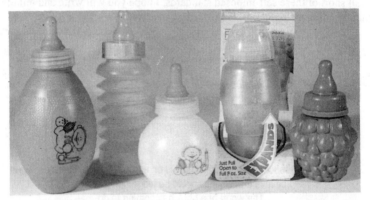

Nor do we test formula and bottle when babies come to hospital with gastroenteritis..

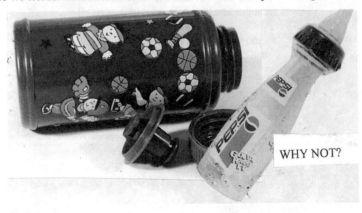

WHY NOT?

GLOSSARY OF ACRONYMS

AAP – American Academy of Pediatrics
ABM – Academy of Breastfeeding Medicine
ACA – Australian Consumers' Association
ACCC – Australian Competition & Consumer Commission
ACHS – Australian Council for Hospital Standards
ACMI – Australian College of Midwives Inc.
ACOIF – Australian Coalition for Optimal Infant Feeding
ACTU – Australian Council of Trades Unions
AGPS – Australian Government Printing Service
ALCA – Australian Lactation Consultants' Association
 ALCA News/Galaxy – ALCA's official journal, *ALCA News*, was renamed
  ALCA Galaxy in 1997
AMA – Australian (or American) Medical Association
ANF – Australian Nursing Federation or Australian Nutrition Foundation
ANZFA – Australian & New Zealand Food Authority. Formerly NFA (National Food
 Authority)
APMAIF – Advisory Panel on the Marketing in Australia of Infant Formula
BFA(G) – BabyFood Action (Group)
BFHI – Baby-Friendly Hospital Initiative
 NAC – National Advisory Council (Australia) First met August 1996.
 NSG – National Steering Group. Operated Feb 1993 – June 1995
 ACMI given control by UNICEF Australia, August 1995
BFPU – Baby-Friendly Paediatric Unit
BMJ – *British Medical Journal*
BPA – Baby Products Association (Australia)
CAA – Community Aid Abroad
CERP – (IBLCE) Continuing Education Representative Point
Code/International Code/WHO Code – The International Code of Marketing of
 Breastmilk Substitutes, 1981
FBCA – Federal Bureau of Consumer Affairs
FDA – Food & Drug Administration (USA)
IBCLC – International Board Certified Lactation Consultant
IBFAN – International Baby Food Action Network
IBLCE – International Board of Lactation Consultant Examiners
ICCR – Interfaith Centre for Corporate Responsibility

ICIFI – International Council of Infant Food Industries
IFM – Infant Formula Manufacturers' association, which replaced ICIFI
ILCA – International Lactation Consultant Association
INBC – International Nestlé Boycott Committee
JHL – Journal of Human Lactation (official journal of ILCA)
LLL(I) – La Leche League (International)
LLLNZ - La Leche League New Zealand
MAIF AGREEMENT – Marketing in Australia of Infant Formula Agreement
MCH(N) – Maternal & Child Health (Nurse)
MIDIRS – Midwives' Information and Resource Service (International, run from UK)
NABA – National Alliance for Breastfeeding Action (USA)
NH&MRC – National Health and Medical Research Council (Australia)
NMAA – Nursing Mothers' Association of Australia
NZLCA – New Zealand Lactation Consultants' Association
QIC – Quality Improvement Council
TGA – Therapeutic Goods Administration (Australia)
UNICEF – United Nations International Children's Emergency Fund
WABA – World Alliance for Breastfeeding Action
WHA – World Health Assembly.
WHO/OMS – World Health Organization
WHO CREF – WHO Common Review and Evaluation Framework (for monitoring Code)

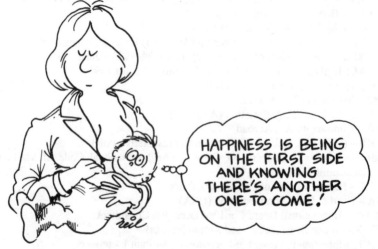

Courtesy of Neil Matterson, from *Is he biting again?* (Marion Books, 1984)

*Complete indexing is virtually impossible:
on this page add any other references
 you want to be able to locate*